Questions & Answers

Exam-Oriented

ANATOMY

Above Diaphragm

Questions & Answers

Exam-Oriented

ANATOMY

Above Diaphragm

**(Gross Anatomy, Systemic Histology, Systemic Embryology
of Superior Extremity, Thorax, Head, Face & Neck,
and Neuroanatomy)**

(With Colour Diagrams)

Shoukat N. Kazi

M.S. (Anatomy), D.T.C.D., B.Sc., L.L.B., M.B.A. (Hospital Admin.)

Professor, Dr. D.Y. Patil Medical College
(Dr. D.Y. Patil Vidhyapeeth—deemed university),
Pune - 411 018 (India)

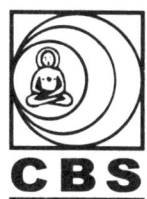

CBS

CBS PUBLISHERS & DISTRIBUTORS PVT. LTD.

NEW DELHI • BENGALURU • CHENNAI • KOCHI • MUMBAI • PUNE

ISBN : 81-239-1211-0

First Edition : 2005
Reprint : 2006, 2007, 2008, 2009, 2010,
          2011, 2012, 2013, 2014

Published by Satish Kumar Jain and produced by V.K. Jain for
CBS Publishers & Distributors Pvt. Ltd.,
CBS Plaza, 4819/XI Prahlad Street, 24 Ansari Road, Daryaganj,
New Delhi - 110002, India. • Website: www.cbspd.com
e-mail: delhi@cbspd.com, cbspubs@airtelmail.in
Ph.: 23289259, 23266861, 23266867 • Fax: 011-23243014

Branches:

• *Bengaluru:* Seema House, 2975, 17th Cross, K.R. Road,
  Bansankari 2nd Stage, Bengaluru - 560070
  • Ph.: +91-80-26771678/79 • Fax: +91-80-26771680
  • E-mail: cbsbng@gmail.com, bangalore@cbspd.com
• *Pune:* Bhuruk Prestige, Sr. No. 52/12/2+1+3/2,
  Narhe, Haveli (Near Katraj-Dehu Road By-pass), Pune - 411041
  • Ph.: +91-20-64704058/59, 020-32392277 • E-mail: pune@cbspd.com
• *Kochi:* 36/14, Kalluvilakam, Lissie Hospital Road,
  Kochi - 682018, Kerala • Ph.: +91-484-4059061-65
  • Fax: +91-484-4059065 • E-mail: cochin@cbspd.com
• *Chennai:* 20, West Park Road, Shenoy Nagar, Chennai - 600030
  Ph.: +91-44-26260666, 26208620 • Fax: +91-44-42032115
  • E-mail: chennai@cbspd.com
• *Mumbai:* 83-C, Ist Floor, Dr. E. Moses Road, Worli, Mumbai-400 018,
  Maharashtra Ph.: +91-9833017933, 022-24902340/24902341
  • E-mail: mumbai@cbspd.com

Printed at :
SDR Printers Pvt. Ltd., Delhi

Dedicated

To

my Parents

Haji Nizamsaheb K. Kazi
Mrs. Jainnabbi N. Kazi

&

Students

FOREWORD

Prof. S. N. Kazi's book is intended to help medical and dental students rapidly master complex intricacies of human anatomy that is essential to clinical care.

It is also of practical value to nurses and paramedical personnel who are confronted with anatomical problems. This book is written to fulfill the need for a brief but readable summary of the relevant anatomy, with succinct notes on applied anatomy wherever indicated. It addresses the diverse and mounting needs of medical students preparing for professional examinations. The text will not only enhance the knowledge to an extent sufficient to satisfy the examiners but will equip the readers with the necessary understanding of applied anatomy for future practice. A recurring problem in medical education is the common inability of the students to relate the large body of factual knowledge to practical application in their future clinical training. A commendable endeavour has been made by Pro. Kazi to bridge the gap between rote anatomy and clinical relevance. The mnemonics and humour in this book do not intend any disrespect for anyone, rather they are employed as an educational device, as it is well known that the best memory techniques involve the use of ridiculous association. Stephen Goldberg in his unique book titled. "Clinical Neuroanatomy made ridiculously simple", has already demonstrated their efficacy superbly. **Further more, this book is very well-illustrated with 93 LAQs, 20 SAQs & 156 SNs, 91 Keywords, 254 line diagrams and elegantly constructed 47 tables.**

This book is not designed to replace standard reference texts, but rather is to be read as a companion text before appearing in an examination. This will enable the student to gain an overall perspective of essential anatomy.

My best wishes for the success of this endeavor which merits appreciation.

Formerly:-
Professor & Chairman
Department of Anatomy &
Founder Director,
Inter Disciplinary Brain Research Center,
Dean, Principal & Chief medical Suptdt.
Jawaharlal Nehru Medical College,
Aligarh Muslim University
Aligarh 202 002 U. P. (India)

Prof. Dr. Mahdi Hasan
M.B.B.S., M.S. (Hons.) FICS, FAMS., Ph. D., D.Sc., FNA
Professor Emeritus
INSA Senior Scientist
Department of Anatomy
King George's Medical College
Lucknow-226 003
U. P. India.

FOREWORD

All the Medical Colleges in the state of Maharashtra were affiliated to eight different conventional universities in the state up to 1997. After the establishment of *Maharashtra University of Health Sciences* in the state in 1998, all of them were affiliated to this single State level University. Previously, syllabi and pattern of examinations were different, but now it is same for all undergraduate students.

The university accepted the new pattern (1+1½ + 2 yrs.) of curriculum recommended by the Medical Council of India, while the conventional universities were following the old (1½ + 1½ + 1½ yrs.) pattern. *First time in the examination LAQ, SAQ and MCQ patterns were introduced by MUHS.*

On the background of the reduced duration for both students (for learning) and teachers (for teaching) of I MBBS, there was a need for examination oriented revision book.

It is really a great pleasure for me to introduce this book *"EXAM-ORIENTED ANATOMY - Above diaphragm"* written by one of my ex-colleague Dr. Shoukat. N. Kazi.

I have gone through the manuscript of this book and the previous book *"EXAM-ORIENTED ANATOMY - Below diaphragm"* which adequately covers the subject. Usually students have to purchase separate books for Anatomy, Histology, Embryology, Gen. Anatomy, Genetics, etc. Dr. Shoukat N. Kazi has tried to cover all these branches in simple language with the help of computerized line diagrams. It is designed to meet the need of the undergraduate students appearing the exams. *Most of the information is given in tabular forms, easy to compare and remember and clinical applications of the subject have been touched adequately.*

The book speaks the long experience of the author in the subject and will minimize the stress and strain of a medical student during pre-examination period. I congratulate the author for this venture and wish the book great success.

Dr. Shingare P. H.
M.S.

Dean Grant Medical College &
Sir J. J. Group of Hospitals
Byculla, Mumbai 400 008.

- Prof. & former Head, Dept. of Anatomy Grant Medical College, Sir. J.J. Group of Hospitals
- Ex. Dean, Faculty of Medicine North Maharashtra University.
- Ex-Controller of Exam - MUHS, Nashik.
- Ex-Chairman BOS Preclinical -MUHS.
- Member of BOS Preclinical Faculty of Medicine & Faculty of Dentistry - MUHS.
- Ex-Vice Dean U. G. - Grant Medical College, Mumbai.
- Ex. Vice Dean P. G. - Grant Medical College, Mumbai.

ABOUT THE BOOK

Medical Council of India has reduced the duration of first year M.B.B.S. by 6 months and introduced new pattern of questions which include long answer question, short notes, short answer question, clinical problems and multiple choice question. The students are expected to know all the topics as well as specific information and minute, relevant details having clinical importance.

There is no source for the definition and the extent of the contents of the various terms used in the theory questions. The author has extensively discussed these terms with eminent anatomist in India and attempted to define these terms. He is aware of the limitations and has high regard about others views.

To all above problems the author has given a solution by a book **'Exam Oriented Anatomy'**.

The salient features of the book are

- The book is written using short and simple sentences.
- Three types of questions are discussed 47 LAQs (Long Answer Questions), 125 SN (Short Notes) & 38 SAQs (Short Answer Questions).
- The information given in italic is the information required to answer the MCQs.
- The answers are written in the form of points by using indentation.
  1.
     A.
        a.
           I.
              i.
                 -
  2.
- Tables are used to save the time and display the information for immediate references for the students and examiners.
- The relevant, simple, linear, informative diagrams are drawn with the respective colours.
- Histology diagrams are drawn by pink and violet colour.
- The question of the development of organ is discussed by applying rule of five wives and one husband by using key word NORTHY (When, Who, Where, What, How & Why).
  - o Chronological age: When.
  - o Germ layer: Who.
  - o Site: Where.
  - o Source: What and how.
  - o Anomalies: Deviation from normal. Anomalies are described depending upon the incidence.
- Important key words, which help to memorize the subject without taxation to the memory.
- **'Key to memory'** is displayed at the end of the book, which help the student to revise important points.

The author humbly request all the students, teachers and well wishers to point out any corrections, which will be rectified in the next edition. He is very much free for correction and welcomes all sorts of criticism.

Special thanks

I am extending my sincere and special thanks to following persons, without whom the book would not have been completed.

♦ **Dr. P. H. Shingare** (Professor & Head, Department of Anatomy, Grant Medical College, Mumbai) has meticulously corrected the text and has given solutions to diagrams. He has tolerated my disturbance at odd hours in his busy schedule.

♦ **Dr. Mrs. Kanaklata Iyer** (Professor of Anatomy at Somaiya Medical College, Sion, Mumbai.) has really given a breakthrough to the problems of diagrams. She has helped outrightly by sparing her valuable time through her busy schedule by taking keen interest. She has contributed for diagrams of gross anatomy of abdomen, inferior extremity and general embryology.

♦ **Dr. Savgaonkar** (Professor of Anatomy at B. J. Medical College, Pune) has drawn histology diagrams of abdomen section. He being my close friend, understood the difficulties and offered his help by completing the diagrams in very short time.

♦ **Dr. Anjali Dhamangaonkar** (Associate Professor, in Anatomy at G. S. Medical College, Mumbai) has contributed to the general embryology diagrams. It was very difficult for her to give some time. But her desire to help me has solved the problems.

♦ **Dr. Manvikar Purushottam Rao** (Lecturer in Anatomy at Dr. D. Y. Patil Medical College, Pimpri) has drawn some of the histology diagrams.

♦ **Dr. Kadasne D. K.** has allowed me to use some of the diagrams from his book.

♦ *Lt. Col. (Retd)* **Dr. P. K. Verma** M.B.B.S., M.S., (Professor & Head, Department of Anatomy, MIMER'S Medical College, Talegaon, Dabhade) for critical evaluation and valuable suggestions.

♦ **Dr. Mrs. U. P. Dubhashi** Professor of Dr. D. Y. Patil Medical College, Pimpri, for her valuable guidance in histology diagrams and constant encouragement.

♦ **Dr. Mrs. K. A. Rangari** Professor of D. Y. Patil Medical College, Pimpri for her valuable correction in gross anatomy.

Acknowledgment

Writing acknowledgment is a sign of sigh of relief. It is the last leaf of the process of book writing. Though there is a feeling that the phenomenon of book writing has ended, in reality it is the beginning of shouldering the responsibility of the contents. Though I have authored the contents, it was indeed a teamwork. Many of my friends, colleagues and students have contributed immensely. It is great pleasure to acknowledge them.

When I proposed the idea of writing an 'Exam Oriented Anatomy' book to late **Dr. Indra Bhargava**, he patted on my back and gave an encouragement to take the first step in this direction. My sincere and humble salutations to the great soul.

Prof. Dr. Mahdi Hasan (Professor & Chairman, Department of Anatomy & Founder Director, Inter Disciplinary Brain Research Center, Dean, Principal & Chief Medical Superintendent, Jawaharlal Nehru Medical College, Aligarh Muslim University) has agreed to write a preface without any hesitation and guided me regarding the approach to the subject. I think myself fortunate to have the preface of such eminent professor in Anatomy. I salute to him from the bottom of my heart.

Dr. Inderbir Singh (Professor Emeritus, Rohtak) has thrown light upon the definition of each term used in the examination and warned to use the original diagrams. I am really thankful for cautioning me about the consequences. I am indebted to his valuable guidance. **Dr. V. Balasubramanyam,** (Professor and head department of anatomy St. John's Medical College, Bangalore) thoroughly went through the general lay out of the book and gave me very valuable suggestions regarding alteration of diagrams and copy right regulations.

My sincere and heartfelt thanks to following colleagues.

Dr. P. H. Shingare (Professor & Head, Department of Anatomy, Grant Medical College, Mumbai) for preparing the preface and guidance in all respects.

Dr. Kadasne (Civil Surgeon & Professor of Anatomy at Government Medical College, Nagpur), **Dr. Mrs. S. L. Pathak** (Associate Professor at Government Medical College, Nagpur) and **Dr. Mrs. Palikundwar** (Professor at Government Medical College, Nagpur) have given their invaluable guidance in drawing diagrams.

My sincere thanks are to **Dr. P. L. Jahagirdar** (Professor at Al-Amin Medical College, Bijapur) for encouragement in the initial stage of writing the book.

I am very much thankful to **Dr. Miss. A. N. Nandedkar** (former Professor & HOD) for understanding me and making me free from departmental activities. She has knowingly unknowingly helped me a lot in bringing up the book. I am also thankful to **Dr. Mrs. V. Arole**, Professor & HOD at D.Y. Patil Medical College, Pimpri, for inspiring me from time to time. I am also thankful to **Dr. D. L. Ingole** (Dean & Pro Vice Chancellor of Dr. D. Y. Patil Vidyapeeth - Deemed University) & **Mr. B. S. Mane** (Registrar of Dr. D. Y. Patil Medical College, Pimpri) for their constant and continued encouragement.

Dr. Herekar (Professor at Government Medical College, Miraj), Dr. Mrs. Aruna Mukherji (Ex. Deputy Dean & Professor at M. G. M. Medical College, New Mumbai), Dr. Bhatnagar (Professor Emeritus) & Dr. Sadhna Roy Chaudhary for inspiring me to write the book.

I must thank my core group who were associated with the metamorphosis of the book since inception. I thank Dr. Manvikar Purushottam Rao, Dr. R. J. Patil (Professor at Dr. D. Y. Patil Medical College) for their contribution to every section of the book in each stage of the process of writing.

My heartfelt thanks are to Ms. Benazeer Mujawar who had worked odd hours tirelessly for secretarial help. Her contribution has been indispensable. Mr. Sanjay Raut, our artist who has drawn the diagrams and patiently done numerous corrections as suggested. I must thank Mrs. Geeta Pomaji and Mr. Dinesh Kelji for immense help. I sincerely acknowledge with gratitude the patience, skill and zeal of Mr. Pradeep Tamse for proofreading and gearing-up the things faster.

I should not fail to mention the name of my better half Mrs. Kamartaj S. Kazi who is my silent and constant inspiration. She has kept me free from all our domestic and family problems. I express my grateful appreciation for her love, patience and understanding. I also appreciate my daughter Ms. Sadiya for tolerating my absence from home. I am indebted for the support and blessings of my parents. I constantly get charged by the moral boosting by my brothers Shikandar, Kabir, Allabax and Nazir. I am also thankful to my brother Mr. Badshah Kazi for his continuous feedback and support. I extend my thanks to my elder brother Mr. Akbar Kazi who has constantly encouraged me to write the book. I would like to extend my thanks to Mrs. Shama Kazi for understanding me and allowing to remain absent in real time.

Last and most important are the students, without whose feed-back the book would not have taken the shape.

It has been my pleasure to work with the staff of CBS Publication and Distributors (Delhi), Mr. Satish Kumar Jain, Mr. Vinod Jain, Mr. Wajid Khan & Mr. B. R. Sharma, for their keen interest and devotion in getting this book published.

Dr. S. N. Kazi
60, Atlas colony,
Mahesh Nagar, Pimpri,
Pune - 411 018.
Mobile - 94220 27718.

Syllabus of Maharashtra University of Health Sciences, Dr. D. Y. Patil Medical College, Deemed University, Pimpri

Paper II (Below Diaphragm)

Includes gross anatomy, systemic histology, systemic embryology of upper limb, thorax, head-face-neck & neuro anatomy.

Pattern of Question Papers :
(The syllabus and the pattern of question paper of MUHS and Dr. D. Y. Patil Medical College, Deemed Vidyapeeth is same)

Maharashtra University of Health Sciences & Dr. D. Y. Patil Vidyapeeth Deemed University

Total Marks 50   {30 Minutes}

Section A
  Q. No. 1   Multiple choice questions (MCQ)   : 15 Marks
Section B
  Q. No. 2   Write in brief (five out of six)   : 10 Marks (2 marks each)
  Q. No. 3   On applied anatomy (two out of three)   : 8 marks   (4 marks each)
Section C
  Q. No. 4   Long Question OR
  Q. No. 4   Long Question   : 9 Marks
  Q. No. 5   Write Short Notes (two out of three)   : 8 Marks (4 Marks each)

Rajiv Gandhi University of Health Sciences

Paper I   Total Marks 100

Contents   Types & No. of Questions   **Marks**

Section - I

1. Long Essays :   : 20 Marks (2 x 10 marks)
    Head and Neck, Brain and spinal cord, Thorax including
    diaphragm and upper limbs.

2. Long Essays :   : 50 Marks (10 x 5 marks)
    Head and Neck, Brain and spinal cord, Thorax including
    diaphragm and upper limbs.

3. Short answers :   : 30 Marks (15 x 2 marks)
    General Anatomy, Histology and Embryology and also
    Head and Neck, Brain and Spinal cord, Thorax including
    diaphragm and upper limbs.

Section - II
1. Short Essays   : 50 Marks (10 x 5 marks)
Section - III
1. Short Answers   : 32 Marks (16 x 2 marks)

Bharati Vidyapeeth Medical College

Marks 100   **{3 Hrs.}**

Instruction: Answer **any five** from each section.

Section-I

Q. No.1	Short notes on	:10 marks (2 x 5 marks)
	a. General anatomy	
	b. General embryology	
Q. No.2	LAQ from superior extremity.	:10 marks
Q. No.3	LAQ from superior extremity.	:10 marks
Q. No.4	LAQ from inferior extremity.	:10 marks
Q. No.5	LAQ from inferior extremity.	:10 marks
Q. No.6	Notes on	:10 marks
	a. General anatomy.	
	b. General embryology.	

Section II

Q. No.7	Write short notes on	:10 marks (2 x 5 marks)
	a. General anatomy	
	b. Genetics	
Q. No.8	LAQ on abdomen	: 10 marks
Q. No.9	LAQ on abdomen	: 10 marks
Q. No.10	LAQ on pelvis	: 10 marks
Q. No.11	LAQ on pelvis	: 10 marks
Q. No.12	Notes on	: 10 marks (2 x 5 marks)
	a. General anatomy	
	b. Genetics	

Prototype description of the questions

LAQ on joint
1. **Introduction :**
2. **Classification**
   A.   Structural classification
      a.   Depending upon the number of bones
      b.   Depending upon the presence of intra articular structure
      c.   Depending upon the shape of the articular surface of the bone
      d.   Depending upon the presence & absence of the features of typical synovial joint
      e.   Depending upon the axis
   B.   Functional classification
      a.   Depending upon the mobility
3. **Bones taking part in the joint**
4. **Ligaments**
   A.   Fibrous capsule
      a.   Attachments of the capsule to the proximal and distal bones
      b.   Variation of the thickness of the capsule
      c.   Areas where the capsule is deficient
      d.   Factors (muscles, ligaments) strengthening (reinforcing) the capsule
   B.   Other ligaments
5. **Bursae in relation to joint**
6. **Movements**
   A.   Name of the movement
   B.   Range of the movement
   C.   Axis of the movement
   D.   Limiting factors (bones and ligaments)
   E.   Muscles bringing movement
7. **Intra articular structures**
8. **Relations**
   A.   Anterior
   B.   Posterior
   C.   Lateral
   D.   Medial
   E.   Superior
   F,   Inferior
9. **Blood supply**
   A.   Arterial supply
   B.   Venous drainage
10. **Nerve supply**
11. **Applied anatomy.**
   A.   Functions :
      a.   Maintenance
      b.   Common diseases of the joint

B. Disease :
  a. Dislocation or fracture of the joint
  b. Deformity
  c. Ankylosis

―――――◇―――――

LAQ on Artery
1. **Introduction :**
   Region supplied
2. **Origin**
3. **Termination**
4. **Extent**
5. **Course and relations**
6. **Distribution**
7. **Branches**
   A. Muscular branches,
   B. Cutaneous branches,
   C. Nutrient branches,
   D. Articular branches,
   E. Branches to nerve,
   F. Anastomosing branches,
   G. Terminal branches,
8. **Applied anatomy**
   A. Pressure points
   B. Ligation and exposure
   C. Vulnerable points
   D. Collateral circulation
   E. Arteriography
9. **Development :**
10. **Variations :**

―――――◇―――――

LAQ on Vein
1. **Introduction :**
   Areas drained
2. **Formation**
   A. How?
   B. Where?
3. **Termination**
   A. How?
   B. Where?
4. **Course and relation**
5. **Subdivision**
6. **Peculiarities**

7.   **Tributaries**
8.   **Applied anatomy**
    A.   Obstruction and collateral circulation
    B.   Vulnerable points
    C.   Surgical procedure

—◇—

LAQ on cranial nerve
1.   **Introduction** : Brief information about the nerve.
2.   **Nature :**
    A.   Sensory or
    B.   Motor or
    C.   Mixed
3.   **Functional components**
4.   **Nuclei related to the nerve and their location :**
    A.   Sensory
    B.   Motor
    C.   Salivatory
    D.   Lacrimatory
    E.   Parasympathetic
5.   **Exit of the nerve :**
    A.   Part of the brainstem
    B.   Site of the exit
    C.   Surface of the exit
6.   Course of the nerve
    A.   Intracranial
        a.   Intraneural
        b.   Extraneural
    B.   Extracranial
7.   Important relations
8.   Branches
    A.   Sensory
    B.   Motor
    C.   Articular
    D.   Cutaneous
    E.   Vascular
    F.   Communicating
    G.   Glandular
    H.   Ganglionic
9.   Applied anatomy
    A.   Lesion of the nerve
        a.   Site and effect of upper motor neuron
        b.   Site and effect of lower motor nerve
    B. Syndromes

—◇—

LAQ on peripheral nerve

1. **Introduction :** Region of distribution
2. **Nature**
3. **Origin and root value :**
   A. Level
   B. Mode of origin
4. **Course and relations**
5. **Branches :**
   A. Sensory branches,
   B. Motor branches,
   C. Articular branches,
   D. Vascular branches,
   E. Communicating &
   F. Miscellaneous.
6. **Applied anatomy :**
   A. Functions and testing of the nerve
   B. In disease
      a. Sensory - loss or pain
      b. Motor - paralysis deformity
   C. Vulnerable points for injury

SN on ganglion
1. Introduction
2. Gross anatomy
   A. Shape and size
   B. Situation
   C. Relation
3. Components
   A. Sensory
   B. Secretive motor / parasympathetic
   C. Sympathetic
4. Applied anatomy

LAQ on space / triangle
Axilla, cubital fossa and triangles of neck (anterior, posterior, suboccipital).
1. **Introduction :**
   A. Location
   B. Shape

2. **Boundaries :**
   A. Lateral border / wall
   B. Medial border
   C. Superior border
   D. Inferior border
   E. Roof / anterior wall
      a. Skin,
      b. Cutaneous vein, artery, nerve
      c. Superficial fascia
      d. Deep fascia
   F. Floor
3. **Content :**
   A. Neurovascular
   B. Glands
   C. Other structures
4. **Applied anatomy**
   A. Function
      a. Protection of the contents
      b. Accommodate for movements
   B. Disease
      a. Vulnerable structures
      b. Collection of pus
      c. Path of spread
      d. Incision drainage

LAQ on hollow organ

1. **Gross anatomy (e.g. Heart) :** It includes everything about a particular organ excluding *Histology, Development and Applied anatomy*
   A. Introduction :
      a. General introduction : Brief information about the organ.
      b. Location
      c. Size
      d. Peculiarity(ies)
      e. Dimension
   B. External features :
      a. Parts : Subdivision
      b. Situation, extent &
      c. Capacity.
   C. Internal features (orifices)
   D. Site of the normal constriction and curvatures
   E. Relations
      a. Peritoneal &
      b. Visceral.

F. Blood supply
   a. Arterial supply
      I. Main artery of the organ,
      II. Origin of the artery,
      III. Important relations,
      IV. Peculiarities if any,
      V. Relevant applied anatomy.
   b. Venous drainage
      I. Main veins &
      II. Draining veins.

G. Nerve supply
   a. Sympathetic
      I. Origin of the fiber
      II. Function
      III. Action on
         i. Smooth muscle
         ii. Blood vessels
         iii. Sphincter
   b. Parasympathetic
      I. Origin of the fibers
      II. Function
      III. Action on
         i. Smooth muscle
         ii. Glands
         iii. Sphincter
      IV. Movement
   c. Somatic
      I. Origin of the fibers
      II. Action at various site

H. Lymphatic
   a. Lymph nodes draining the organ and situation
   b. Afferent lymphatic
   C. Efferent lymphatic

2. **Histology**
   A. Identifying features
   B. Structures and their functions
   C. Correlation at micro (cellular) level
   D. Staining peculiarities

3. **Development**
   A. Chronological age
   B. Germ layer
   C. Site
   D. Source
   E. Anomalies

4. **Applied anatomy**
    A. Obstruction : Congenital or acquired
        a. Cause
        b. Effect
    B. Vulnerable blood supply
    C. Important relations of the structure helping to diagnose the disease.
    D. Operative procedures
        a. Removal or resection
        b. Anastomosis
        c. Exposures
    E. Diagnostics methods of examination

LAQ on solid organ
1. **Gross anatomy (e.g. Lung and tonsil):** It includes everything about a particular organ excluding *Histology, Development and Applied anatomy*.
    A. Introduction : Brief information about the organ.
        a. Location and orientation
        b. Shape
        c. Dimension :
            I.   Length,
            II.   Breadth and
            III. Weight of the organ.
    B. External features :
        a. Subdivision
        b. Ends or poles
        c. Borders
        d. Surfaces
        e. Lobes
        f. Capsule / coverings
        g. Hilum / structures in the hilum and the position of the hilum
        h. Side determination (for paired organ)
        i. Fissure
        j. Bare area
    C. Relations
        a. Peritoneal
        b. Visceral
        c. Neurovascular
        d. Fascial
    D. Blood supply
        a. Arterial supply
            I.   Main artery of the organ
            II.   Origin of the artery
            III. Important relations
            IV.   Peculiarities if any
            V.   Relevant applied anatomy

    b.   Venous drainage
            I.   Main veins
            II.   Draining veins
E.   Nerve supply
    a.   Sympathetic
            I.   Origin of the fiber,
            II.   Functions of the nerve &
            III. Action on.
                    i.   Smooth muscle,
                    ii.   Blood vessels &
                    iii. Sphincter.
    b.   Parasympathetic
            I.   Origin of the fibers,
            II.   Function &
            III. Action on
                    i.   Smooth muscle,
                    ii.   Glands,
                    iii. Sphincter.
    c.   Somatic
            I.   Origin of the fibers
            II.   Action at various site
F.   Lymphatic
    a.   Lymph nodes draining the organ and situation,
    b.   Afferent lymphatic &
    c.   Efferent lymphatic.
G.   Duct system

2.   **Histology**
    A.   Staining character,
    B.   Type of the cell,
    C.   Position of nuclei &
    D.   Identifying features.

3.   **Development**
    A.   Chronological age,
    B.   Germ layer,
    C.   Site,
    D.   Source &
    E.   Anomalies.

4.   **Applied anatomy**
    A.   Relations of the structure helping to diagnose the disease.
    B.   Diagnostic methods of examination
    C.   Operative procedure

1. **Gross anatomy of tubular, Long structure (e.g. Oesophagus, Ureter, vas deferens fallopian tube, thoracic duct):** It includes everything about a particular organ excluding *Histology, Development and Applied anatomy*

   It includes

   A. Introduction : Brief information about the organ.
      a. General introduction
      b. Measurement :
         I. Length,
         II. Diameter &
      c. Constrictions,
   B. Internal features (interior)
   C. Course
   D. Relations
      a. Peritoneal,
      b. Visceral.
   E. Blood supply
      a. Arterial supply
         I. Main artery of the organ,
         II. Origin of the artery,
         III. Important relations,
         IV. Peculiarities if any &
         V. Relevant applied anatomy.
      b. Venous drainage
         I. Main veins &
         II. Draining veins.
   F. Nerve supply
      a. Sympathetic
         I. Origin of the fiber,
         II. Function(s) &
         III. Action on.
            i. Smooth muscle,
            ii. Blood vessels &
            iii. Sphincter.
      b. Parasympathetic
         I. Origin of the fibers,
         II. Function(s),
         III. Actions on
            i. Smooth muscle,
            ii. Glands &
            iii. Sphincter.

c. Somatic
  I.   Origin of the fibers &
  II. Action at various site.
G. Lymphatic
  a. Lymph nodes draining the organ and situation,
  b. Afferent lymphatics &
  c. Efferent lymphatics.

2. **Histology**
  A. Identifying features
  B. Structures and their functions
  C. Correlation at micro (cellular) level
  D. Staining peculiarities

3. **Development**
  A. Chronological age,
  B. Germinal layer,
  C. Site,
  D. Source &
  E. Anomalies.
    a. Common anomalies
    b. Sex,
    c. Incidence.

4. **Applied anatomy**
  A. Relations of the structure helping to diagnose the disease.
  B. Investigation carried out diagnose the disease.

———————————◇———————————

SN on muscle
1. **Introduction :**
  A. Position
  B. Compartment
2. **Peculiarity(ies)**
  A. Subcutaneous
  B. Intra capsular
  C. Synovial attachment
  D. Comminuting to joint space
  E. Divides the artery
  F. Peripheral heart
  G. Contents (venous sinus)
3. **Morphology**
  A. Shape
  B. Direction of fibers
  C. Type of fibers

4. **Origin**
   A. Site
      a. Bone
      b. Ligament and/or
      c. Fascia
   B. Mode
      a. Fleshy
      b. Tendinous or aponeurotic
5. **Insertion**
   A. Site
   B. Mode
6. **Relations**
   A. Superficial surface
   B. Deep surface
   C. Upper border
   D. Lower border
   E. Bursae
   F. Sesamoid bone
7. **Nerve supply**
   A. Segments, root value
   B. Source
   C. Point of entry
8. **Actions**
   A. As a prime mover
   B. As a synergist
   C. As an antagonist
   D. As a fixator
9. **Applied anatomy**
   A. Position of the part after paralysis of the muscle
   B. Testing the muscle

Histology lymphatic organ (palatine tonsil, thymus, lymph node)
1. **About capsule**
2. **Division of the gland : cortex medulla**
3. **Types of cell**
4. **Lining epithelium**
5. **Arrangement of cell**
6. **Specific cells of the organ**
7. **Particular features of the organ**
8. **Staining characters**

SN on gland

1. **Type of the gland**
2. **Classification of the exocrine gland based on**
   A. Number of cells
   B. Way of expulsion of secretion
   C. Nature of secretion
   D. Depending upon the shape of the acinus
3. **Gross anatomy**
   A. **Morphology**
      a. Size, shape and weight
      b. Location
      c. Extent
   B. **Relations**
      a. Superficial and deep
      b. Superior, inferior, medial and lateral
4. **Blood supply**
   A. Arterial supply
   B. Venous drainage
5. **Nerve supply**
6. **Lymphatic**
7. **Histology**
   A. Identification features
   B. Staining peculiarities
   C. Structure and function
   D. Correlation at micro (cellular) level

LAQ on ventricles

1. Gross anatomy
   A. Introduction
   B. Extent
   C. Communication
2. Boundaries
   A. Roof
   B. Floor
   C. Anterior wall
   D. Posterior wall
   E. Lateral wall
3. Recesses
4. Applied anatomy

CONTENTS

Section One
SUPEX

Section Two
THORAX

Section Three
HEAD, FACE AND NECK

Section Four
NEURO

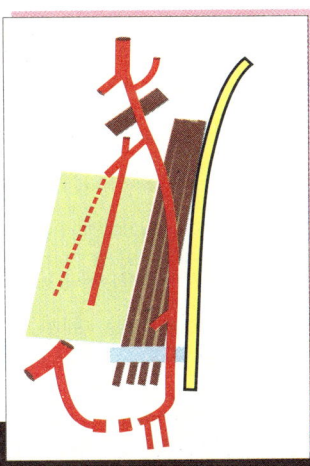

INDEX

SN-1   Coracoid process

(*Coracos* crow's beak)

1. **Introduction :** It is a process of a scapula projecting forward and slightly laterally.

2. **Evolution :** It represents the ventral element of scapula and is homologous to the ischium of hip bone. It is a type of atavistic epiphysis.

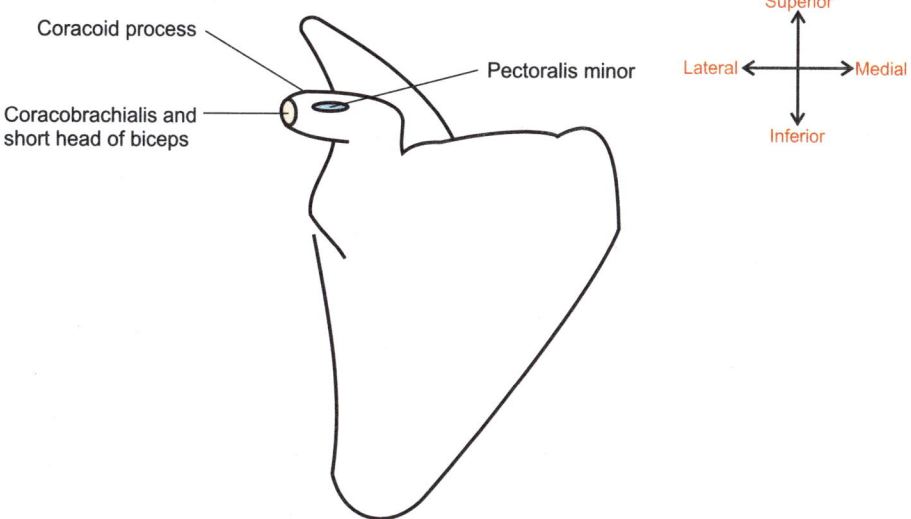

Fig. 1.1 : Muscles attached to coracoid process.

3. **Attachments :**
   A. It gives attachment to following <u>muscles</u>
      a. Short head of biceps and coracobrachialis which are attached to the tip of coracoid process.
      b. Pectoralis minor gets inserted into the superior surface of the medial border of the coracoid process.
   B. It gives attachment to following <u>ligaments</u>
      a. Coracohumeral ligament which extends from lateral border of coracoid process to anatomical neck of humerus.
      b. Coracoacromial ligament : It is attached to coracoid and acromial process of scapula.
      c. Coracoclavicular ligament : It is a strong band between coracoid process and clavicle. It consists of
         I. Conoid part : It is vertical triangular band. The base is attached to the conoid tubercle of clavicle and apex is attached to the root of the coracoid process.
         II. Trapezoid part is attached to trapezoid line.
      d. Costocoracoid ligament : It extends from the coracoid process to the first rib. It is a thickening of clavipectorial fascia.

4. **Applied Anatomy :** *The weight is transmitted to the medial 2/3rd of clavicle through coracoclavicular ligament.*

LAQ-1 — Describe mammary gland as under
1. **Gross anatomy**   2. **Histology**
3. **Development and**   4. **Applied anatomy.**

1.   Gross anatomy :

A.   **Introduction :**
   a.   General introduction : It is a modified sweat gland, rudimentary in male, well developed in female after puberty.
   b.   Situation : It is present in the superficial fascia except the tail part which pierces deep fascia of axilla through foramen of Langer. It is called tail of Spence.
   c.   Extent :
      I.   Vertically : It extends from 2nd to 6th rib.
      II. Horizontally : It extends from the lateral border of sternum to mid axillary line.

B.   **External features :**
   Structures :
   a.   Skin consists of nipple and areola.
      I.   Nipple : It is a blackish, conical projection of skin situated in the 4th intercostal space. It is pierced by 10-15 lactiferous ducts and contains smooth muscles.
      II. Areola : It is circular blackish discolouration around the nipple. It contains plenty of modified sebaceous glands, which enlarge during pregnancy and are called tubercles of Montgomery. They secrete oily secretion, which lubricates and prevents cracking of the skin over the nipple. It is devoid of hair and fat.
   b.   Parenchyma : It consists of
      I.   Glandular part : It consists of alveoli, lactiferous duct and dilated part called lactiferous sinus.

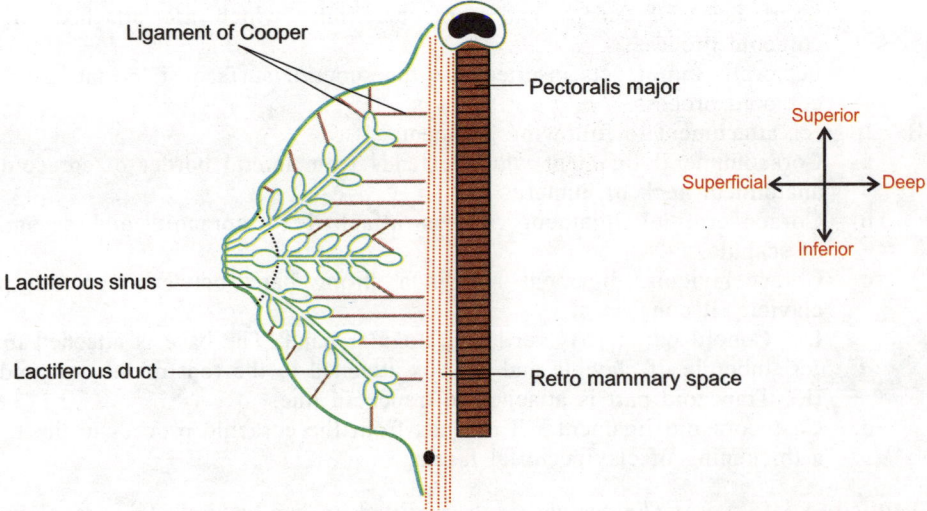

Fig. 1.2 : Structure of the mammary gland.

II. Fibrous stroma : It consists of fibrous septa, which extends from skin to the deep fascia and divides gland into 10 to 15 lobes by ligament of Cooper.

III. Fatty stroma : It lies between septum and glandular part.

C. Relations :

a. Superficial relations are : Skin, superficial fascia.

b. Deep relations are :

I. Retro mammary space : It is traversed by lymph and blood vessels. *The breast prostheses are usually inserted in this space.*

II. Pectoral fascia.

III. Muscles : The base of the gland rests on the following muscles

   i. Pectoralis major in medial $2/3^{rd}$

   ii. Serratus anterior in lateral $1/3^{rd}$

   iii. External oblique in inferomedial quadrant.

c. Structures deep to above muscles are : Subclavius, clavipectoral fascia, pectoralis minor and suspensory ligament of axilla.

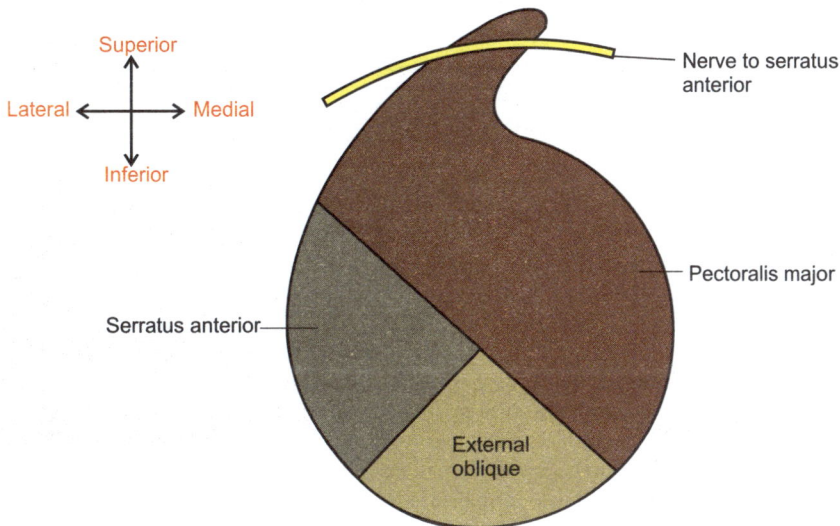

Fig. 1.3 : Deep relations of the mammary gland and its tail.

D. Blood supply : The mammary gland is extremely vascular.

a. Arterial supply :

I. Lateral thoracic artery (second branch of axillary artery) **is the main artery supplying the mammary gland**, that curls around the lateral border of pectoralis major and supplies lateral part of mammary gland.

II. Internal thoracic artery (branch of first part of subclavian artery) sends branches through intercostal spaces. It supplies medial half of the mammary gland. *The branches in the second and third intercostal space are largest.*

III. Lateral branches of posterior intercostal arteries (branch of descending thoracic aorta) give perforating branches which also supply mammary gland.

IV. Acromio thoracic, a branch of axillary artery supplies upper lateral quadrant of the gland.

    b.   Venous drainage : The main veins draining the area around areola and glandular tissue are deep veins. These veins run with the corresponding arteries. The veins are
       I.   Internal thoracic vein drains into - subclavian vein.
       II. Acromiothoracic vein
       III. Superior thoracic vein   } drains into - axillary vein.
       IV. Lateral thoracic vein
       V. Posterior intercostal veins are important link to the internal venous plexus and to the vertebral veins. This is a pathway for metastatic spread to bone.

E. Nerve supply :
    a.   Sensory and sympathetic : 4th to 6th intercostal nerve.
    b.   Hormonal control :
       I.   Oestrogen stimulates duct system.
       II. Progesterone stimulates the formation of alveoli.
       III. Oestrogen and progesterone are responsible for the formation of true (secretory) alveoli during pregnancy.
       IV. Prolactin maintains lactation and
       V. Oxytocin helps in ejection of milk.

SN-2   Lymphatic drainage of mammary gland   V. Imp.

F. Lymphatic drainage
    a.   Lymphatic drainage is important because of the following reasons :
       I.   The malignancy of mammary gland is common in females particularly in post menopausal age.
       II. It almost spreads to the regional lymph nodes and to the opposite side.
       III. Early diagnosis has better prognosis.
    b.   Lymph nodes : 75 % lymphatics drain into axillary nodes.
       I.   20 % lymphatics drain into internal mammary nodes.
       II. 5 % lymphatics drain into posterior intercostal nodes.
    c.   Superficial and deep of lateral half of mammary gland drain into anterior group of axillary lymph nodes, central and apical group of axillary lymph nodes.
    d.   Medial half is divided into upper medial and lower medial quadrants.
    e.   Now a days, simpler nomenclature is adapted
       I.   Low nodes (level 1) : Below pectoralis minor muscle.
       II. Medium nodes (level 2) : Behind pectoralis minor muscle.
       III. High node (level 3) : Above pectoralis minor muscle.

Note : Please write the applied anatomy of lymphatic from the applied anatomy of mammary gland.

2. Histology :

2. Histology :

A. Classification : Apocrine, serous, modified, tubuloalveolar gland.

B. Microscopy : It consists of

    a. Glandular tissue which are lined by cuboidal epithelium and encloses large lumina.

    b. Large amount of fibrofatty tissue.

    c. A duct which is lined by two layers of cuboidal or flattened cells.

    d. In active stage, the lumen contain secretion.

Table 1.1 : The table shows 'lymphatic drainage of mammary gland'.

Particulars	Superficial (except skin over Nipple and areola)	Deep (Parenchyma+skin over nipple and areola)
Medial I. Upper medial	Drains into any one of the following lymph nodes : i. Parasternal group of lymph nodes on the same side (which are situated along the internal mammary artery) ii. Opposite parasternal group of lymph nodes. iii. Supraclavicular lymph nodes present above the clavicle	Drains into one of following nodes : i. Apical nodes and ii. Internal mammary lymph nodes.
II. Lower medial	Drains into any one of the lymph nodes mentioned below : i. Parasternal group of lymph nodes on the same side (which are situated along the internal mammary artery) ii. Opposite parasternal group of lymph nodes. iii. Drains into lymph node in the rectus sheath → Liver → ovary (Krukenberg's tumor).	

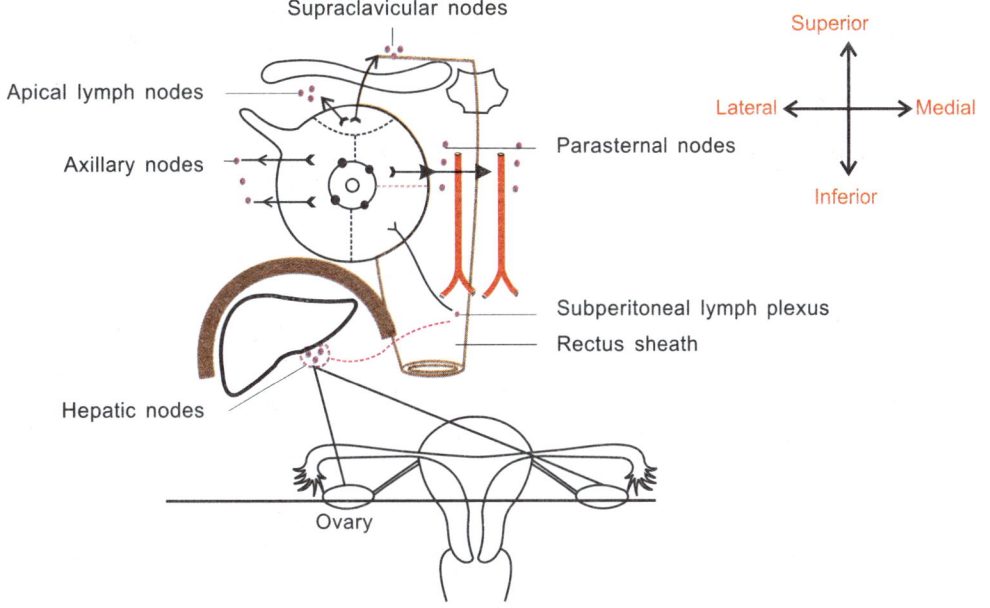

Fig. 1.4 : Lymphatic drainage of mammary gland.

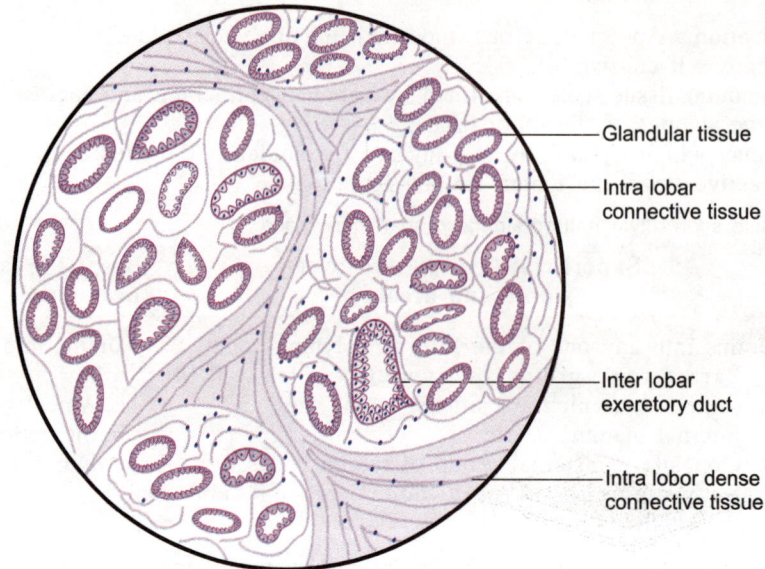

Fig. 1.5 : Mammary Gland (Active).

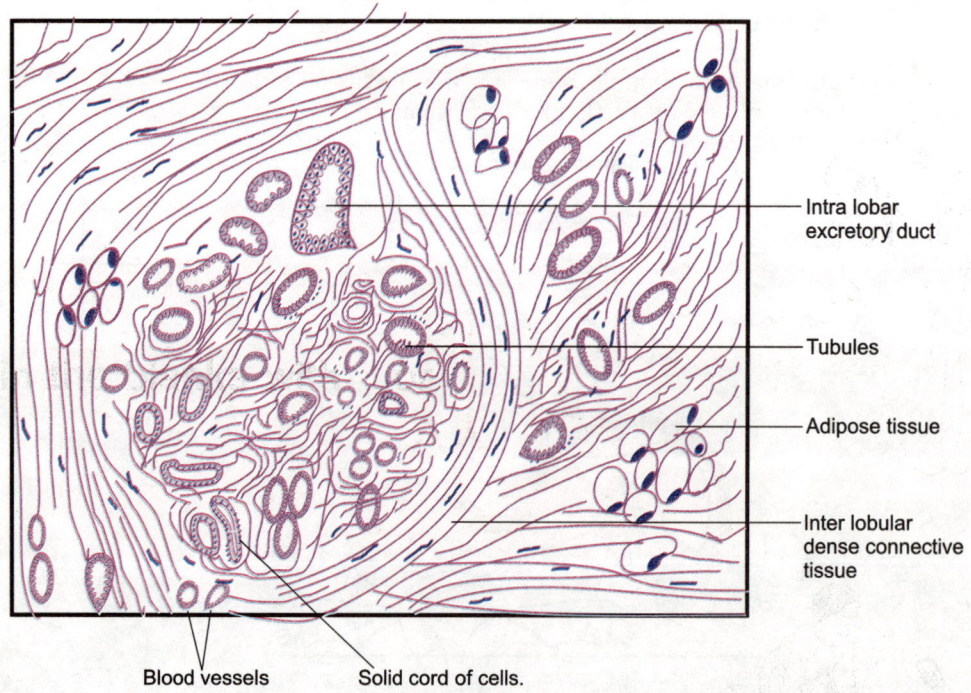

Fig. 1.6 : Histology of mammary gland.

SN-3   Development of mammary gland

3. **Development :**
    A. Chronological age : It develops in the fourth week of intrauterine life.
    B. Germ layer :
        a. Ectoderm and
        b. Mesoderm.
    C. Site : It develops in the region of milk line which extends from axilla to inguinal region on ventral side of body.
    D. Source :
        a. Epithelial lining of duct and alveoli are developed from surface ectoderm.
        b. Fibrofatty stroma is developed from underlying mesoderm.
    E. Anomalies :
        a. Polymastia : Supernumerary breast.
        b. Amastia : Absence of breast.
        c. Athelia : Absence of nipple.
        d. Polythelia : Supernumerary nipples.

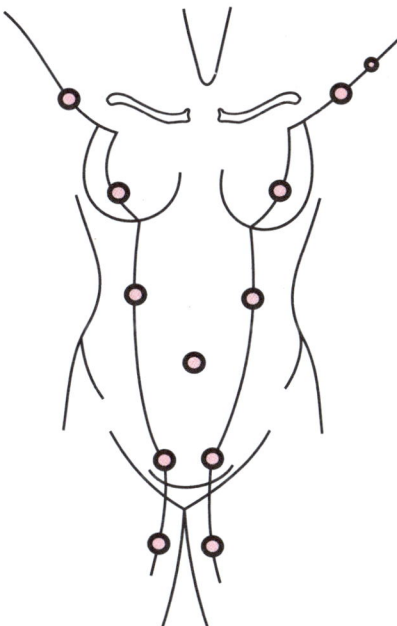

Fig. 1.7 : Diagram showing milk line.

4. **Applied anatomy :**
    A. In breast abscess, the incision is taken radially to avoid damage to the lactiferous duct.
    B. Applied anatomy of lymphatics :
        a. Axillary lymphadenopathy is frequently due to the infection and malignant diseases of mammary gland. In malignant disease the lymph node is hard, irregular and fixed to the deeper structures.
        b. Lymphatics from upper and lower medial quadrants go to opposite side and therefore a tumor arising from the medial half of mammary gland is dangerous.

c. Back door exit : The malignant cells may penetrate pectoralis major and go to Reiters lymph node, which drain into apical group of axillary lymph nodes.
d. Carcinoma usually arises from epithelium of larger ducts.
e. Suspensory ligaments of Cooper are infiltrated by malignant cells and produce dimples overlying skin.
f. Peau D'orange is a condition where the hair follicles over the lump appear to be retracted, and is caused by obstruction of the cutaneous lymphatics with stagnation of lymph and oedema of skin around the hair follicles. This resembles the skin of an orange, hence the name.

SN-4   Pectoralis major

1. **Origin** : It is a spiral muscle and has two heads
    A. Clavicular head : It arises from medial half of anterior surface of clavicle.
    B. Sternocostal head : It arises from
        a. Lateral part of anterior surface of sternum upto 6th costal cartilages.
        b. Second to sixth costal cartilages.
        c. Aponeurosis of external oblique muscle.

2. **Insertion** : By a flat bilaminar tendon (5 cms long) into the lateral lip of bicipital groove of humerus in 'U' shaped manner.
    A. Upper fibers are inserted in lower part.
    B. Lower fibers are inserted in upper part.
    C. Tendon is twisted by 180° and has two laminae which are described in the table 1.2.

Table 1.2 : The table shows detailed insertion of anterior and posterior lamina of pectoralis major.

Anterior lamina	Posterior lamina
A. Thick and shorter.	A. Thin and longer.

B. It receives 3 layers of muscle fibers
   a. Superficial fibers arises from clavicle
   b. Middle fibers arise from manubrium
   c. Deep fibers arises from margin of
      Sternum and 2nd to 6th rib.
	B. It receives fibers from
	   a. Front of sternum
	   b. 2nd to 6th rib
	   c. 6th costal cartilage
	   d. Aponeurosis of external oblique
	      a. and b. fibers are twisted and
	      forms the anterior axillary fold.

3. **Nerve supply :**
    A. Medial pectoral nerve (C_8 & T_1) : *It pierces pectoralis minor and supplies the muscle.*
    B. Lateral pectoral nerve (C_5, C_6 & C_7) : *It pierces clavipectoral fascia.*

4. **Action :**
    A. The clavicular fibers of pectoralis major combine with the anterior fibers of deltoid and bring flexion of the shoulder joint.
    B. The sternal fibers of pectoralis major combine with latissimus dorsi and bring adduction and medial rotation of the shoulder joint.
    C. It is also an accessory muscle of inspiration.
    D. It is well developed in climbing and flying animals.

SN-5   Clavipectoral fascia

1. **Introduction :** It is the strong sheet of fascia extending from pectoralis minor to the inferior surface of clavicle.

2. **Attachments :**
   A. Medially : It fuses with anterior intercostal membrane of upper two intercostal spaces and attaches to the first rib.
   B. Laterally : It is thick and dense and attaches to coracoid process.

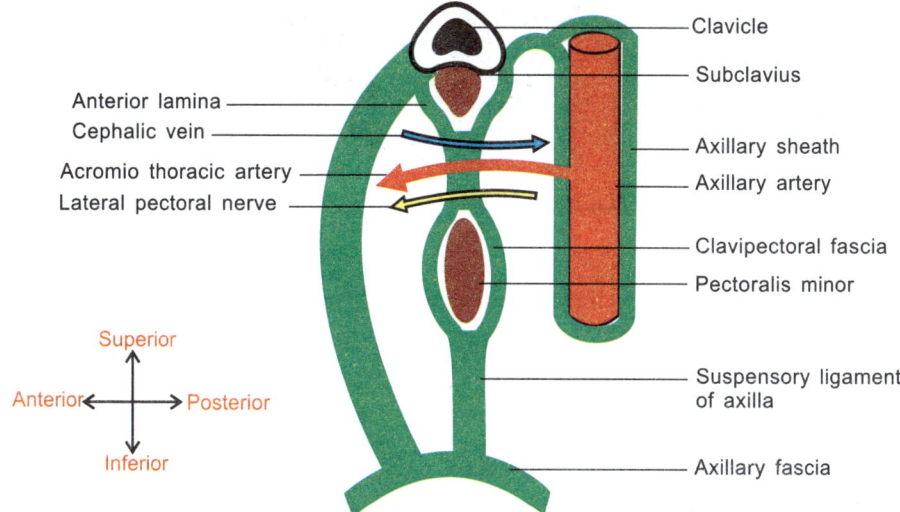

Fig. 1.8 : Vertical disposition of clavipectoral fascia.

   C. Above : It splits to enclose subclavius and attaches to the lips of the subclavian groove of clavicle. Its posterior layer has medial and lateral part. The medial part fuses with deep cervical fascia which connects the omohyoid to clavicle. Its lateral part fuses with the axillary sheath.
   D. Below : It splits to enclose pectoralis minor and ends laterally into short head of biceps.

3. **Modifications :**
   A. Costo-coracoid ligament : The fascia thickens along lower border of subclavius between coracoid process and first costo-chondral junction and is called costo-coracoid ligament.
   B. Suspensory ligament of axilla : The part of the fascia below the pectoralis minor.

4. **Structures piercing :**
   A. *Passing outwards*
      a. *Thoraco acromial artery and its branches*
      b. *Lateral pectoral nerve.*
   B. *Passing inwards*
      a. *Cephalic vein*
      b. *Lymphatics from*
         I. Infraclavicular nodes and
         II. Mammary gland.

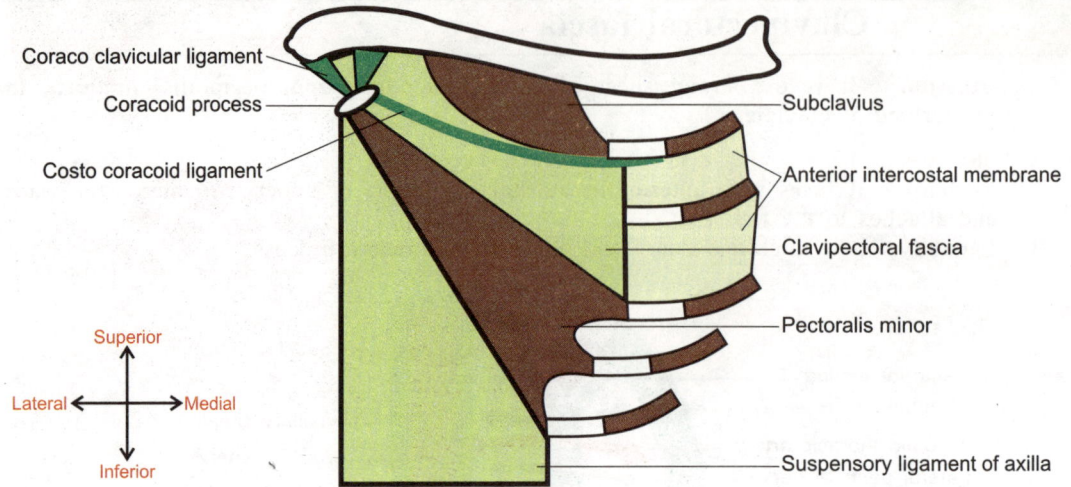

Fig. 1.9 : Horizontal disposition of clavipectoral fascia.

5. **Action :** It acts as a suspensory ligament of axilla and maintains the dome of axilla.

6. **Applied :** The malignant cells of breast may pierce clavipectoral fascia and go to Reiters and to the apical group of lymph nodes. This is called back-door exit.

LAQ-2 **Describe axilla under**
1. **Boundaries** 2. **Walls**
3. **Contents &** 4. **Applied anatomy.**

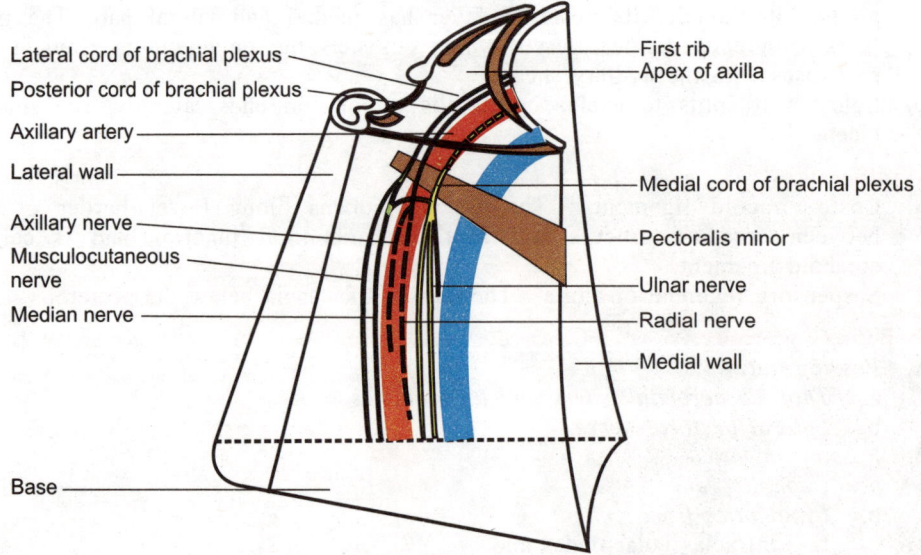

Fig. 1.10 : Boundaries and contents of right axilla.

Axilla (armpit) :
Introduction : It is pyramid. It is present in the medial side of upper part of arm.

1. **Boundaries :**
    A. Apex is also called cervico-axillary canal and is formed
        a. Medially : By outer border of 1st rib.
        b. Laterally : By superior border of scapula.
        c. Anteriorly : By posterior border of clavicle.
    B. Base is formed by
        a. Skin,
        b. Superficial fascia and
        c. Deep fascia extending from anterior axillary fold to posterior axillary fold.

2. **Walls :**
    A. Anterior wall is formed by following structures :-
        a. Superficial layer is formed by pectoralis major.
        b. Deep layer is formed by subclavius, clavipectoral fascia, pectoralis minor and suspensory ligament of axilla from above downwards.
    B. Posterior wall is formed by
        a. Subscapularis muscle,
        b. Latissimus dorsi muscle and
        c. Teres major muscle.
    C. Lateral wall is formed by
        a. Intertubercular sulcus of the shaft of humerus which contains long head of biceps brachii and
        b. Coracobrachialis and short head of biceps.
    D. Medial wall is broad and formed by
        a. Upper 4 to 5 ribs & their intercostal muscles,
        b. Upper part of serratus anterior covered by a strong fascia,
        c. Long thoracic nerve and
        d. Intercostobrachial nerve (T_2).

3. **Contents of axilla :**
    A. Axillary artery and its branches,
    B. Axillary vein and its tributaries,
    C. Cords of brachial plexus and their branches, long thoracic and intercostobrachial nerves,
    D. Axillary lymph nodes and their afferent and efferent connections and
    E. Axillary fat.

4. **Applied anatomy :**
    A. Abscess in axilla may occur
        a. Superficial to pectoralis minor muscle. Here abscess appears at the edge of anterior axillary fold or in the deltopectoral groove.
        b. Deep to pectoralis minor muscle. Here pus would surround vessels and nerves and ascend into neck or may track along the vessels in arm.
    B. Axillary abscess is drained by putting the knife at the base of axilla midway between anterior and posterior axillary fold and move towards thoracic side.
    C. One should be careful of the relations of vessels while removing lymph nodes.

LAQ-3   Describe brachial plexus

1. **Introduction :** It is the network of nerves present at the junction of neck and thorax. It supplies the muscles, joints, skin and blood vessels of the anterior wall of thorax, scapular region and upper limb. It is formed by ventral divisions of C_5, C_6, C_7, C_8 & T_1.

2. **Brachial plexus :** It may be fixed by two ways
   A. Prefixed : When C_4 root joins with C_5. Here C_4 is large T_2 is often absent.
   B. Postfixed : When T_2 root joins with T_1. Here C_4 root is absent. The contribution by T_1 is large.

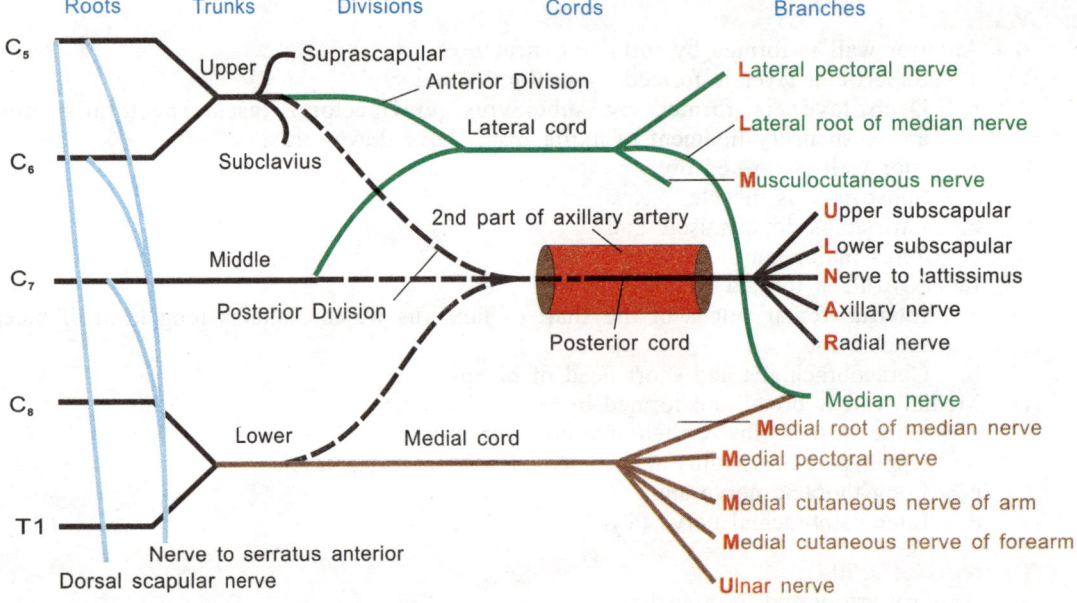

Fig. 1.11 : Roots, trunks, divisions, cords & branches of brachial plexus.

3. **Situation :** Roots of brachial plexus emerge between the scalenus anterior and scalenus medius muscles.
   A. Trunks appear in the lower part of posterior triangle of neck.
   B. Divisions lie behind the clavicle.
      a. Anterior divisions supply all the muscles present on the ventral part of thorax and upper limb.
      b. Posterior divisions supply the muscles present on dorsal part of thorax and upper limb.
   C. The Cords are present in axilla. *The names of the cords are in relation with the second part of axillary artery.* The cords give branches around 3rd part of axillary artery.

4. **Relations of brachial plexus :**
   A. Supra clavicular part : The roots and trunks of the brachial plexus lie above clavicle.
   B. Retroclavicular part : The divisions of brachial plexus lie behind the clavicle.
   C. Infra clavicular part : The cords and branches of cords lie below the clavicle.

5. **Branches :**
   A. The nerves arising from roots supply the muscles which bring protraction and retraction of shoulder girdle i.e.
      a. Nerve to rhomboids (dorsal scapular nerve) (C_5).
      b. Nerve to serratus anterior (long thoracic) (C_5, C_6 & C_7).
   B. Trunks
      a. Suprascapular nerve (C_5 & C_6) supplies
         I. Supraspinatus,
         II. Infraspinatus,
         III. Shoulder joint,
         IV. Acromioclavicular joint and
         V. Scapula.
      b. Nerve to subclavius (C_5 & C_6) supplies subclavius muscle.
   C. Cords : Following are the branches from respective cords.
      a. Lateral : 🔑 **L**aila **L**oves **M**ajnu
         I. **L**ateral pectoral nerve
         II. **L**ateral root of median nerve
         III. **M**usculo cutaneous nerve
      b. Medial 🔑 The word "medial" and the branches of the medial cord begin with the letter "**M**" except ulnar nerve
         I. **M**edial pectoral
         II. **M**edial root of median nerve
         III. **M**edial cutaneous nerve of arm
         IV. **M**edial cutaneous nerve of forearm
         V. **U**lnar nerve
      c. **Posterior** 🔑 **ULNAR**. The letters of the word "Ulnar" give the branches of the posterior cord.
         I. **U**pper subscapular.
         II. **L**ower subscapular.
         III. **N**erve to latissimus dorsi.
         IV. **A**xillary nerve.
         V. **R**adial nerve.

6. **Applied anatomy :**
   A. **Horner**'s syndrome : It is due to involvement of sympathetic nerve, which is contributed by T_1 through white rami communicans. It usually occurs due to injury at the root of brachial plexus.
   B. Erb's paralysis : Injury to upper trunk usually at the Erb's point causes Erb's paralysis.
   C. Klumpke's paralysis : Injury to the lower trunk of brachial plexus.
   D. Winging of scapula : Injury to the nerve to serratus anterior.
   E. Claw hand : Injury to the ulnar nerve.

SN-6   Horner's syndrome   V. Imp

Horner's syndrome : It is due to involvement of sympathetic nerve, which is contributed by T_1. It usually occurs due to injury at the root of brachial plexus.

🗝   HORNER. The letters of the word "Horner" give the information about clinical manifestations of Horner's syndrome.

1. **H**ypohydrosis (*hypo* less, *hydrosis* sweating) is due to involvement of sympathetic nerves, which arise from first thoracic nerve. These are secretomotor fibers supplying the sweat glands of the skin of the face and forehead.

2. **O**pening of eye is lost due to ptosis (drooping of the upper eyelid). It is caused by paralysis of Muller's muscle (smooth muscle of levator palpebrae superioris). In fact it is pseudo ptosis.

3. Argyll **R**obertson pupil [constricted pupil] due to paralysis of dilator pupillae (unopposed action of sphincter pupillae).

4. **N**arrowing of palpebral fissure.

5. **E**levation of lower eyelid.

6. **R**etraction of eyeball. (Sunken eyeball) - Enophthalmus is due to involvement of orbitalis muscle.

SN-7   Erb's paralysis

1. **Introduction :** Injury occurring at Erb's point is called Erb's paralysis. The junction of six nerves is called as Erb's point. The following are the nerves contributing in the formation of
   A. Ventral division of fifth cervical nerve.
   B. Ventral division of sixth cervical nerve.
   C. Suprascapular nerve.
   D. Nerve to subclavius.
   E. Anterior division of upper trunk and
   F. Posterior division of upper trunk.

2. **Site of injury :** Injury to upper trunk usually at the Erb's point causes Erb's paralysis.

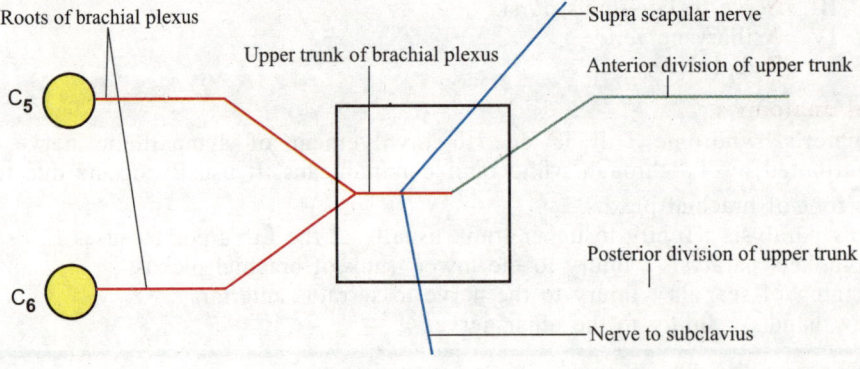

Fig. 1.12 : Erb's point.

3.   Causes of injury : It is caused by undue separation of the head from the shoulder. It results from
   A.   Birth injury (Pulling by forceps during forceps delivery)
   B.   Fall on the shoulder
   C.   Anaesthesia

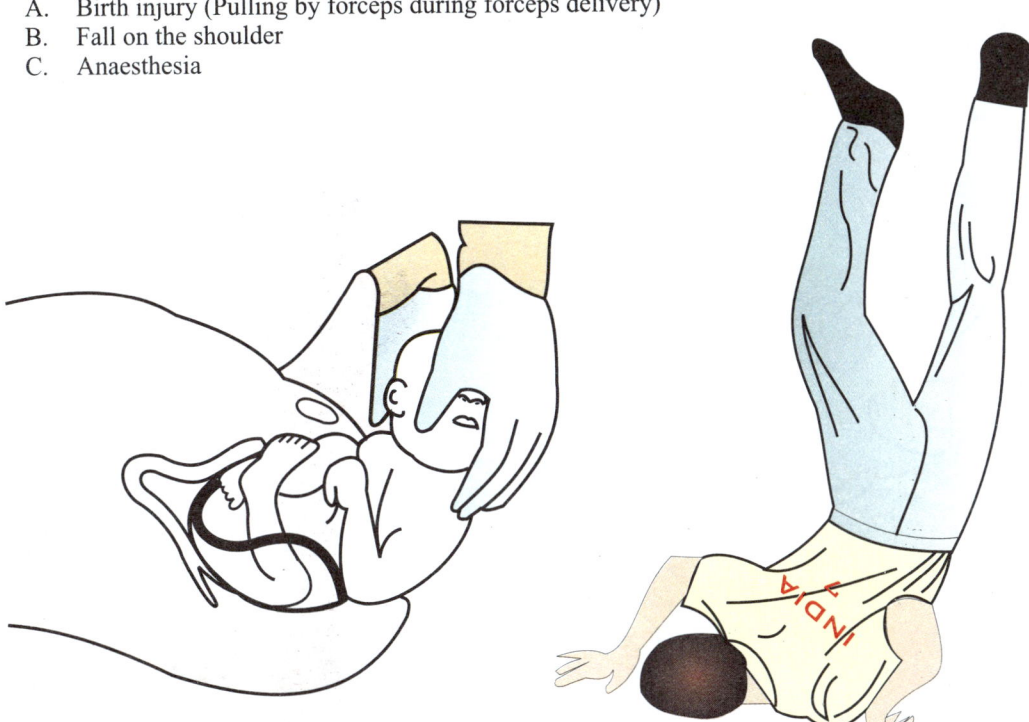

Fig. 1.13 : Erb's paralysis due to birth injury.   Fig. 1.14 : Injury due to falling on the shoulder.

Table 1.3 : Table shows affected nerves, muscles paralysed and the clinical manifestations of Erb's paralysis.

   🗝 The muscles paralysed in Erb's Palsy can be recollected by the mnemonics. "Damaged brachial plexus should be treated intelligently".

Trunk	Nerves	Muscle	Clinical features
Upper trunk C₅ & C₆	Suprascapular	Supraspinatus, infraspinatus.	Position of arm A. Hangs by the side B. Adducted C. Medially rotated forearm extended and pronated
Lateral cord	Musculo cutaneous	Biceps, Brachialis, Coracobrachialis.	
Posterior cord	Upper subscapular Lower subscapular	Subscapularis, teres major	
	Nerve to latissimus dorsi	Latissimus dorsi	
	Axillary nerve	Deltoid, teres minor	

SN-8   # Klumpke's paralysis

A. Site of injury : Lower trunk of brachial plexus.
B. Cause of injury
    a. Birth injury.
    b. In a person falling from the height.
C. Nerve roots involved.

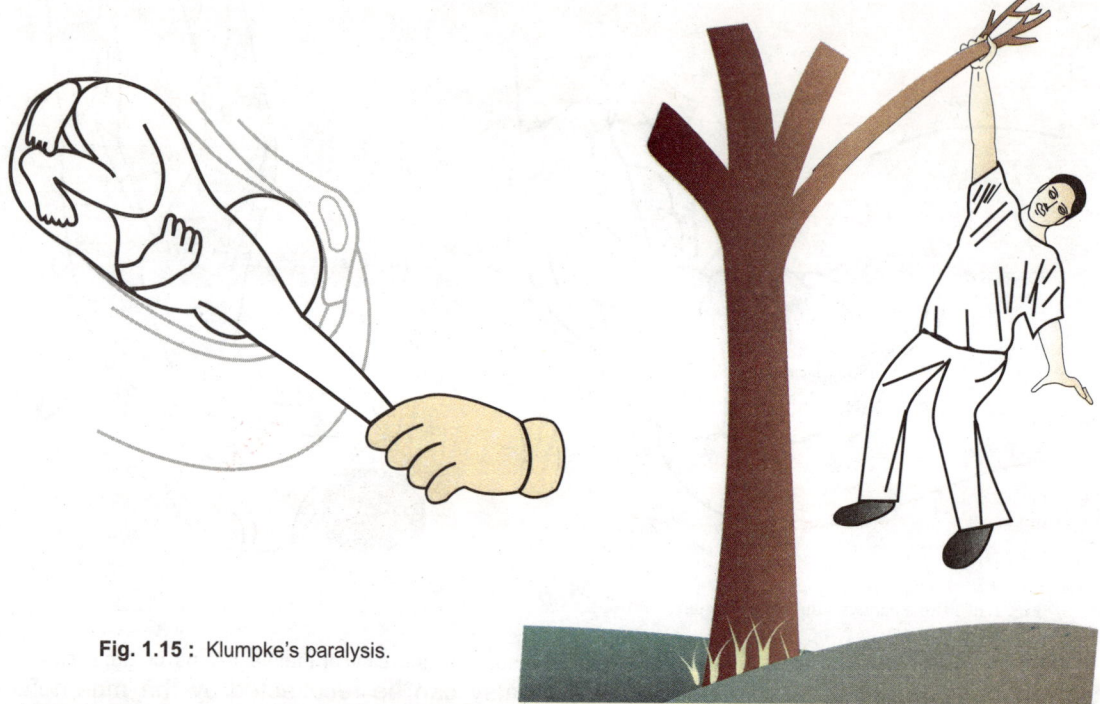

Fig. 1.15 : Klumpke's paralysis.

Fig. 1.16 : Klumpke's paralysis due to falling from the height.

Table 1.4 : Table showing muscles paralysed in ulnar nerve injury.

Nerve	Muscles	Clinical condition
Ulnar nerve	Intrinsic muscles of hand, a. Dorsal and palmar interossei, b. Lumbrical, C. Flexors of wrist and fingers.	Claw hand

Table 1.5 : Table showing muscles paralysed due to nerve to serratus, lateral cord

Particulars	Muscles paralysed and nerves involved	Clinical features
D. Nerve to serratus anterior	Injury during radical mastectomy muscle - serratus anterior	Winging of scapula
E. Lateral cord	a. Coraco brachialis, biceps. b. All muscles are supplied by median nerve except those of the hand.	a. Midprone forearm b. Loss of flexion of forearm and wrist c. Sensory loss on the radial side of forearm.
F. Medial cord	a. Ulnar nerve. b. Medial root of median nerve.	a. Claw hand b. Sensory loss on the ulnar side of forearm and hand.

LAQ-4 Describe axillary artery under
1. Origin 2. Course and relations
3. Branches and 4. Applied anatomy.

Introduction : It is the artery of axilla.
1. **Origin :** It is the continuation of third part of subclavian artery
   Extent : It extends from outer border of first rib to the lower border of teres major.
2. **Course and relations :** Axillary artery is divided into three parts by pectoralis minor muscle
   A. First part : Medial to pectoralis minor.
   B. Second part : Deep to pectoralis minor.
   C. Third part : Lateral to pectoralis minor.

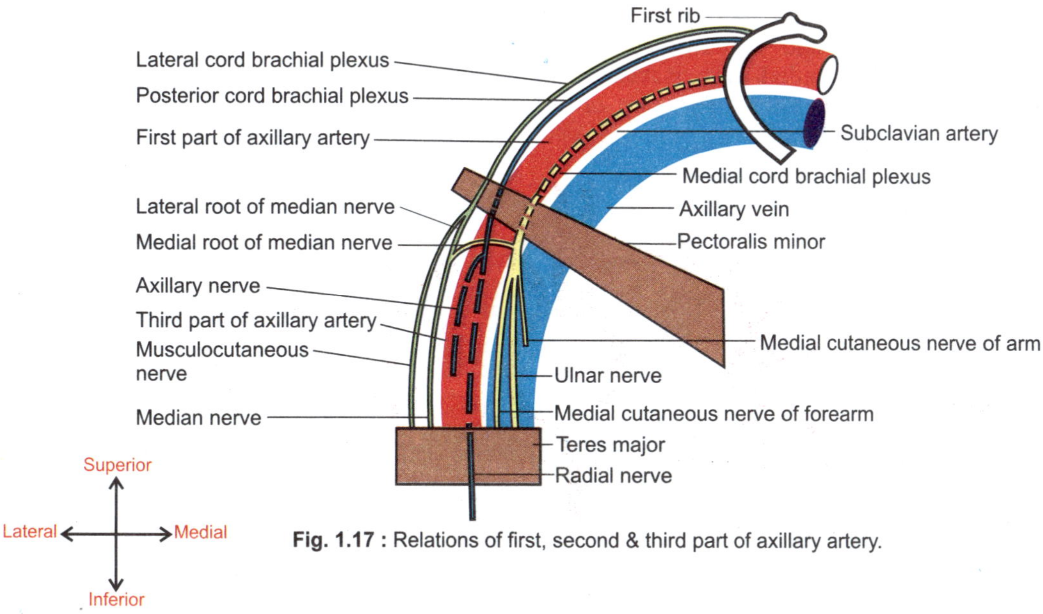

First rib

Lateral cord brachial plexus

Posterior cord brachial plexus

First part of axillary artery

Subclavian artery

Medial cord brachial plexus

Lateral root of median nerve

Axillary vein

Medial root of median nerve

Pectoralis minor

Axillary nerve

Third part of axillary artery

Musculocutaneous nerve

Medial cutaneous nerve of arm

Ulnar nerve

Median nerve

Medial cutaneous nerve of forearm

Teres major

Radial nerve

Superior

Lateral

Medial

Inferior

Fig. 1.17 : Relations of first, second & third part of axillary artery.

Table 1.6 : Table showing relations of the axillary artery.

Part	Anterior	Posterior	Medial	Lateral
1st	a. Skin, b. Superficial fascia, c. Platysma, d. Supra clavicular nerves, e. Deep fascia, f. Pectoralis major & g. Lateral pectoral nerve	a. Medial cord of brachial plexus, b. Nerve to serratus anterior, c. Serratus anterior, d. Ribs and e. Intercostal muscles	Axillary vein	Lateral and posterior cord of brachial plexus
2nd	a. Skin b. Superficial fascia c. Deep fascia d. Pectoralis major e. Pectoralis minor	A. Posterior cord of brachial plexus & b. Subscapularis	A. Axillary vein b. Medial cord c. Medial pectoral nerve	Coracobrachialis and lateral cord
3rd	a. Skin b. Superficial fascia c. Deep fascia d. Pectoralis major e. Medial root of median nerve	A. Upper sub-scapular nerve b. Lower sub-scapular nerve c. Nerve to latissimus dorsi d. Axillary nerve e. Radial nerve	a. Axillary vein b. Medial cutaneous nerve of arm c. Medial cutaneous nerve of arm of forearm d. Ulnar nerve	Coracobrachialis

Clue :

A. The lateral, medial and posterior cord of brachial plexus are related at the respective positions of second part of axillary artery.

B. The branches of the respective cords of brachial plexus are related to the third part of axillary artery.

C. Lateral cord of brachial plexus is related on the lateral side of first part of axillary artery. The medial and posterior cords are clockwise rotated in 90° and occupy the position, i.e. The medial cord is related on the posterior side and posterior cord is related on the lateral side of first part of axillary artery.

3. Branches :

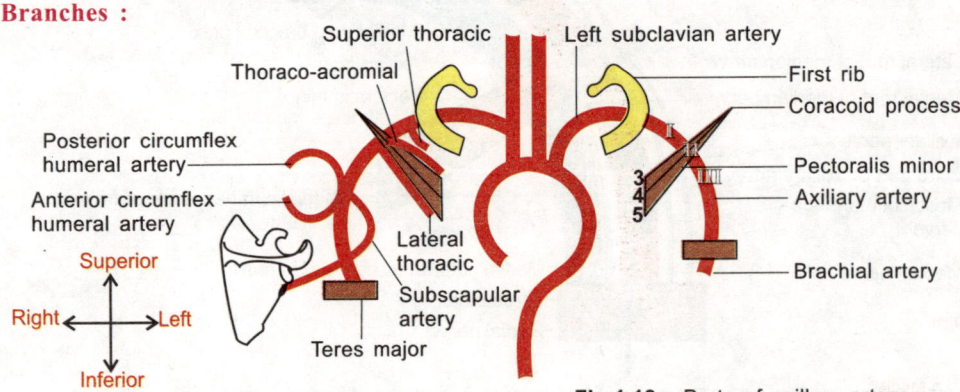

Fig.1.18 : Parts of axillary artery.

Table 1.7 : The table shows branches of the axillary artery and their distribution.

Part	Branches	Course and relation	Remarks	Area of distribution
1st	A. Superior thoracic	Runs on upper border of pectoralis minor muscle	It is a small branch. It anastomoses with a. Internal thoracic b. Upper intercostal	Supplies mammary gland and pectoralis major and minor Muscle.
2nd	A. Thoraco-acromial

B. Lateral thoracic | a. It *pierces clavi-pectoral fascia* b. It runs on the upper border of pectoralis minor Accompanies lower border of pectoralis minor | a. Bones : clavicle, acromion Process of scapula b. Muscles : pectoralis Major and deltoid Mammary gland | Supplies sterno-clavicular joint. |
3rd	A. Subscapular - circumflex scapular	a. Largest branch b. Runs on lower border of subscapularis	Anastomoses with posterior circumflex humeral.	Forms important anastomosis around the scapula, humerus and shoulder joint. Forms anastomoses with the deltoid branch of profunda brachii artery.
	B. Anterior circumflex humeral-ascending branch	--	Anastomoses with a. Lateral thoracic b. Intercostal c. Deep branch of transverse cervical	--
	C. Posterior circumflex humeral a. Descending I. Infra-scapular b. Thoraco- dorsal		II. Small branches	--

4.   Applied anatomy :

A.   Axillary artery can be effectively compressed against the humerus.

B.   Axillary artery is likely to rupture during reduction of an old dislocated head of humerus.

SN-9   Axillary lymph nodes

The lymph nodes of the axilla are described in following ways

Table 1.8 : The table shows situation of axillary lymph nodes.

Type	Situation	Receives from	Drains into	Draining area
1. Anterior	Along inferior border of pectoralis minor	Lateral half of breast	Central	Drains most of the lymphatic of breast
2. Posterior	Situated along subscapular vessels	Axillary tail	Central	Dorsal part of trunk above the iliac crest
3. Lateral	Situated posteromedial to axillary vein	Upper limb	Central	Drains entire upper limb except those accompanying cephalic vein
4. Central	Present at the base of axilla	A. Anterior B. Posterior C. Lateral	Apical	From A, B & C.
5. Apical	Present in the apex of axilla medial to axillary vein	Central	A. Subclavian trunk B. Thoracic	A. Drains a. Upper limb b. Mammary gland B. Axillary lymph node

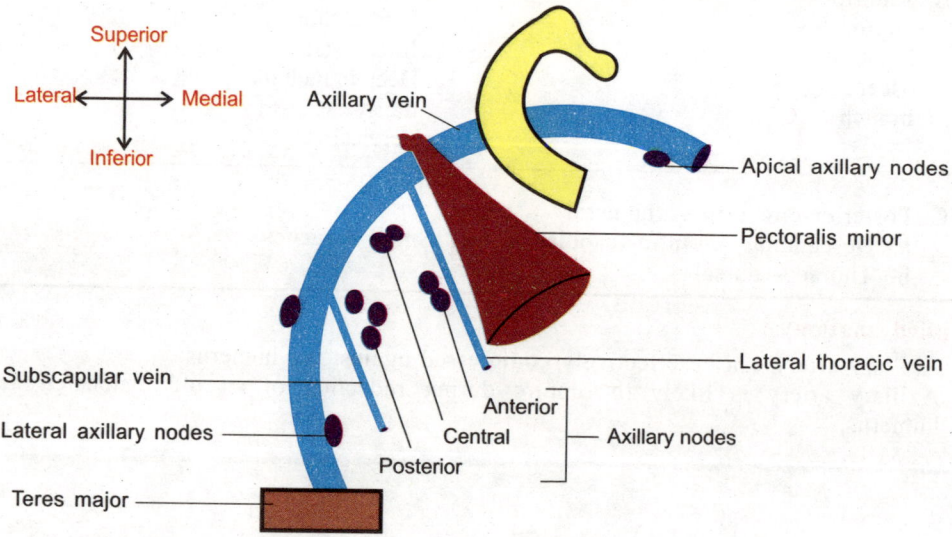

Fig. 1.19 : Situation of axillary lymph nodes.

Applied anatomy : There is an enlargement of the anterior axillary group of lymph nodes in malignancy of lateral half of superficial and deep structures of mammary gland.

SN-10   Deltoid

1. **Introduction :** It is a triangular, multi pennate muscle present in the shoulder region.

Table 1.9 : Table showing origin, insertion and action of different fibers of deltoid.

Particulars	Anterior	Middle	Posterior

Synonymous
A. Morphology
  a. Type of fibers
  b. Range of Movement
  c. Force of pull
	Clavicular
	
	Long and parallel
	More
	
	Less
		Acromial
		
		Multi pennate
		Less
		
		More
			Scapular
			
			Long and parallel
			More
			
			Less

B. Origin	Anterior and upper surface of lateral $1/3^{rd}$ of clavicle	Lateral border of acromion process of scapula	Lower lip of crest of spine of scapula
C. Insertion	Deltoid tuberosity on a V shaped impression extending on lateral surface of middle third of shaft of humerus.		
D. Action	Anterior fibers are flexors and medial rotators of shoulder joint.	Middle fibers are strong abductors of shoulder joint from 15° to 120°.	a. Posterior fibers are extensors and lateral rotators of shoulder joint.

2. **Nerve supply :**
   Axillary nerve : C_5 & C_6 of posterior cord of brachial plexus.

3. **Structures under cover of deltoid :**
   A. Bones :
      a. Upper end of humerus with greater and lesser tuberosities, intertubercular sulcus, upper part of shaft and surgical neck of humerus.
      b. Coracoid process of scapula.
   B. Muscles attached to
      a. Greater tubercle : Supraspinatus, infraspinatus, teres minor.
      b. Lesser tubercle : Subscapularis.
      c. Coracoid process : Origins of coracobrachialis and short head of biceps.
      d. Glenoid cavity : Long head of biceps (supraglenoid tubercle), long head of triceps (infraglenoid tubercle).
   C. Vessels : Anterior and posterior circumflex humeral.
   D. Nerve : Axillary.
   E. Joints and ligaments : Shoulder joint and coracoacromial ligaments.
   F. Bursae : Subacromial and subdeltoid bursae and bursae of shoulder joint.

4. **Applied anatomy :**
   A. Fracture of surgical neck of humerus, causes lesion of the axillary nerve. It results in paralysis of deltoid. This affects the movement of shoulder joint especially abduction from 15° to 90°.
   B. Paralysis of deltoid results into loss of rounded contour of shoulder region.

SN-11   Median cubital vein

It is a large communicating vein, which shunts blood from the cephalic vein to the basilic vein.

1. **Origin :** From cephalic vein, which is present 1" below bend of elbow. It runs obliquely upward and medially.

2. **Termination :** It ends in basilic vein, 1" above the medial epicondyle.

3. **Relations :** Superficial to deep
    A. Skin and fascia.
    B. Bicipital aponeurosis.
    C. Brachial artery.

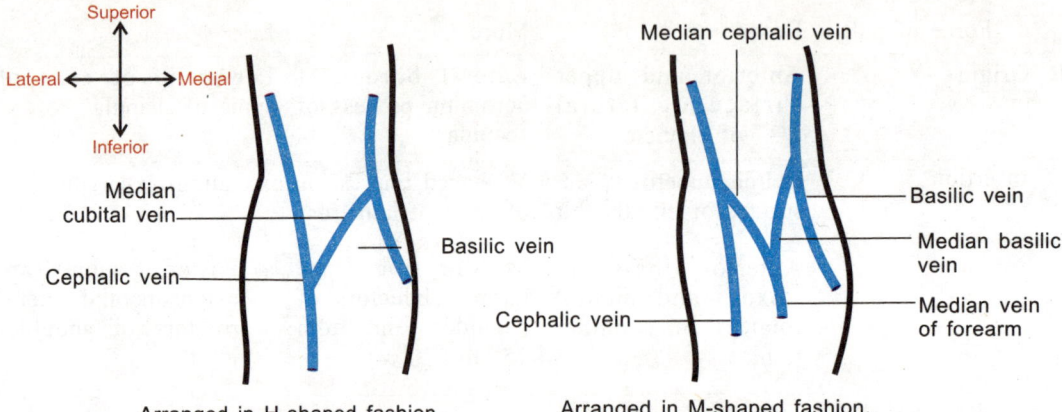

Fig. 1.20 : Arrangement of median cubital vein.

4. **Tributaries :** Median anti brachial vein.

5. **Applied anatomy :**
    A. It is commonly used vein for withdrawal of blood for investigation and therapeutic purposes (intra venous injection, intra venous fluid, blood).
    B. This vein is fixed by perforator vein.

SAQ-1   Rotator cuff

1. **Introduction :** It is musculotendinous cuff of shoulder joint. This is a fibrous sheath formed by four flattened tendons namely
    A. Supraspinatus,
    B. Infraspinatus,
    C. Teres minor,
    D. Subscapularis and lateral part of capsule of shoulder joint.

2. **Features :** 🗝 S
    A. **S**its on tuberosities
    B. **S**ticks to capsule of shoulder joint
    C. **S**teadies head of humerus
    D. **S**trengthens the capsule.

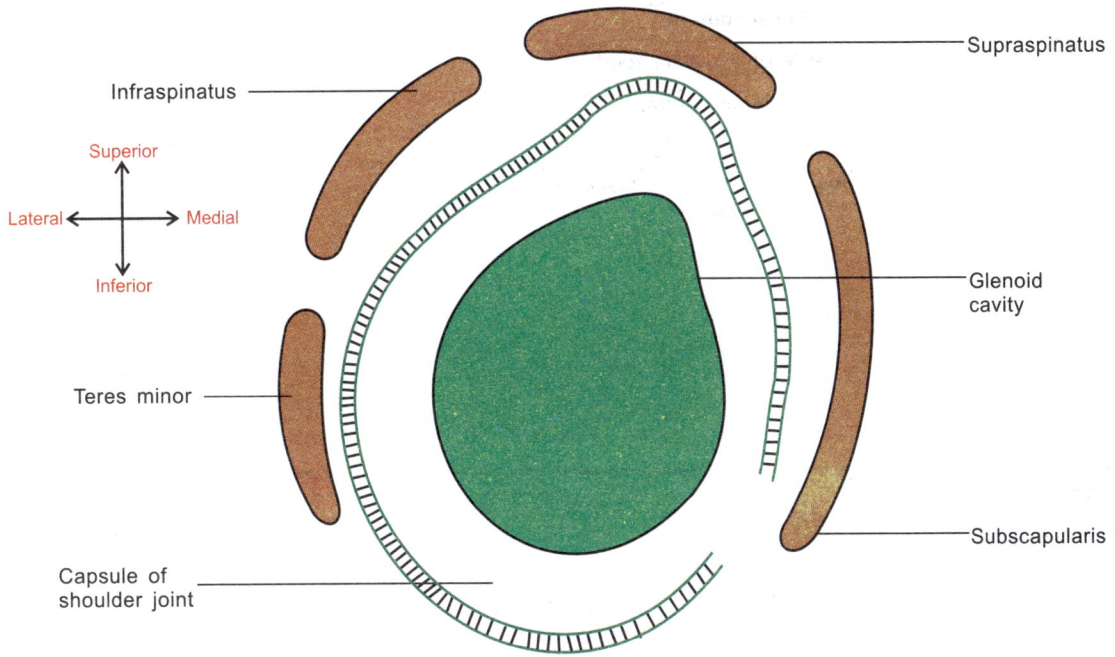

Fig.1.21 : Rotator cuff of the shoulder.

3. **Applied anatomy :** *Dislocation of the shoulder joint is more commonly in a downward direction.* Because capsule is lax inferiorly.

SAQ-2   Quadrangular space

1. **Introduction :** It is an intermuscular space present in the axilla.

2. **Boundaries :**
   A. Above (from anterior to posterior) :
      a. Subscapularis in front.
      b. Capsule of the shoulder joint.
      c. Teres minor behind.
   B. Below : Teres major.
   C. Medial : Long head of the triceps.
   D. Lateral : Surgical neck of the humerus.

3. **Structures passing :**
   A. Axillary nerve
   B. Posterior circumflex humeral vessels.

4. **Applied anatomy :** Fracture of surgical neck of humerus causes lesion of axillary nerve leading to paralysis of deltoid muscle.

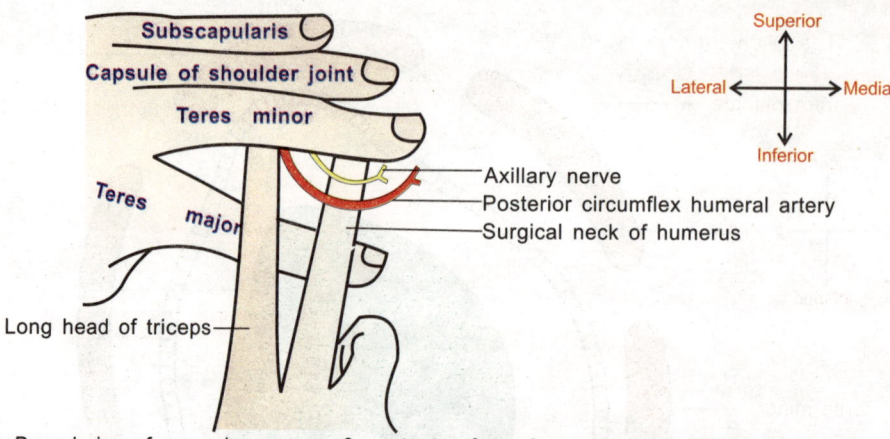

Fig. 1.22 : Boundaries of muscular spaces & contents of quadrangular space (Posterior view).

SAQ-3   Upper triangular space

1. **Introduction :** It is an upper intermuscular triangular space present in the axilla.

2. **Boundaries :**
    A. Above : Teres minor
    B. Lateral : Long head of the triceps
    C. Below : Teres major
    D. Apex : Lateral border of scapula where teres major and minor muscles converge.

3. **Structures passing :** Circumflex scapular artery.
    It pierces the origin of the teres minor and reaches the infraspinatus fossa to anastomose with the suprascapular artery.

4. **Applied anatomy :** The circumflex scapular artery anastomoses with descending branch of transverse cervical artery and forms important anastomosis around the scapula.

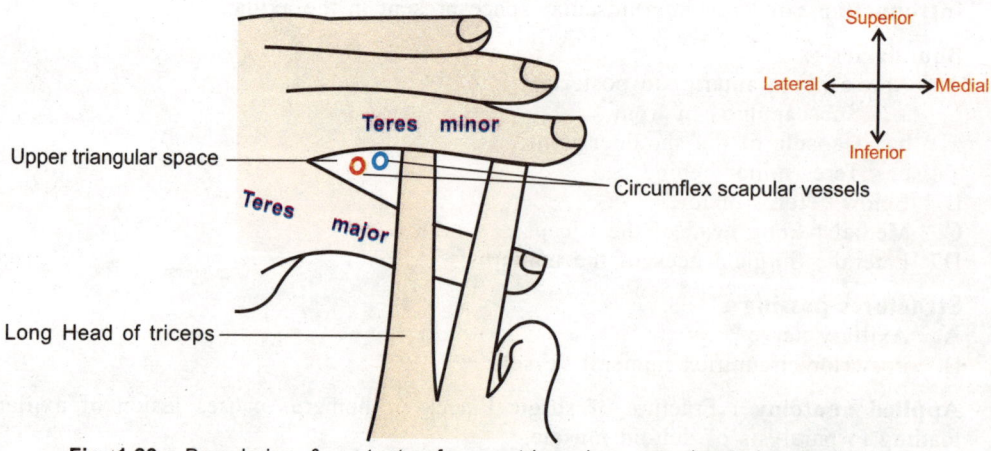

Fig. 1.23 : Boundaries & contents of upper triangular space (posterior view).

SAQ-4   Lower triangular space

1. **Introduction :** It is a lower intermuscular triangular space present in the axilla.

2. **Boundaries :**
   A. Medially by long head of the triceps.
   B. Laterally by shaft of humerus.
   C. Above by teres major.

3. **Structures passing :**
   A. Radial nerve.
   B. Profunda brachii vessels.

4. **Applied anatomy :** Fracture of middle third of humerus causes injury to radial nerve and results in wrist drop.

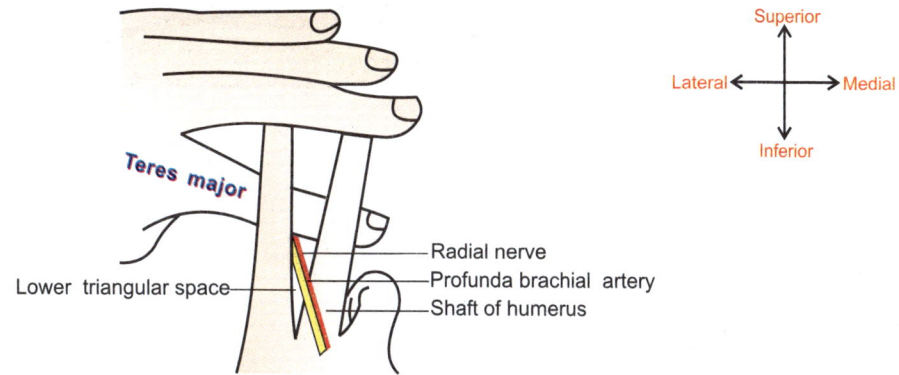

Fig. 1.24 : Boundaries & contents of lower triangular space (posterior view).

LAQ-5   Describe axillary nerve under
     1.   Root value   2.   Course and relations
     3.   Branches   &   4.   Applied anatomy.

1. **Root value :** Ventral rami of C_5 & C_6.
   Peculiarities :
   A. Posterior division of axillary nerve bears pseudo ganglion.
   B. Axillary nerve is the ideal example of Hilton's Law i.e. The nerve supplying the muscles acting on the joint supplies the joint and skin over the joint.

2. **Course and relations :** It arises from posterior cord of brachial plexus. The posterior cord lies posterior to the second part of axillary artery. The axillary nerve lies posterior to third part of axillary artery.
   A. In axilla : It lies on lateral side of radial nerve.
   B. In quadrangular space : It divides into anterior and posterior division.
   C. Anterior division is accompanied by posterior circumflex humeral artery (branch of 3rd part of axillary artery). It runs deep to deltoid muscle and supplies deltoid and skin over its anterior part of deltoid muscle.

D. Posterior division supplies teres minor which bears pseudoganglion. It also supplies posterior part of deltoid muscle. It pierces deep fascia to become **u**pper **l**ateral **c**utaneous **n**erve of arm. 🗝 **ULC**

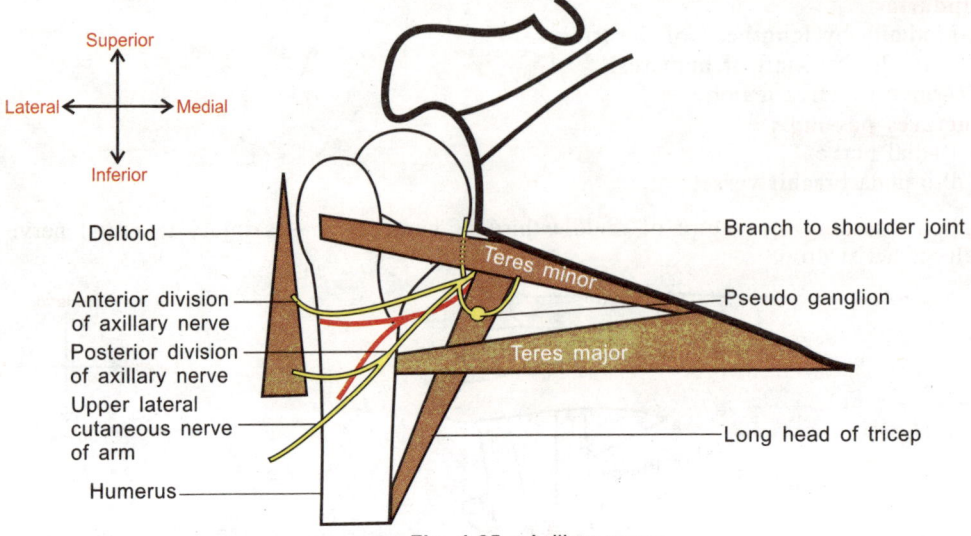

Fig. 1.25 : Axillary nerve.

3. **Branches and distribution :**
A. Muscular :
   a. Deltoid from both divisions.
   b. Teres minor from posterior division.
B. Cutaneous : **U**pper **l**ateral **c**utaneous **n**erve of arm arises from posterior division of axillary artery and supplies skin over posterior
   a. Border of deltoid and
   b. Upper part of long head of triceps.
C. Articular branch to shoulder joint arises from trunk of the axillary nerve.
D. Vascular branch to posterior circumflex humeral artery arises from anterior division.

4. **Applied anatomy :**
A. The damage to axillary nerve is caused by
   a. Inferior dislocation of shoulder joint and
   b. Fracture of surgical neck of humerus.
B. The damage to the axillary nerve results into
   a. Loss of roundness of shoulder.
   b. Prominence of greater tubercle of humerus.
   c. Loss of abduction of shoulder joint.
   d. Loss of sensations of the skin over lower half of deltoid.
   e. Overhead abduction of shoulder joint is prevented by reflex inhibition of deltoid through axillary nerve (Hilton's law).

LAQ-6 | Describe musculocutaneous nerve under
1. Root value 2. Course and relations
3. Branches and 4. Applied anatomy.

Introduction : It is a branch of lateral cord of brachial plexus and is the motor nerve of flexor compartment of arm and sensory nerve of skin of forearm.

1. **Root value :** C_5, C_6 & C_7.

2. **Course and relations :** It arises from lateral cord of brachial plexus.

   A. The lateral cord of brachial plexus lies lateral to the 2nd part of axillary artery.

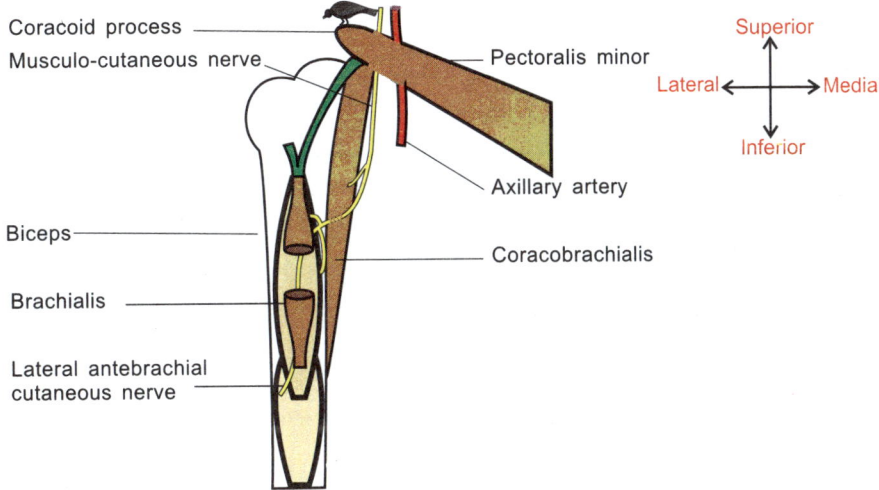

Fig. 1.26 : Musculo-cutaneous nerve.

   B. The nerve lies lateral to 3rd part of axillary artery. It arises at lower border of pectoralis major

   a. In axilla it is related to following structures.

   I. Anteriorly : Pectoralis major.

   II. Posteriorly : Subscapularis.

   III. Medially : Axillary artery.

   IV. Laterally : Coracobrachialis.

   It leaves axilla, pierces coracobrachialis and enters front of arm.

   b. In arm : It runs downwards and laterally.

   I. It passes between biceps and brachialis.

   II. It pierces deep fascia just below the elbow and continues as lateral cutaneous nerve of forearm.

3.   Branches and distribution :

Table 1.10 : Table showing distribution of musculocutaneous nerve.

Muscular	Cutaneous	Articular	Branch to
A. Coracobrachialis B. Biceps brachii C. Brachialis	Lateral cutaneous nerve of forearm supplies skin of lateral side of forearm	A. Elbow joint B. Shoulder joint C. Superior radioulnar joint	Humerus which accompanies nutrient artery.

4.   Applied anatomy :

   A.   Isolated lesion of musculocutaneous nerve is rare.

   B.   The lesion is due to fracture of neck of humerus.

   C.   Myotrophy : Marked weakness of flexion of elbow is due to paralysis of bicep brachii and coracobrachialis.

   D.   Lesion of the nerve causes anesthesia on anterolateral surface of forearm. The pain and anesthesia may be aggravated by the extension of elbow.

   E.   The nerve may be involved in Erb's paralysis.

LAQ-7   **Describe brachial artery under**
   1.   **Origin**   2.   **Course and relations**
   3.   **Branches   &**   4.   **Applied anatomy.**

1.   Origin : It is the continuation of axillary artery below the lower border of teres major.

2.   Course and relations :

   A.   Peculiarities : It is superficial throughout its course. It is accompanied by

      a.   Veins : Venae commitants (brachial veins).

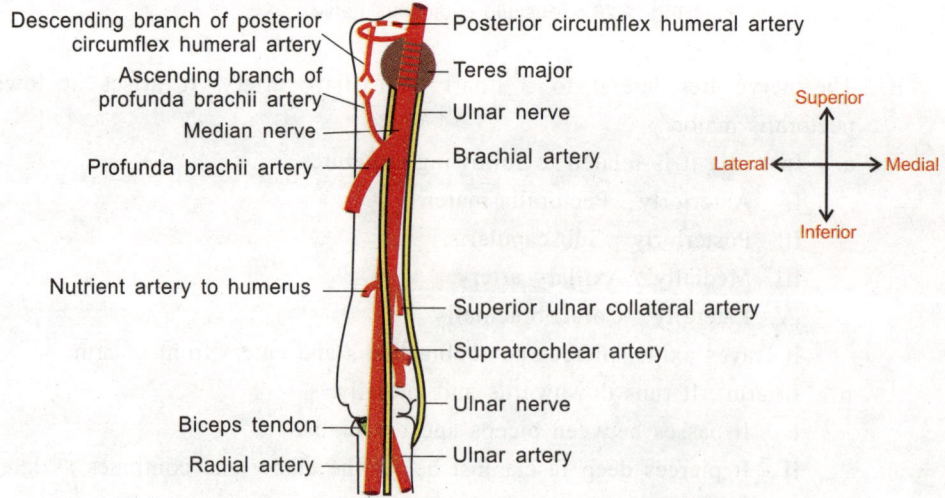

Fig. 1.27 : Course, branches & relations of brachial artery.

   b.   Nerves:
      I.   *Brachial artery accompanies median nerve.*
      II. *Profunda brachii (a branch of brachial artery) accompanies radial nerve.*
      III. *Anterior descending artery (a branch of profunda brachial artery) accompanies radial nerve.*
      IV. *Superior ulnar collateral artery (a branch of brachial artery) accompanies ulnar nerve.*
B. Relations :
   a.   Anterior :
      I.   Skin,
      II.   Superficial fascia,
      III. Deep fascia,
      IV.   Biceps brachii and
      V.   Bicipital aponeurosis at the bifurcation.
   b.   Posterior :
      I.   Long head of triceps,
      II.   Medial head of triceps,
      III. Coracobrachialis and
      IV.   Brachialis.
   c.   Lateral : Upper part median nerve.
   d.   Medial :
      I.   Medial cutaneous nerve of arm.
      II.   Lower part of median nerve.
C. Termination : The artery divides at the neck of radius into radial and ulnar artery.

3. **Branches :**
   A. Cutaneous to skin over arm.
   B. Muscular : Muscles of arm (Deltoid, biceps, brachialis, coracobrachialis).
   C. Articular branches to
      a.   Shoulder joint,
      b.   Elbow joint by superior ulnar collateral and
      c.   Inferior ulnar collateral artery.
   D. Nutrient branch to humerus.
   E. Anastomotic branch to posterior circumflex humeral artery.
   F. Terminal branches : Radial and ulnar arteries.

4. **Applied anatomy :**
   A. The brachial artery is ruptured in supra condylar fracture of humerus leading to Volkman's ischaemic contracture.

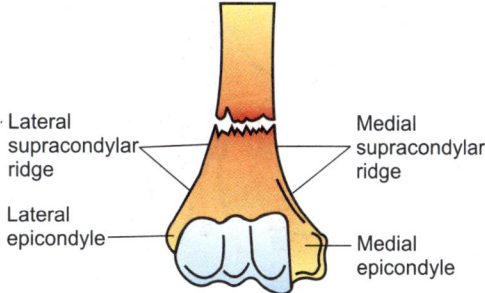

Lateral supracondylar ridge

Medial supracondylar ridge

Lateral epicondyle

Medial epicondyle

Fig. 1.28 : Supracondylar fracture

B. *Haemorrhage due to brachial artery can be controlled by direct compression of brachial artery in the middle of arm on the tendon of coracobrachialis and medial to humerus.*

C. Blood pressure is recorded by auscultation of the pulsations of brachial artery in cubital fossa.

D. The blood for blood gas analysis is collected from brachial artery.

E. The pulsations of brachial artery are felt or auscultated in front of the elbow.

SN-12   Anastomosis around the elbow joint

1. **Introduction :** It is an important communication between brachial and the terminal branches of brachial artery (radial and ulnar arteries).

2. **Distribution :** It supplies
   A. Ligaments and
   B. Bones of the elbow region.
   C. Elbow joint,
   D. Superior radioulnar joint.

3. **Division :**
   A. In front of the lateral epicondyle of the humerus : The radial collateral artery branch of profunda brachii anastomoses with the radial recurrent branch of radial artery.

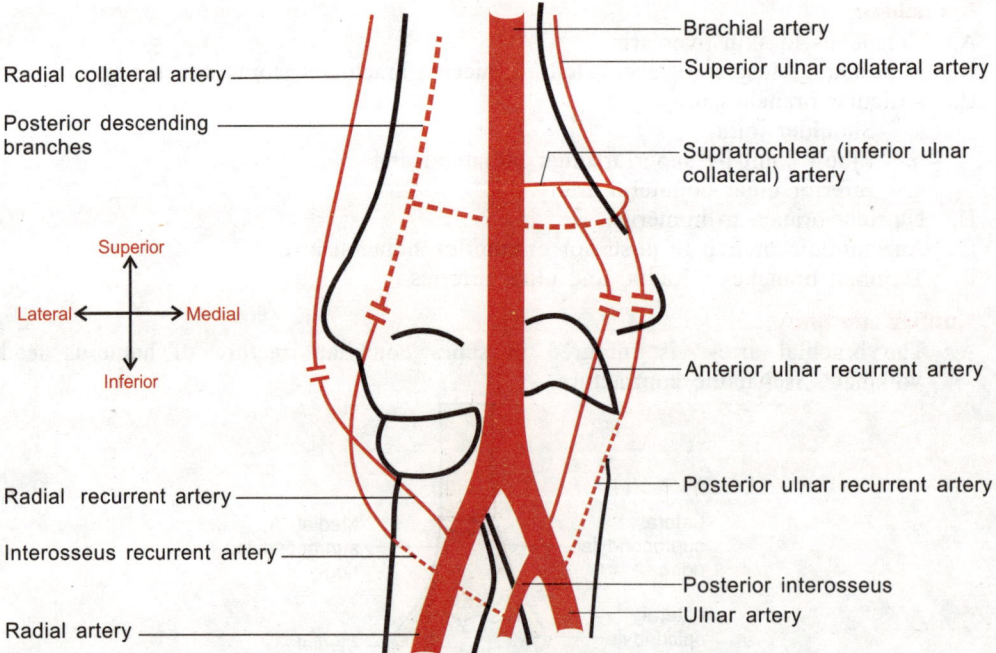

Fig. 1.29 : Anastomosis around the elbow joint.

B. Behind the lateral epicondyle of the humerus : The posterior descending branch of the profunda brachii artery, anastomoses with the interosseous recurrent branch of the posterior interosseous artery.

C. In front of the medial epicondyle of the humerus : The inferior ulnar collateral branch of the brachial artery, anastomoses with the anterior ulnar recurrent branch of ulnar artery.

D. Behind the medial epicondyle of the humerus : The superior ulnar collateral branch of the brachial artery, anastomoses with the posterior ulnar recurrent branch of ulnar artery.

E. Just above the olecranon fossa : A branch from posterior descending branch of the profunda brachii artery, anastomoses with the branch from the inferior ulnar collateral artery.

LAQ-8 Describe radial nerve under
1. Root value   2. Course and relations
3. Branches and   4. Applied anatomy.

1. **Root value :** C_5, C_6, C_7, C_8 & T_1.

2. **Course and relations :** It arises from posterior cord of brachial plexus. The posterior cord lies posterior to the 2nd part of axillary artery and radial nerve lies posterior to 3rd part of axillary artery. *It lies medial to axillary nerve.*

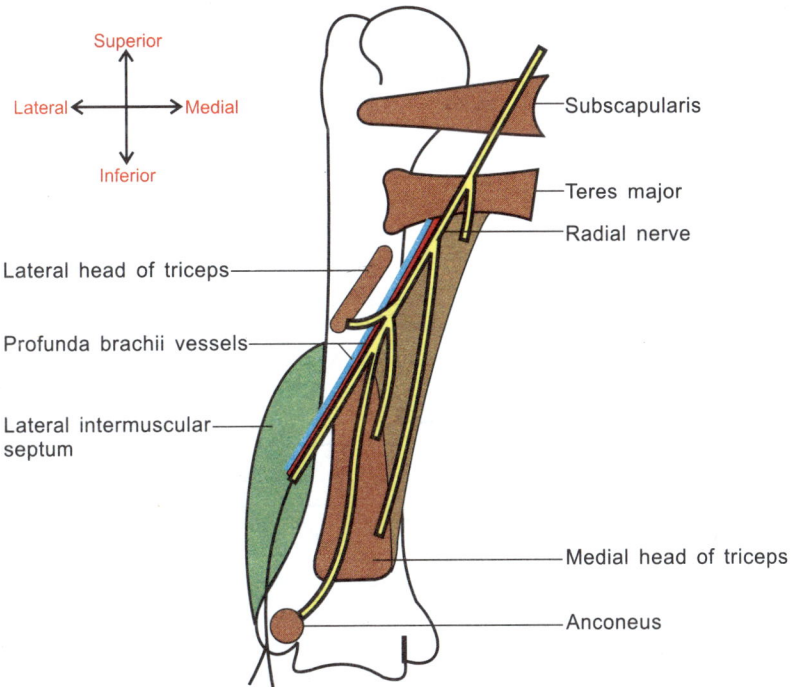

Fig. 1.30 : Course, branches & relations of radial nerve in arm.

A. In lower part of axilla, the nerve passes downwards and has following relations
   a. Anteriorly : Axillary artery and pectoralis major.
   b. Posteriorly : Subscapularis, teres major and latissimus dorsi.
   c. Medially : Axillary vein
   d. Laterally : Coracobrachialis muscle. It passes through lower triangular space and enters the radial groove along with profunda brachii artery.

B. In radial groove : It runs downwards between lateral and medial head of triceps. At lower end of radial groove it pierces the lateral intermuscular septum and enters into anterior compartment of arm.

C. In anterior compartment of arm it passes in an intermuscular interval between the brachioradialis and extensor carpi radialis longus and supply these muscles.

D. In forearm : At the level of lateral epicondyle it gives off posterior interosseous branch which leaves the fossa by piercing supinator muscle and enters back of forearm.

E. At elbow joint, the radial nerve divides into superficial and deep terminal branches. The superficial terminal branch reaches the dorsum of forearm and divides into 4 to 5 branches.

3. **Branches :**
   A. In arm :

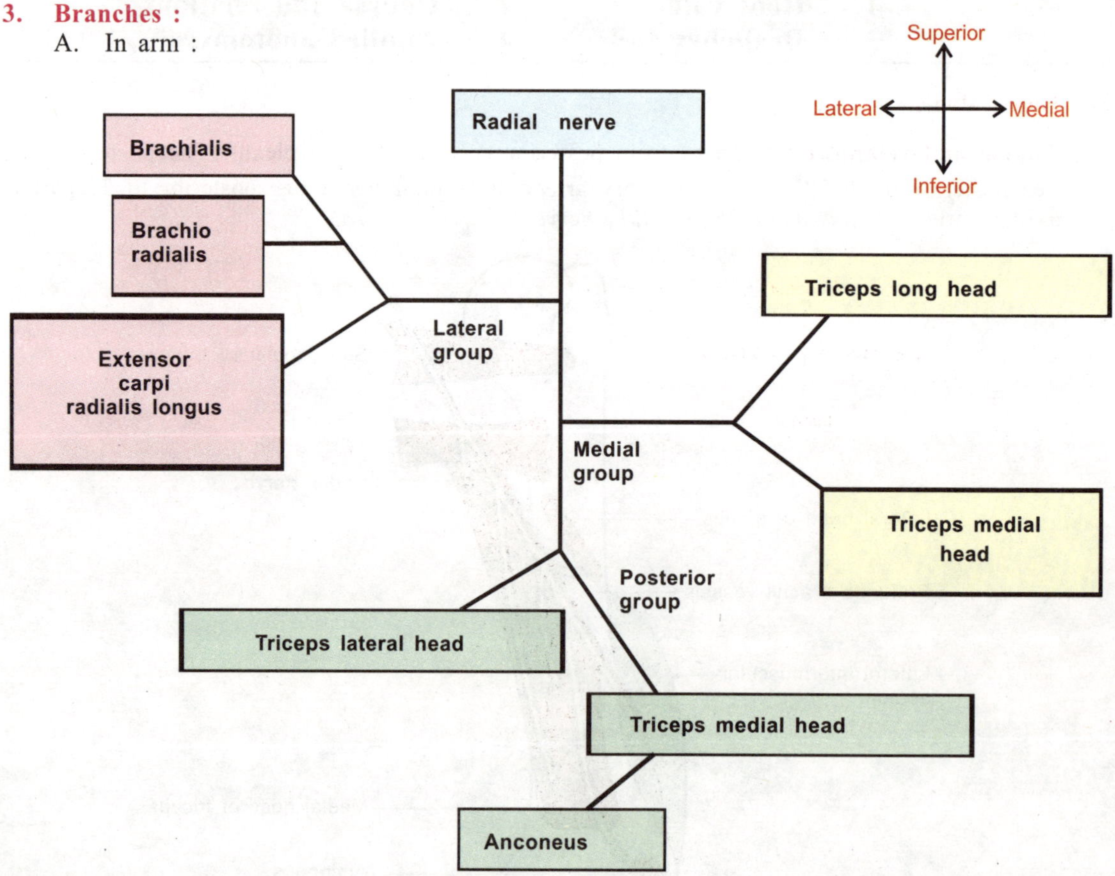

Fig. 1.31 : Motor branches of the radial nerve in the arm.

Table 1.11 : Table showing distribution of radial nerve in the arm.

Particulars	Muscular	Cutaneous	Joint
a. Above radial groove (medial group)	Long and medial head of triceps.	Posterior cutaneous nerve of arm.	Elbow
b. In the groove (posterior group)	a. Medial head of triceps. b. Lateral head of triceps. c. Anconeus.	a. Lower lateral cutaneous nerve of arm. b. Posterior cutaneous nerve of forearm.	-- --
c. Below radial groove (lateral group)	a. Brachioradialis. b. Extensor carpi radialis longus. c. Brachialis (proprioceptive branch).	-- -- --	-- -- --

B.   In the forearm it gives two terminal branches.

Table 1.12 : Table showing distribution of branches of radial nerve in the forearm.

Superficial branch	Deep (posterior interosseous nerve) branch

Superficial terminal branch (cutaneous) divides into :
  a. Digital and
  b. Communicating.
	Muscular branches to
	  a. Extensor carpi radialis brevis (branch is given before piercing supinator).
	  b. Supinator.
	  c. Muscles forming anatomical snuff box.
	    I. Abductor pollicis longus,
	    II. Extensor pollicis brevis &
	    III. Extensor pollicis longus.
	  d. Extensor indices.
	  e. Extensor digitorum.
	  f. Extensor digiti minimi.
	  g. Extensor carpi ulnaris.

SN-13   Applied anatomy of radial nerve

4.   **Applied anatomy :** Injury to radial nerve at different levels.

Table 1.13 : The table shows injury to radial nerve and the effects at different region.

	Site	Cause	Effect	
			Motor	**Sensory**
A.	Axilla	a. Saturday night palsy b. Crutch palsy	Extensor muscles of arm, forearm and wrist are paralysed.	Loss of sensations of a. Posterior surface of arm b. Dorsum of hand
B.	Middle of arm	a. Fracture of shaft of humerus b. Injection in radial groove	Paralysis of extensors of forearm and wrist.	Loss of sensations of dorsum of hand.

(cont.) Table 1.13 : The table shows injury to radial nerve and the effects at different region.

	Site	Cause	Effect	
			Motor	**Sensory**
C.	Proximal part of forearm	Fracture of proximal $1/3^{rd}$ of radius	Paralysis of extensors of wrist and hand.	Loss of sensation of radial side of dorsum of hand.
D.	Wrist joint	Lesion of superficial radial nerve at wrist.	No muscles are paralysed.	Loss of sensation of radial side of dorsum of hand.

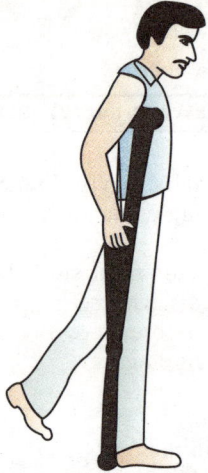

Fig. 1.32 :Crutch palsy.

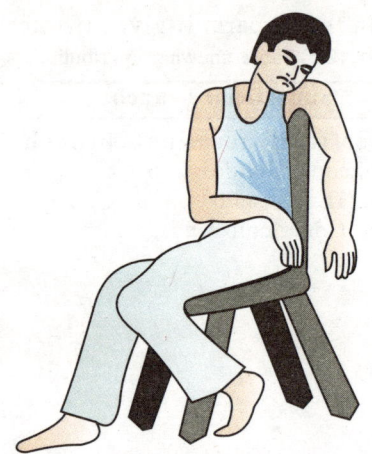

Fig. 1.33 : Saturday night palsy.

SN-14   Wrist drop

1. **Introduction :** It is loss of extension of wrist due to paralysis of extensor muscles of the wrist joint.

2. **Nerve involved :** It is produced by the lesion of radial nerve and/or posterior interosseous branch of radial nerve.

3. **Causes of the injury :**
   A. In the axilla :
      a. Saturday night palsy.
      b. Crutch palsy.
   B. In the middle of the arm :
      a. Fracture of middle $1/3^{rd}$ of the shaft of humerus.
      b. Injection in radial groove.
   C. In the proximal part of forearm : Fracture of proximal $1/3^{rd}$ of radius.

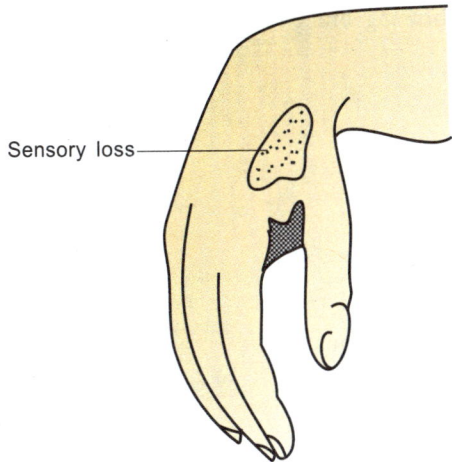

Sensory loss

Fig. 1.34 : Wrist drop.

4. **Muscle paralysed :**
   A. Extensor carpi radialis brevis (a branch of posterior interosseous nerve which is g i v e n before piercing supinator).
   B. Supinator.
   C. Muscles forming anatomical snuff box.
      a. Abductor pollicis longus,
      b. Extensor pollicis brevis &
      c. Extensor pollicis longus.
      d. Extensor indices.
      e. Extensor digitorum.
      f. Extensor digiti minimi.
      g. Extensor carpi ulnaris.

5. **Clinical manifestations :**
   A. Motor : The patient is unable to extend the wrist and results into wrist drop.
   B. Sensory : A variable small area of anesthesia is present over the dorsal surface of the hand and dorsal surface of the roots of the lateral three and one half fingers.

SN-15   Posterior interosseous nerve

1. **Introduction :** It is a deep terminal branch of radial nerve and arises in front of the lateral epicondyle.

2. **Peculiarity :** It bears a pseudo ganglion.

3. **Course and relation :** The nerve appears in the back of the forearm by piercing the supinator muscle and winds round the lateral side of the radius.

4. **Branches :**
   A. Before piercing the supinator :
      a. Extensor carpi radialis brevis.
      b. Supinator.

B. After piercing the supinator following branches are given
   a. Muscular branches
      I. Short branches to
         i. Extensor digitorum,
         ii. Extensor digiti minimi and
         iii. Extensor carpi ulnaris.
      II. Long branches are divided into
         i. Medial set, which supplies
           - Extensor pollicis longus and
           - Extensor indicis.
         ii. Lateral set, which supplies
           - Abductor pollicis longus and
           - Extensor pollicis brevis.
   b. Articular branches to
      I. Wrist joint,
      II. Inferior radioulnar joint,
      III. Intercarpal joints.
   c. Sensory branches
      I. Interosseous membrane,
      II. Radius and
      III. Ulnar.

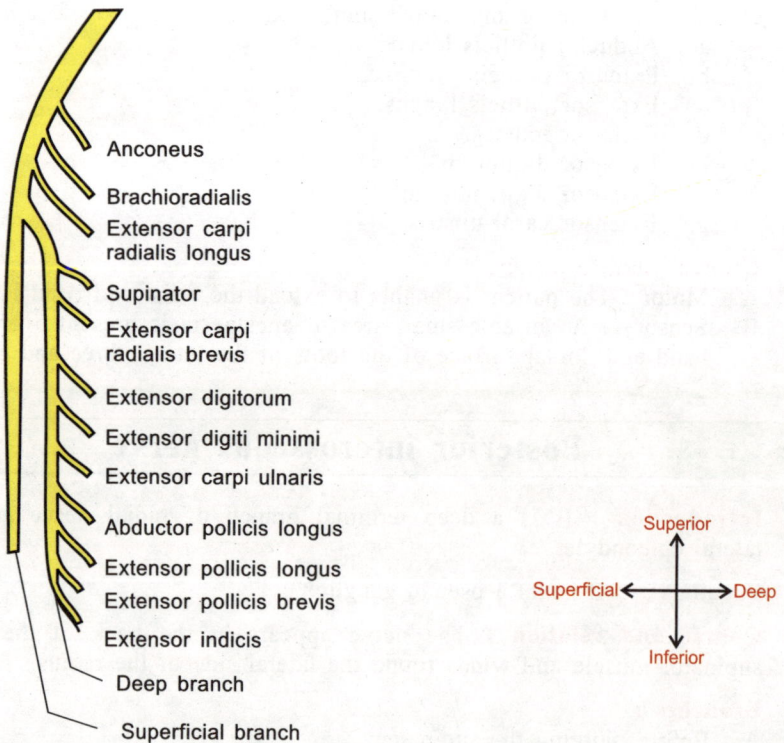

Fig. 1.35 : Branches of posterior interosseous nerve.

SN-16   Profunda brachii artery

1. **Origin :** It is a large branch of the brachial artery.

2. **Course and relations :** It accompanies the radial nerve in the lower triangular space and radial groove. It pierces the lateral intermuscular septum and divides into branches.

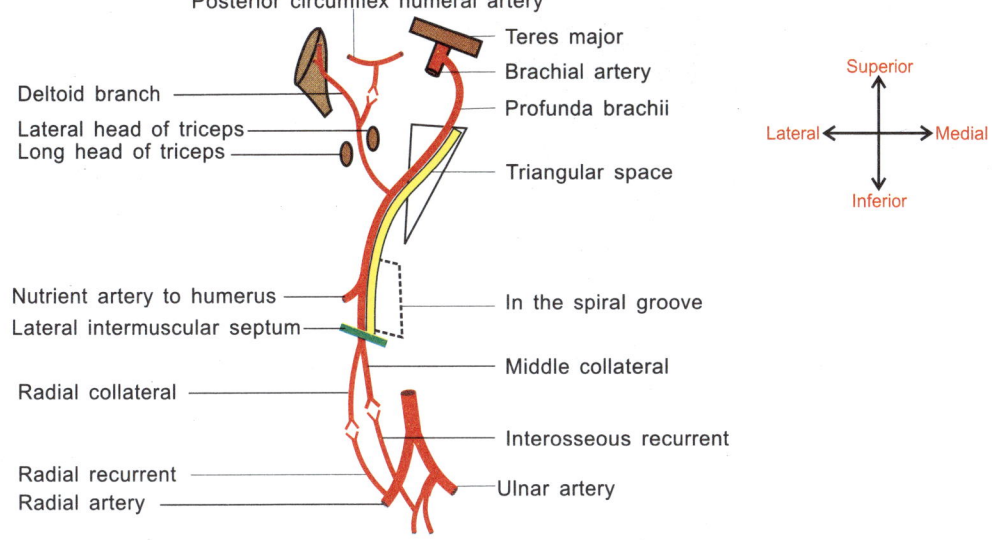

Fig. 1.36 : Course, branches and relations of profunda brachii artery.

3. **Branches :**
   A. The radial collateral artery is one of the terminal branch and represents the continuation of the profunda artery. It ends by anastomosing with the radial recurrent artery.
   B. The middle collateral artery is the larger terminal branch. It ends by anastomosing with the interosseous recurrent artery.
   C. Deltoid branch ascends between the long and lateral head of tricep and anastomoses with the descending branch of posterior circumflex humeral artery.
   D. Nutrient artery to the humerus.

LAQ-9   Describe cubital fossa under
1. Boundaries   2. Contents &   3. Applied anatomy.

1. **Boundaries :**
   A. Medial boundary is formed by lateral border of pronator teres.
   B. Lateral boundary is formed by medial border of brachioradialis.
   C. Roof : It is formed by
      a. Skin and superficial fascia containing
         I. Medial cutaneous nerve of forearm.
         II. Lateral cutaneous nerve of forearm

III. Medial cubital vein which is joined by
   i. Cephalic vein
   ii. Basilic vein
b. Deep fascia and bicipital aponeurosis

D. Floor :
   a. In upper part : It is formed by lower part of brachialis.
   b. In lower part : It is formed by supinator.

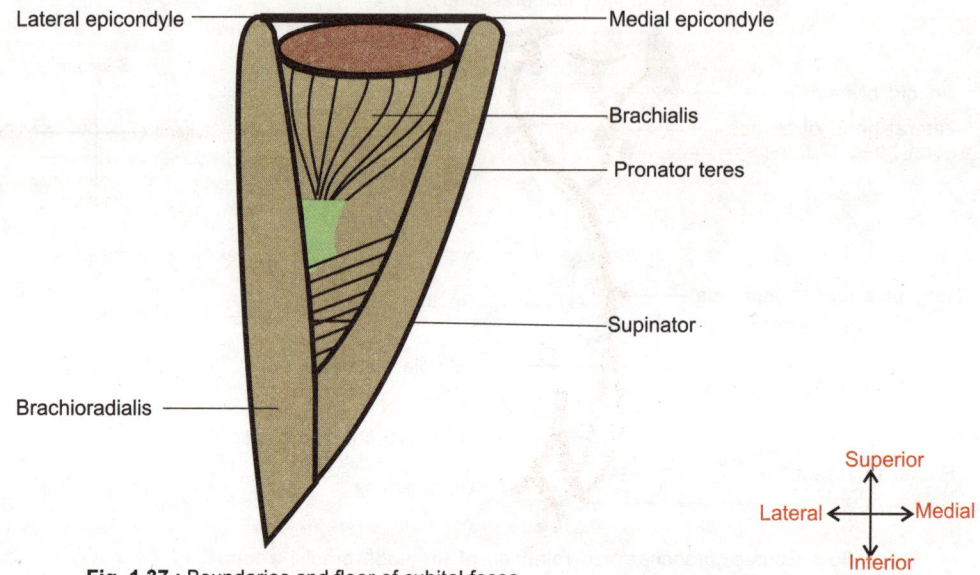

Fig. 1.37 : Boundaries and floor of cubital fossa.

E. Base is formed by imaginary line joining the medial and lateral epicondyle.
F. Apex is formed by meeting point of medial border of brachioradialis and lateral border of pronator teres.

2. **Contents :** From medial to lateral are 🔑 **M B B S**
A. **M**edian nerve passes between two heads of pronator teres
B. The **b**rachial artery divides into two terminal branches in the cubital fossa namely radial and ulnar artery. The radial artery passes through the apex of cubital fossa and runs superficially in the forearm. The ulnar artery is the larger artery runs deep to deep head of pronator teres.
C. Tendon of **b**iceps.
D. Radial nerve divides into
   a. **S**uperficial branch of radial nerve and
   b. Deep branch of radial nerve : It continues as posterior interosseous branch, which passes through supinator and supplies all extensor muscles of forearm except those already supplied by trunk of radial.

3. **Applied anatomy :**
A. Median cubital vein is the most fixed vein. Hence it is used for withdrawal of blood for investigation purposes and giving intravenous fluid.
B. The brachial artery is auscultated for recording blood pressure.
C. The brachial artery is selected for withdrawal arterial blood for blood gas analysis.
D. The supracondylar fracture of humerus results into rupture of brachial artery and ends into condition called Volkman's ischaemic contracture.

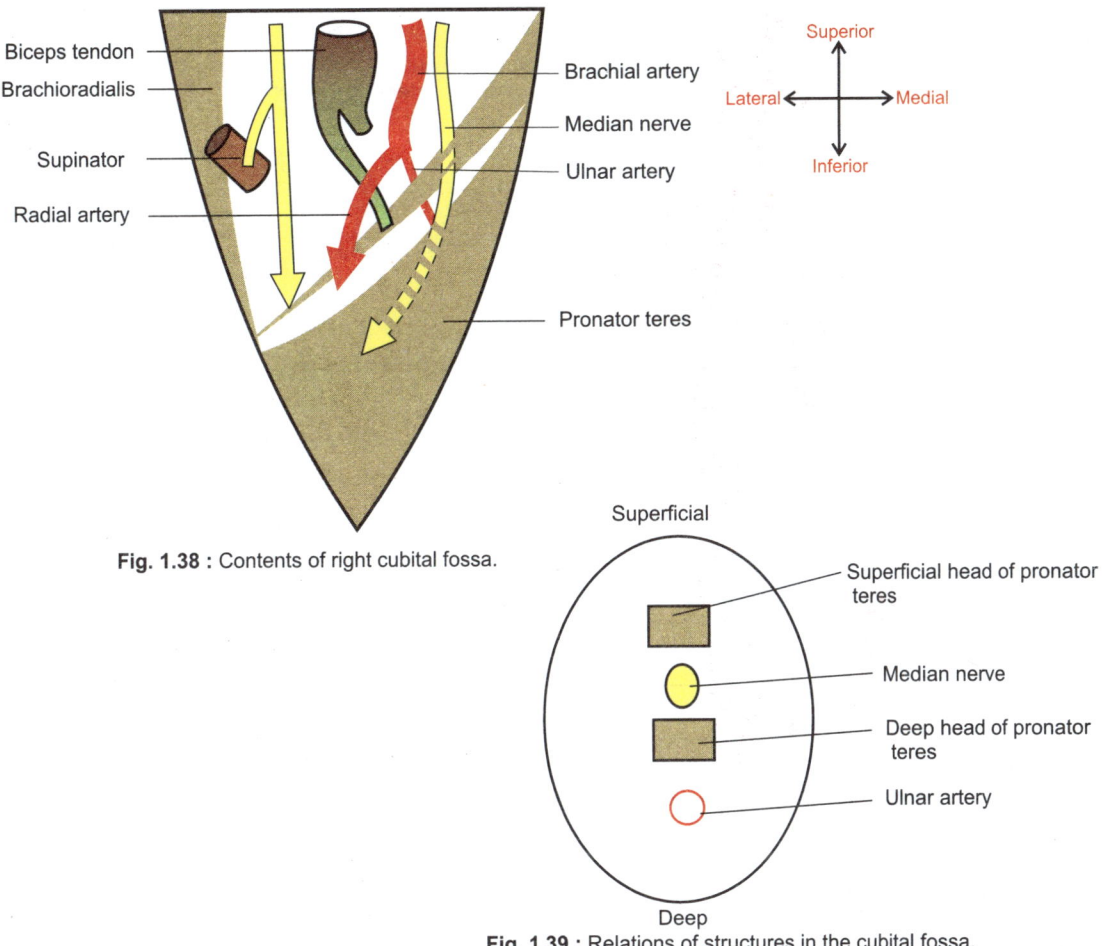

Fig. 1.38 : Contents of right cubital fossa.

Fig. 1.39 : Relations of structures in the cubital fossa.

LAQ-10   **Describe ulnar artery under**
1.   Origin   2.   Course and relations
3.   Branches and   4.   Applied anatomy.

Definition : It is the artery of medial side of forearm.

1.   **Origin :** This larger terminal branch of brachial artery arises 1 cm. below the bend of elbow.

2.   **Course and relations :**
   A.   Peculiarities : It is accompanied by
      a.   Venae comitantes and
      b.   Ulnar nerve in the distal 2/3rd of forearm.
   B.   Extent : It extends from elbow to wrist joint.
   C.   Termination : Ulnar artery forms superficial palmar arch in the hand. It passes downward, medially and leaves cubital fossa deep to ulnar head of pronator teres and lies between two nerves, laterally the median and medially the ulnar nerve.

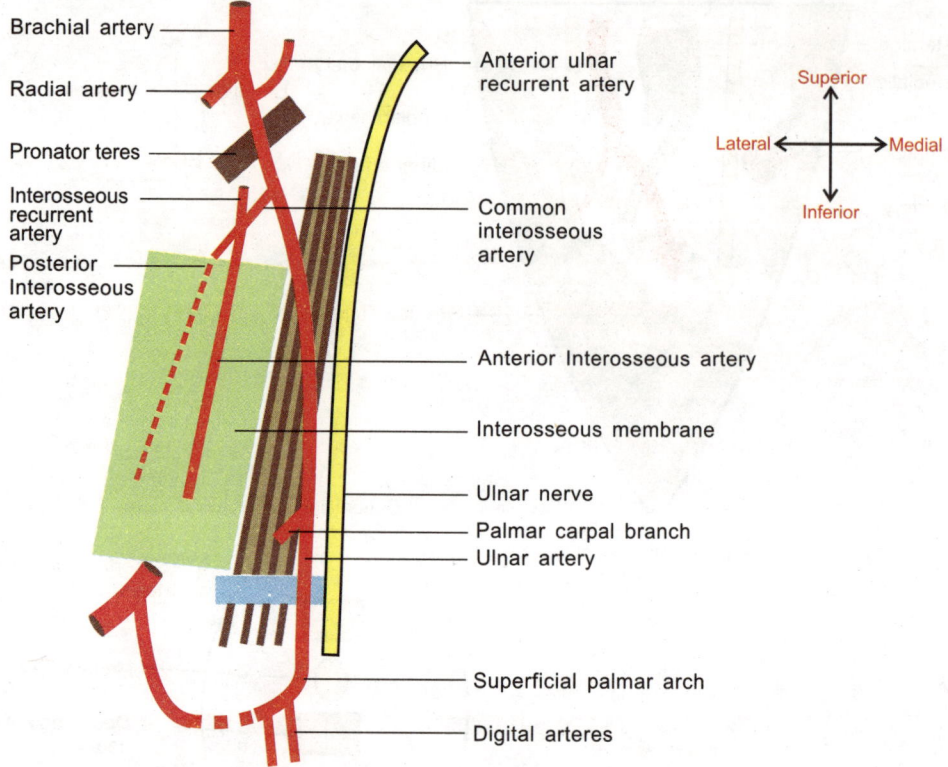

Fig. 1.40 : Course, relations and branches of right ulnar artery.

Table 1.14 : The table shows the relations of ulnar artery in the upper and lower half of the forearm.

Upper half	Lower half
I. Pronator teres. II. Flexor carpi radialis. III. Palmaris longus. IV. Flexor digitorum superficialis. V. Flexor carpi ulnaris.	I. Skin. II. Superficial fascia. III. Deep fascia. IV. Palmar cutaneous branch of ulnar nerve.

   D. Relations :
- a. Anterior
- b. Posterior :
  - I. Flexor digitorum profundus and
  - II. Pronator quadratus.
- c. Lateral : Flexor digitorum superficialis.
- d. Medial : Flexor carpi ulnaris and ulnar nerve.

3. Branches :

   A. Muscular branch to all the superficial group of muscles on medial side of forearm & hand.

B. Cutaneous.
C. Articular branch to
   a. Elbow and
   b. Wrist joint.
D. Branches to nerves :
   a. Ulnar and
   b. Median.
E. Nutrient arteries to :
   a. Radius and
   b. Ulna.
F. Communicating branches to :
   a. Anterior,
   b. Posterior carpal arch &
   c. Superficial palmar arch.
G. Terminates as superficial palmar arch.
H. Branch to synovial sheath.

4. **Applied anatomy :** It is felt lateral to flexor carpi ulnaris and above the pisiform bone.
Note : For easy recalling remember the digit **'2'** 🔑
A. One of **2** terminal branches of brachial artery.
B. Extends between **2** joints namely elbow and wrist joint i.e. Neck (of radius) to head (of ulna).
C. Passes between **2** nerves :
   a. Median and
   b. Ulnar.
D. Relations with **2** groups of muscles
   a. Superficial and
   b. Deep.
E. Lies on **2** muscles
   a. Brachialis and
   b. Flexor digitorum profundus.
F. Branches : 🔑 The letters of the word "BRANCH" provides the information of the structures supplied by the artery.
   a. **2 B**ones
      I. Radius and
      II. Ulna.
   b. **2 R**ecurrent :
      I. Anterior ulnar recurrent and
      II. Posterior ulnar recurrent.
   c. Branches **A**rticular :
      I. Elbow joint and
      II. Wrist joint.
   d. Branches **N**erves :
      I. Ulnar and
      II. Median.
   e. Branches **C**arpal :
      I. Anterior and
      II. Posterior carpal.

    f.   Branches to **H**and
        I.   Superficial palmar arch and
        II. Deep palmar arch.
    g.   Branches to interosseous membrane
    h.   Branches to two group of muscles
        I.   Superficial and
        II. Deep.

SN-17   Anatomical snuff box

1. **Introduction :** It is a depressed triangular area present on the lateral side of wrist and becomes prominent when thumb is fully extended.

2. **Boundaries and contents :** ⚷ Boundaries, floor and contents are formed by **"3"** structures each.
   3 structures form boundaries, **3** structures form floor and **3** structures form the contents.
   A. Laterally : Tendon of abductor pollicis longus and tendon of extensor pollicis brevis.
   B. Medially : Extensor pollicis longus.

3. **Floor :** From proximal to distal three bones
   A. Scaphoid,
   B. Trapezium and
   C. Base of first metacarpal bone.

4. **Contents :** From superficial to deep
   A. Cephalic vein (over the roof),
   B. Superficial branch of radial nerve &
   C. Radial artery.

5. **Applied anatomy :** The fracture of the scaphoid presents with a complaint of pain in the wrist without any gross impairment of function.

SN-18   Flexor retinaculum   Imp

1. **Introduction :** It is a strong fibrous band of deep fascia connecting proximal and distal carpal bones of medial and lateral side.

2. **Gross anatomy :**

Table 1.15 : The table showing attachments of flexor retinaculum.

Particulars	Proximal	Distal
A. Attachment a. Medially	I. To pisiform bone. II. It also gives attachment to extensor retinaculum.	To hook of hamate
b. Laterally	To tubercle of scaphoid	To medial lip of groove of trapezium
B. Termination	I. Antebrachial fascia II. Fascia covering flexor Digitorum superficialis.	Palmar aponeurosis Palmar fascia

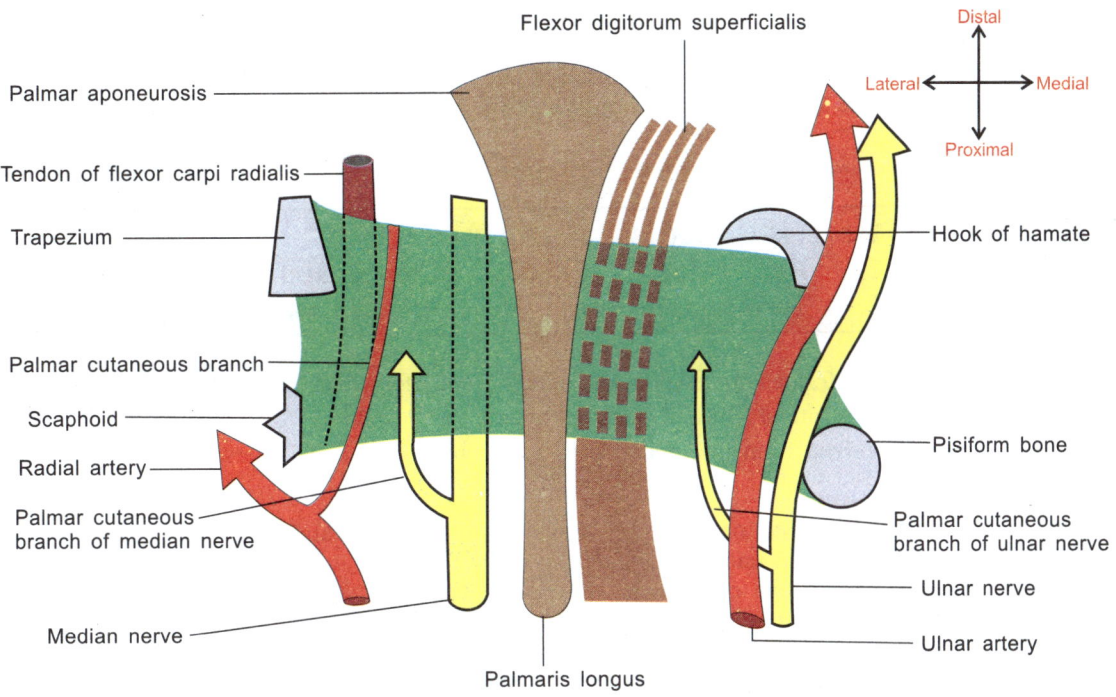

Fig. 1.41 : Left flexor retinaculum.

3.   Relations :

Table 1.16 :   Table showing relations of the flexor retinaculum.

Particulars	Superficial	Deep
A. Tendon	a. Palmaris longus	FDS - Flexor digitorum superficialis - 4 FDP - Flexor digitorum profundus - 4 FPL - Flexor pollicis longus - 1 FCR - Flexor carpi radialis
B. Arteries	a. Ulnar artery b. Superficial palmar branch of radial artery	----------

C. Nerve	a. Ulnar nerve
	b. Palmar cutaneous branch
	    of ulnar nerve
	c. Palmar cutaneous branch
	    of median.
		Median nerve

D. Synovial sheath	------------	For flexor tendons
E. Bursae	------------	a. Radial bursa b. Ulnar bursa

4. **Importance :**
   A. It gives origin to thenar and hypothenar muscles.
   B. The tendon of palmaris longus is fused in the midline.
   C. It keeps all the flexor tendons in position.
   D. It converts bony gutter into tunnel.

LAQ-11 Describe median nerve under
1. Root value 2. Course and relations
3. Termination and 4. Applied anatomy.

1. **Root value :** It is formed by medial and lateral root of median nerve. Lateral root is the continuation of the lateral cord of brachial plexus and contains C_5, C_6 & C_7 fibers. The medial root is derived from the medial cord and contains C_8 & T_1 fibers.

2. **Course and relations :**
   A. Lateral root of median nerve lie on the lateral side and medial root of median nerve lie on the medial side of second part of axillary artery.
   B. Medial root of median crosses the third part of axillary artery anteriorly and joins the lateral root of median nerve and forms the median nerve.
   C. The nerve runs on the lateral side of brachial artery upto middle of the arm. It crosses the brachial artery in the middle of the arm and remains on medial side of the brachial artery.
   D. It lies on medial side of brachial artery in the cubital fossa.
   E. It passes between two heads of pronator teres.
   F. It is separated from ulnar artery by deep head of pronator teres.
   G. In forearm it passes between superficial and deep muscles of forearm.
   H. It is accompanied by median artery (branch of anterior interosseous artery).
   I. In wrist : It passes deep to palmaris longus and lies between flexor digitorum superficialis and flexor carpi radialis. It passes through carpal tunnel and enters the hand. It gives lateral and medial branches.
   J. Before it divides into lateral and medial branch, it gives a recurrent muscular branch, which supplies.
      a. Abductor pollicis brevis.
      b. Opponens pollicis.
      c. Superficial head of flexor pollicis brevis.
   K. The lateral branch subdivides into three palmar digital branches, which supply the skin of both sides of thumb and radial side of index finger.
   L. The branch to index finger provides a muscular branch to first lumbrical.
   M. The medial branch subdivides into two common palmar digital nerves. Lateral common digital nerve gives a branch to 2nd lumbrical.
   N. Median nerve gives anterior interosseous nerve which accompanies anterior interosseous artery and supplies
      a. Flexor pollicis longus,
      b. Pronator quadratus &
      c. Lateral half of flexor digitorum profundus. Medial root of median crosses the artery anteriorly and joins with lateral head to form the median nerve.

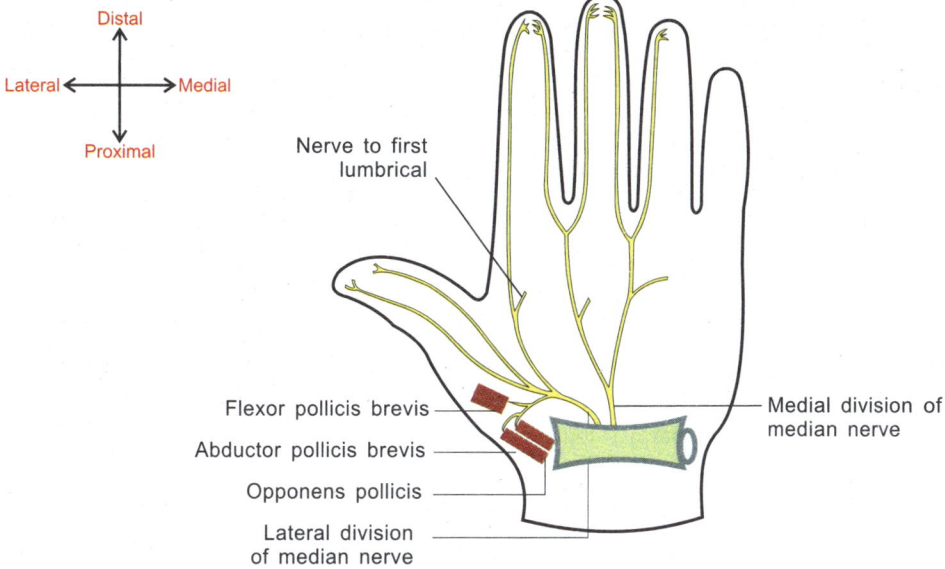

Distal

Lateral ← → Medial

Proximal

Nerve to first lumbrical

Flexor pollicis brevis

Abductor pollicis brevis

Opponens pollicis

Lateral division of median nerve

Medial division of median nerve

Fig. 1.42 : Median nerve in hand.

3. **Termination :** It ends in hand by dividing into two terminal branches.
   A. Medial and
   B. Lateral.

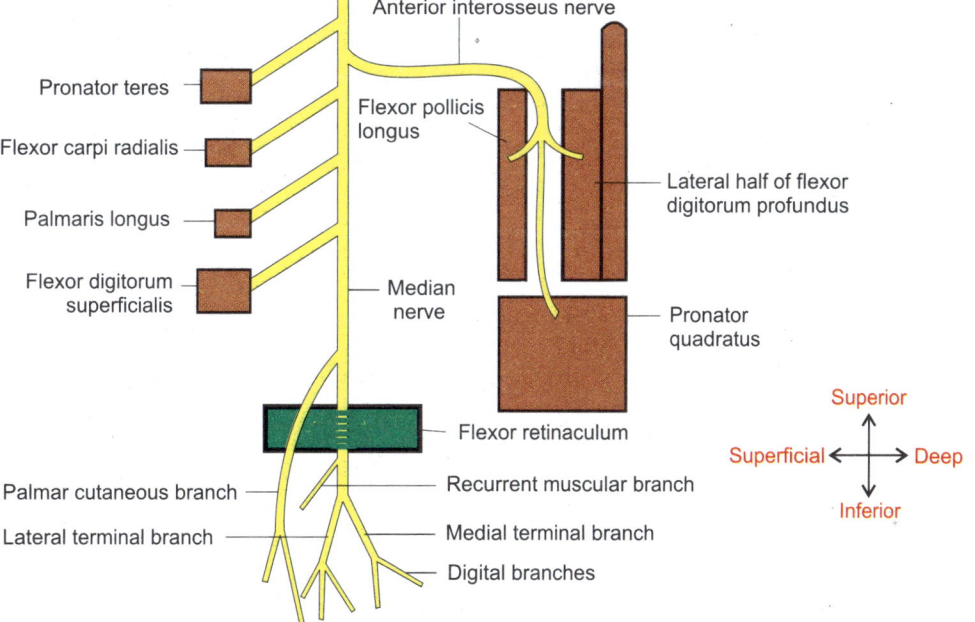

Anterior interosseus nerve

Pronator teres

Flexor carpi radialis

Palmaris longus

Flexor digitorum superficialis

Flexor pollicis longus

Median nerve

Lateral half of flexor digitorum profundus

Pronator quadratus

Flexor retinaculum

Palmar cutaneous branch

Lateral terminal branch

Recurrent muscular branch

Medial terminal branch

Digital branches

Superior

Superficial ← → Deep

Inferior

Fig. 1.43 : Branches of median nerve.

SN-19   **Applied anatomy of median nerve**   **Imp.**

4. **Applied anatomy :**

   A. Injury above the elbow joint : The cause of injury is mainly by supracondylar fracture of the humerus.

Table 1.17 : Table shows distribution of median nerve.

Position of hand	Muscles involved	Testing of nerve
a. Unable to bend terminal phalanx of thumb	Flexor pollicis longus.	Hold the proximal phalanx of thumb and ask to flex the terminal phalanx.
b. Forearm is kept in supine position	Pronator teres and pranator quadratus.	Pronations of the forearm.
c. Hand is adducted	Flexor carpi radialis.	
d. Signs of Benediction	Index and middle fingers cannot be flexed and thumb cannot be opposed.	

Table 1.18 : Table shows details of ape thumb deformity

Position of hand	Muscles involved	Testing of nerve
e. Ape thumb deformity.	I. Flexor pollicis brevis. II. Opponens pollicis. III. Abductor pollicis brevis.	Unable to hold a paper between thumb and index finger.

   B. Injury at the middle of forearm : Flexor digitorum superficialis is paralysed leading to condition called as "Pointing index finger".

   C. At wrist : The main cause is compression of median nerve in the carpal tunnel.

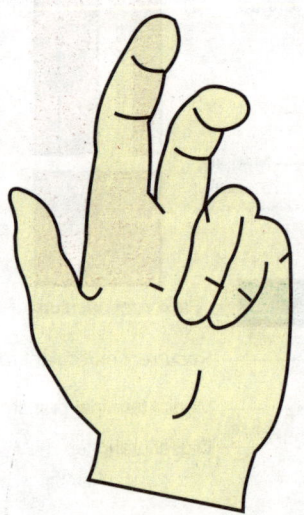

Fig. 1.44 : Hand of benediction.

Table 1.19 : Table shows clinical manifestations of compression of median nerve in the carpal tunnel.

Position of hand	Muscles affected	Testing of nerve
Ape thumb deformity : Thumb is adducted and laterally rotated.	a. Flexor pollicis brevis. b. Opponens pollicis. c. Abductor pollicis brevis.	a. Counting of fingers. b. Index and middle finger is lagging in flexing the index finger while making a fist.

SN-20   Carpal tunnel

1. **Introduction :** It is a fibro osseous tunnel formed by concave palmar surfaces of carpal bones. It is situated in the lower part of anterior surface of forearm.

2. **Location :** It is located near the wrist joint.

3. **Formation :**
   A. Pillars
   Table 1.20 : The table shows bones forming the pillars of carpal tunnel.

Particulars	Laterally	Medially
Proximal row	Scaphoid	Pisiform
Distal row	Trapezium	Hamate

   B. Anterior : Flexor retinaculum.
   C. Posterior : Palmar surfaces of carpal bones.

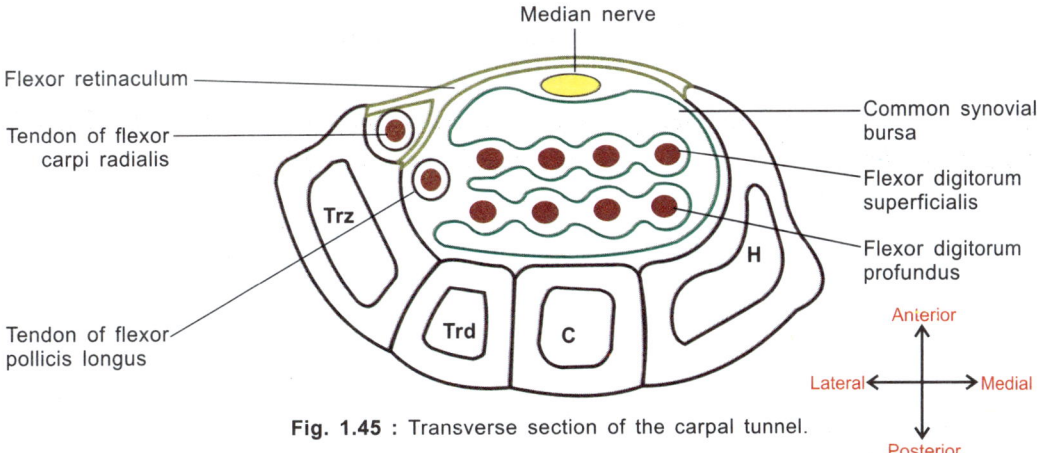

Fig. 1.45 : Transverse section of the carpal tunnel.

4. **Relations :**
   A. Anteriorly :
      a. Skin.
      b. Palmaris longus tendon.
      c. Palmar cutaneous branch of ulnar nerve.

     d. Palmar cutaneous branch of median nerve.

     e. Superficial palmar branch of radial artery.

     f. Ulnar nerve.

     g. Ulnar vessels.

  B. Posteriorly palmar surfaces of carpal bone.

5. **Contents :** (From superficial to deep).
- A. Flexor digitorum superficialis.
- B. Flexor carpi radialis.
- C. Flexor digitorum profundus.
- D. Flexor pollicis longus.
- E. Median nerve.
- F. Radial and ulnar bursa.

6. **Applied anatomy:**   **Imp.**

  A. Carpal tunnel syndrome : Compression of median nerve in the carpal tunnel gives rise to loss of sensations and weakness of the muscles of the thenar eminence, which constitute the carpal tunnel syndrome.

    a. Aetiology : Following are the causes of carpal tunnel syndrome.

       I. Causes due to the involvement of bones :

          i. Arthritis,

          ii. Dislocation of the lunate,

          iii. Old fracture of wrist joint.

       II. Soft tissue pathology

          i. Tenosynovitis,

          ii. Acromegaly,

          iii. Myxaedema,

          iv. Obesity and

          v. Toxaemia of pregnancy.

    b. Sex variation : Carpal tunnel syndrome is common in female.

    c. Age group : Occurs between 40 to 70 years.

  B. Clinical features : It presents as

    a. Intermittent attacks of pain, which are more in the night. It is referred to proximal part of forearm. It may be relieved by dorsiflexion.

    b. Wasting of thenar muscles namely

       I. Flexor pollicis brevis.

       II. Opponens pollicis.

       III. Abductor pollicis brevis.

  C. Treatment :

    a. Pain is relieved by splinting of the wrist in slight dorsiflexion.

    b. The division of flexor retinaculum is required in severe cases.

SN-21   Palmar aponeurosis

It is a flattened tendon of palmaris longus present in the hand.

1. **Features :**
- A. Shape : Triangular.
- B. Apex : Blends with the flexor retinaculum.

C. Base : It is directed distally and divides into four slips opposite the head of metacarpals of the medial four fingers. Each slip divides into two parts which provides the passage for digital vessels, nerves and tendons of lumbricals. The palm is divided into compartments by the slips arising from lateral and medial margins of palmar aponeurosis.

2. **Morphology :** Phylogenetically it represents degenerated tendon of palmaris longus. It is homologous to plantar aponeurosis.

3. **Functions :**
   A. It improves the grip of the hand by fixing the skin.
   B. It protects the vessels and nerves of palmar surface of hand.

4. **Applied anatomy :**
   Dupuytren contracture : It is an inflammation of ulnar side of palmar aponeurosis. There is thickening and contracture of the palmar aponeurosis.

SN-22   Dupuytren contracture

1. **Introduction :** It is an inflammation of ulnar side of palmar aponeurosis. There is thickening and contracture of the palmar aponeurosis.

2. **Cause :** It is due to fibrosis and shortening of the palmar aponeurosis.

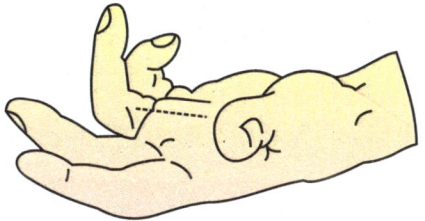

Fig. 1.46 : Dupuytren contracture.

3. **Features :**
   A. Usually the left hand is involved.
   B. It is more severe towards the ulnar side.
   C. There is progressive flexion of the fourth and fifth digit.
   D. There is an involvement of proximal and middle phalanx because of insertion of palmar aponeurosis.
   E. A high correlation exists between Dupuytren contracture and coronary artery disease. It is possibly due to result of vasospasm of the arteries innervated by first thoracic spinal nerve.

SN-23   Dorsal digital expansion

1. **Introduction :** It is a small aponeurosis formed by each extensor tendon which covers the dorsum of proximal phalanx and the sides of its base.

2. **Shape :** It is triangular, base directs proximally and apex directs distally.

3. **Formation :** It is mainly formed by extensor digitorum tendon and it is contributed by interossei and lumbrical muscles. In addition to above tendon
   A. In little finger, it is formed by extensor digiti minimi and
   B. In index finger, by extensor indicis.

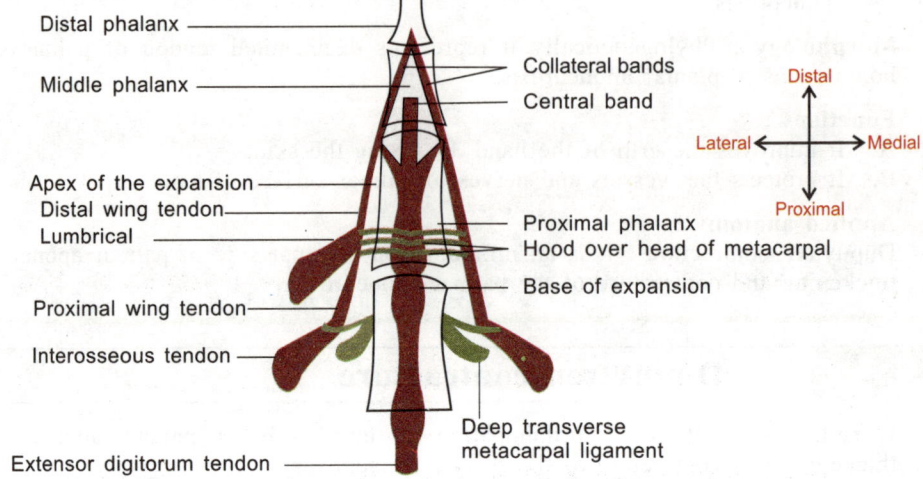

Fig. 1.47 : Dorsal digital expansion.

4. **Features :**
   A. Base of dorsal digital expansion
      a. It covers the dorsal and collateral aspects of metacarpo-phalangeal joint.
      b. It gives attachment to extensor tendon at the centre of base of digital expansion.
      c. It forms hood over head of metacarpal.
      d. It is movable distally and proximally with the flexion, extension of the metacarpo-phalangeal joint.
      e. Each basal angle is attached to deep transverse metacarpal ligament
   B. Margins : The lateral margin is thickened by insertion of tendon of lumbricals and interossei muscles. The medial margin is thickened by the attachments of interossei only.
   C. Wing tendons are of two types
      a. Proximal wings : Formed by dorsal and palmar interossei.
      b. Distal wings : Formed by lumbricals.
   D. Apex of expansion : At the distal end of proximal phalanx, the apex of the expansion is divided into three bands. They are :
      a. One central and
      b. Two collateral.
         The central band is inserted to the base of middle phalanx. The two collateral bands unite and finally are inserted into the dorsal aspect of the base of distal phalanx.

5. **Actions :**
   A. It keeps the extensor tendons in the midline.
   B. It is the only extensor of metacarpophalangeal joints (besides the extensor indices and the extensor digiti minimi) for the medial four fingers.
   C. The collateral bands extend the proximal and distal interphalangeal joint through the dorsal digital expansion.

LAQ-12   Describe interossei

(*Inter* in between, *ossei* bone)

Introduction : These are the small muscles of the hand present in between metacarpals and are divided into palmar and dorsal interossei. They are discussed as :

Table 1.21 : Table showing palmar and dorsal interossei.

Particulars	Palmar interossei	Dorsal interossei
1. Number and morphology	Four in number and are unipennate.	Four in number and are bipennate.
2. Dimension	1st palmar interossei is small.	All dorsal interossei are of uniform size.
3. Interossei for middle finger	Is absent.	They are 2 in number.
4. Origin	A. 1st and 2nd palmar interossei arise from medial or ulnar surface of respective metacarpals. B. 3rd and 4th palmar interossei arise from lateral or radial surface of 4th and 5th metacarpal.	Adjoining metacarpal.

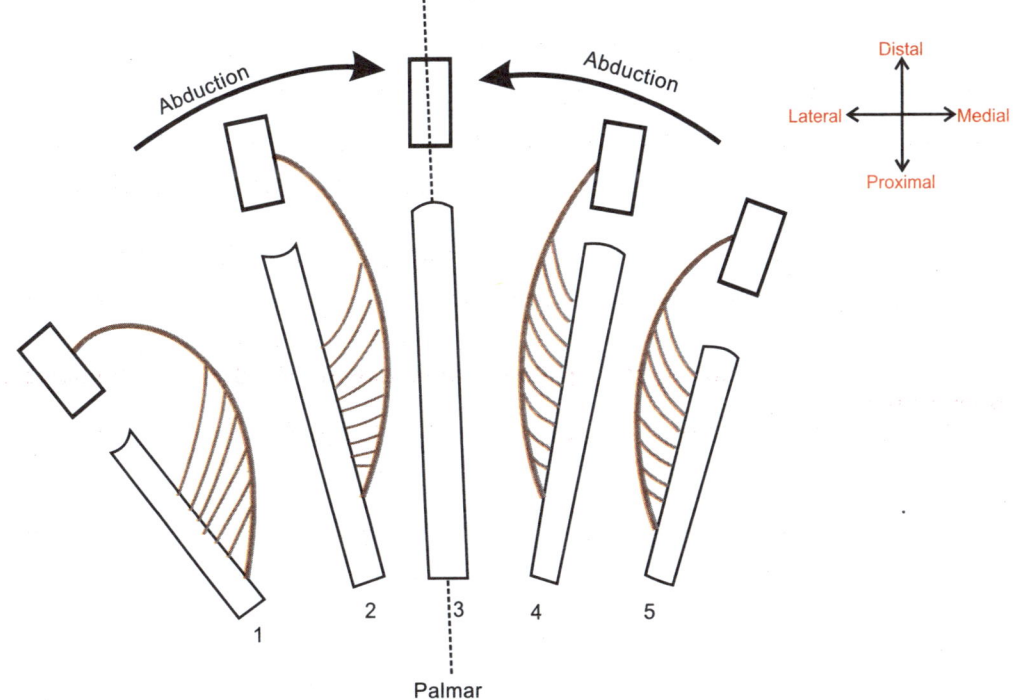

Fig. 1.48 : Palmar interossei.

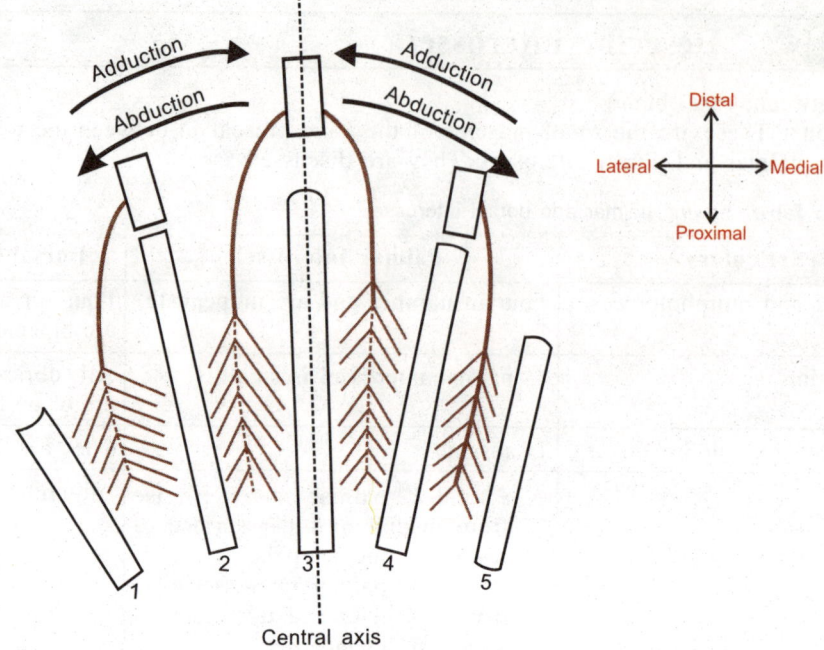

Central axis
Fig. 1.49 : Dorsal interossei.

5. **Insertion :** Both are inserted on
    A. Dorsal digital expansion and
    B. Base of proximal phalanx of respective finger.

6. **Axis :** Passes through middle finger.

7. **Strength :** Palmar interossei are less strong than dorsal interossei.

8. **Relations :**
    A. They are related posteriorly to deep transverse metacarpal ligaments.
    B. Radial artery passes between the gap produced by two heads of 1st dorsal interosseous.
    C. Proximal perforating arteries pass between the gap produced by two heads of 2nd, 3rd and 4th dorsal interossei.

9. **Actions :** 🔑 **PAD, DAB. P=palmar, AD=adductor ; D=Dorsal, AB=abductor, B=bipennate**
    A. *Palmar interossei are adductors, dorsal interossei are abductors.*
    B. They are powerful flexors of metacarpophalangeal joint (M.P.) because their tendons are placed ventrally and distally with respect to metacarpophalangeal joint.
    C. They produce extension of interphalangeal joint. Both these movements are useful for precision work.

10. **Nerve supply :** They are supplied by deep branch of ulnar nerve.

11. **Testing :** Interossei can be tested in following ways.
    A. Dorsal interossei : By asking to spread the fingers against resistance.
    B. Palmar interossei : By asking to hold a piece of paper between the testing finger and normal finger.

SN-24   Lumbricals

1. **Features :**
    A. These are worm like muscles, arise from tendons of flexor digitorum profundus.
    B. They are four in number and are present on palmar aspect.
    C. They are counted from lateral to medial.
    D. First and second lumbricals are unipennate.
    E. Third and fourth lumbricals are bipennate.
    F. They act as link muscles between deep flexor and extensor tendons of hand.

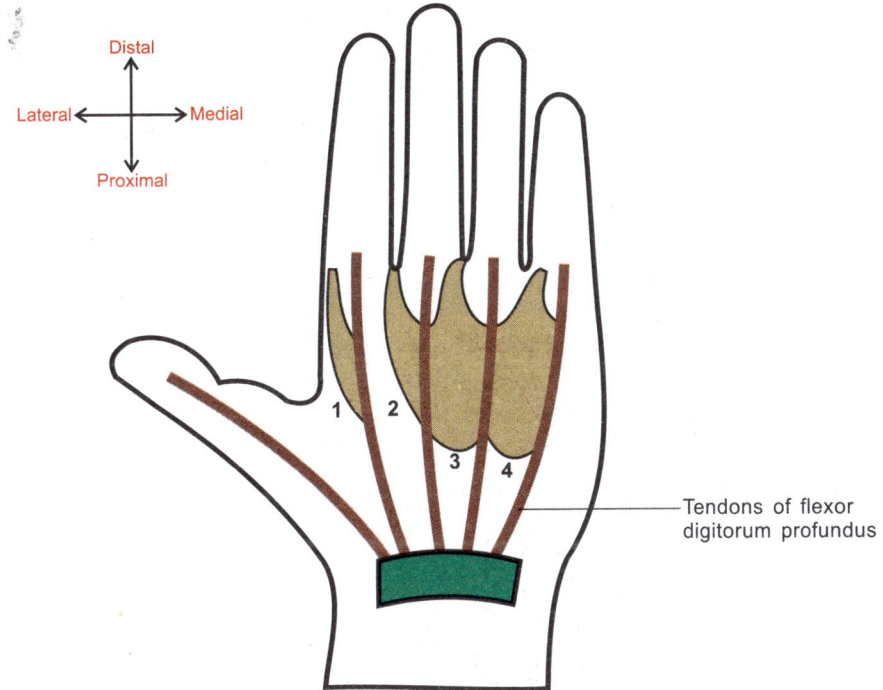

Fig.1.50 : Morphology of lumbricals.

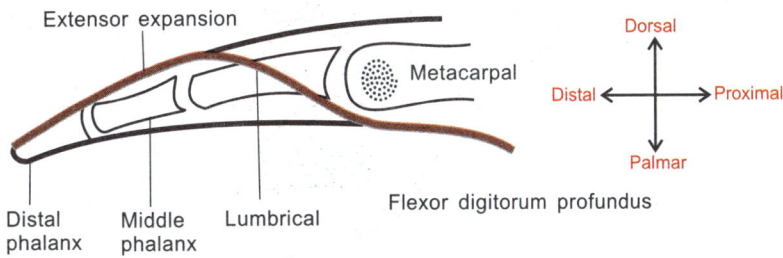

Fig. 1.51 : Origin and insertion of lumbrical.

2. **Origin :**
   A. First and second lumbricals arise from radial side of profundus tendon.
   B. Third and fourth lumbricals arise between neighboring tendons of flexor digitorum profundus.

3. **Insertion :** They are inserted on dorsal surface of base of middle and distal phalanx, through lateral border of dorsal digital expansion.

4. **Action :** They are flexors of metacarpophalangeal joints and extensors of interphalangeal joints.

5. **Nerve supply :** Medial two lumbricals are supplied by deep branch of ulnar nerve and lateral two lumbricals are supplied by median nerve.

6. **Relations :** They are dorsal to digital vessels and nerves.

7. **Functions :** They produce up and down strokes of fingers for skilled work.

8. **Test :** The muscles are best tested by asking the patient to hold a piece of paper between the sides of two adjacent fingers. If the muscles are acting, the paper will be firmly held and some resistance will be offered to its withdrawal.

LAQ-13	Describe superficial palmar arch

1. **Introduction :** It is the arterial arch, formed superficial to all the structures in the palm. It is compared with circle of Willis present at base of brain and plantar arterial arch in the foot.

2. **Arch :** It may be complete.

3. **Location :** It is situated in distal part of palm and corresponds to distal palmar crease.

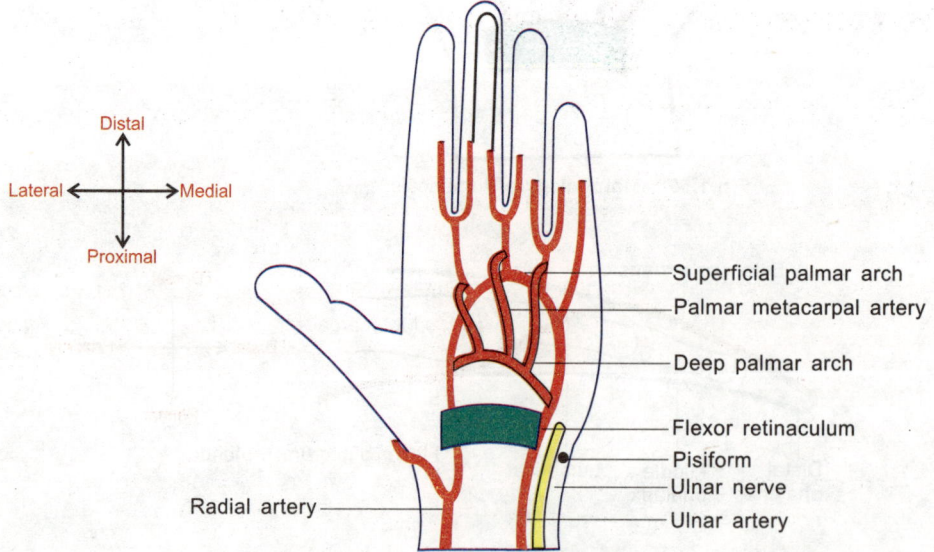

Fig. 1.52 : Superficial palmar arch.

4. **Formation :**
    A. It is formed on medial side of hand as a continuation of ulnar artery.
    B. On lateral side it is completed by one of the following arteries.
        a. Superficial palmar branch of radial artery.
        b. Arteria radialis indicis : Artery of index finger (branch of radial artery).
        c. Arteria princeps pollicis : Artery of thumb (branch of radial artery).
        d. Median artery (branch of anterior interosseous artery which is a branch of common interosseous artery - ulnar artery).

5. **Relations :**
    A. Anterior :
        a. Palmaris brevis and
        b. Palmar aponeurosis.
    B. Posterior : Flexor digitorum superficialis :
        a. Flexor digitorum profundus,
        b. Lumbricals,
        c. Flexor digiti minimi and
        d. Digital branches of median nerve.

6. Branches :   There are four digital branches to supply medial $3\frac{1}{2}$ fingers. Out of these four digital branches, lateral three digital branches join deep palmar arch by palmar metacarpal arteries.

7. Applied anatomy :   It is one of the important anastomotic channel for efficient blood supply of palm, in case of blockage of radial or ulnar artery.

LAQ-14   Describe deep palmar arch

1. **Introduction :** It is an arterial arch present deep to flexor tendons of digits.

2. **Formation :** It is mainly formed by radial artery and completed on medial side by deep palmar branch of ulnar artery.

3. **Location :** It is present at proximal palmar crease

4. **Arch :** It is complete.

5. **Relations :**
    A. Anterior :
        a. Oblique head of adductor pollicis,
        b. Flexor tendons of fingers and
        c. Lumbricals.
    B. Posterior : Shaft of metacarpal and interossei.

6. **Branches :**
    A. From the convexity of the arch, three palmar metacarpal arteries run distally in second, third and fourth spaces. They supply medial four metacarpals, terminate in finger cleft by joining with common digital branch of superficial palmar arch.
    B. From dorsal side three perforating arteries pass through medial three interosseous spaces to anastomose with dorsal metacarpal arteries.
    C. From the convexity of arch, recurrent branch arises to supply carpal bones and ends in palmar carpal arch.

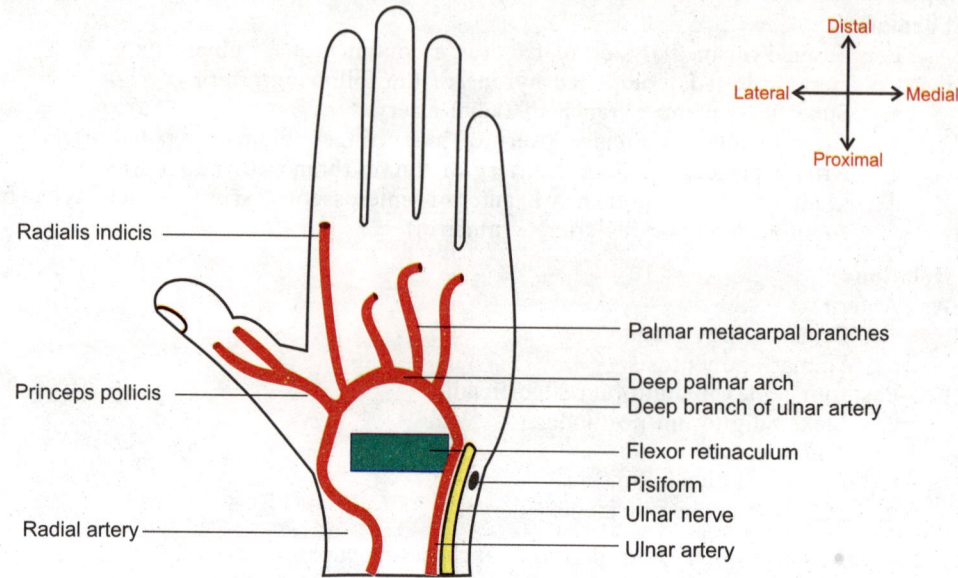

Fig. 1.53 : Deep palmar arch.

7. **Applied anatomy :** It is one of the important anastomotic channel for efficient blood supply of palm, in case of blockage of radial or ulnar artery.

LAQ-15   Describe ulnar nerve under
1. Definition   2. Root value   3. Course & relations
4. Branches &   5. Applied anatomy.

1. **Introduction :** Ulnar nerve is also called musician's nerve, because it supplies all the intrinsic muscles of hand except lateral two lumbricals and muscles of the thenar eminence. It supplies the muscles of forearm and hand. It carries cutaneous sensation from medial 1½ fingers.

2. **Root value :** It arises from medial cord of brachial plexus C_7, C_8 & T_1.

3. **Course and relations :** The structures in the course and relation of ulnar nerve begin with the letter **M**.
    A. The **m**edial cord of brachial plexus lies on **m**edial side of second part of axillary artery.
    B. The ulnar nerve lies **m**edial to third part of axillary artery.
    C. It also lies **m**edial to brachial artery.
    D. In the **m**iddle of the arm, it pierces **m**edial intermuscular septum along with superior ulnar collateral artery.
    E. It enters posterior compartment and lies on **m**edial head of triceps. It passes behind **m**edial epicondyle of humerus and is received by flexor carpi ulnaris.
    F. It lies on **m**edial ligament of elbow joint and rests on **m**edial side of the flexor digitorum profundus under thin blanket of flexor carpi ulnaris in upper $2/3^{rd}$ of forearm.

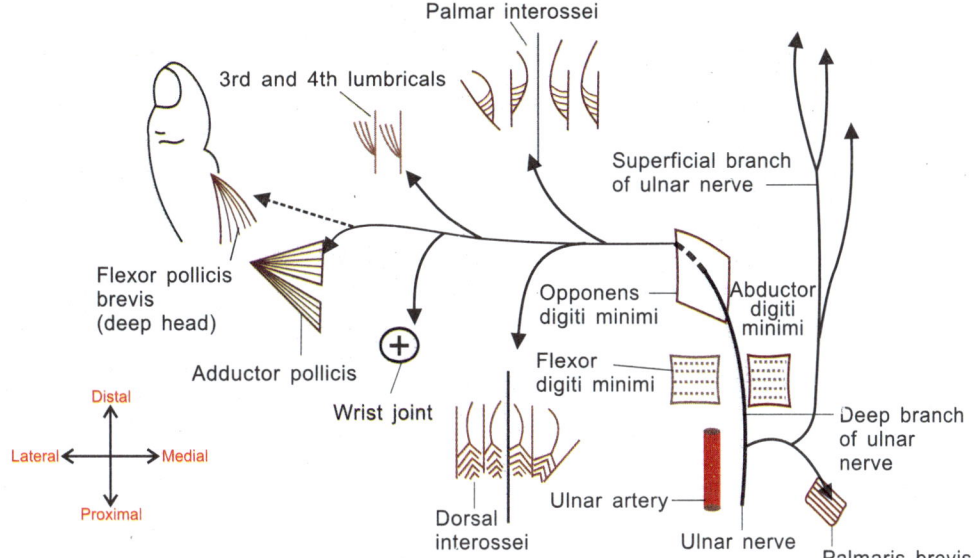

Fig. 1.54 : Ulnar nerve of left hand.

G. It runs on **m**edial side of ulnar artery.

H. In the hand : It lies in front of flexor retinaculum and divides into superficial and deep branch.

I. The deep branch is accompanied by deep branch of ulnar artery and passes in between abductor digiti minimi and flexor digiti minimi, then passes through the substance of opponens digiti minimi.

4. Branches :

Table 1.22 : Table showing distribution of ulnar nerve.

	Muscular	**Cutaneous**	**Joint**
	---	---	---
	a. Flexor carpi ulnaris b. Flexor digitorum profundus (medial half)	---	Elbow

	a. Palm : Palmaris brevis
	 b. Hypothenar
	   I. Abductor digiti minimi brevis
	   II. Flexor digiti minimi
	   III. Opponens digiti minimi
	 c. Thenar :
	   I. Adductor pollicis
	   II. Flexor pollicis brevis (deep head)
	 d. Interossei
	   I. 4 palmar
	   II. 4 dorsal
	 e. Lumbricals : 2 medial
		Skin of hypothenar eminence and skin of medial one and half fingers.	---

5. **Applied anatomy :**
   A. Ulnar nerve is palpated behind medial epicondyle of humerus. This is thickened and is cord like in Henson's disease.
   B. Ulnar nerve is damaged
      a. At elbow joint due to
         I. The cubital tunnel is formed by tendinous arch connecting two heads of flexor carpi ulnaris. The ulnar nerve is often entrapped in this tunnel and this entrapment of ulnar nerve in the cubital tunnel is called cubital tunnel syndrome. It results into radial deviation of hand.
         II. Pressure on the ulnar nerve as it passes along ulnar groove produces funny sensations along the medial border of forearm, hypothenar surface and little finger. Hence 'humerus' is called "funny bone".
      b. At wrist joint by the compression of volar carpal ligament and palmaris brevis muscle.
         I. Here all intrinsic muscles of hand are paralysed resulting into typical claw hand (ulnar claw).
         II. There is a hyperextension of metacarpophalangeal joint of the ring and little finger and flexion of interphalangeal joint. This is because of paralysis of interossei and lumbricals.
         III. There is also loss of sensations on the medial 1½ fingers.
         IV. There is loss of adduction of thumb, as adductor pollicis is paralysed.

SN-25   Pulp space

It is space between palmar skin and distal phalanges of all digits of hand
1. **Situation :** Distal to fibrous sheath of flexor tendon.

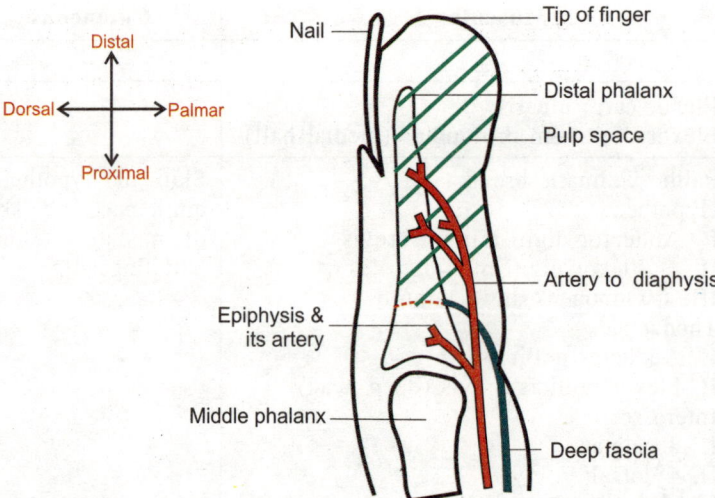

Fig. 1.55 : Digital pulp space.

2. **Formation :** Formed by fibrous septa connecting skin to periosteum of distal phalanx.

3. **Content :**
   A. Subcutaneous fat   B. Blood vessel.

4. **Blood supply of terminal phalanx :** Distal $4/5^{th}$ part by digital arteries and proximal part by epiphyseal artery.

5. **Applied anatomy :**
   A. Infection of pulp space, is called Whitlow, which is associated with severe throbbing pain due to increased tension in spaces.
   B. Abscess is drained by lateral incision and breaking all septa. In neglected cases it may lead to avascular necrosis of terminal phalanx.

SN-26 Palmar spaces

Table 1.23 : Table showing palmar spaces.

Particulars	Mid palmar	Thenar
1. **Introduction:**	Hollow space situated on the inner side of palm	Hollow space situated on outer side of palm
2. **Shape**	Triangular	Triangular
3. **Situation:**	Inner side of palm	Outer side of palm
4. **Communication:** A. Distally	Fascial sheath of 3rd, 4th lumbricals [occasionally 2nd].	Fascial sheath of first lumbrical [occasionally 2nd].
B. Proximally	The space is closed by the attachment of ulnar bursa to the floor of carpal tunnel.	
5. **Boundaries :** A. Anterior	a. Skin and palmar aponeurosis b. Flexor tendons of 3rd, 4th, 5th, fingers c. 2nd, 3rd, 4th lumbricals	a. Skin and palmar aponeurosis. b. Short muscles of thumb, flexor pollicis brevis, opponens pollicis, adductor pollicis. c. Flexor tendon of index finger. d. 1st lumbrical.
B. Posterior	Fascia covering interossei and metacarpal.	Transverse head of adductor pollicis
C. Lateral	Intermediate palmar septum	Lateral palmar septum and radial bursa.
D. Medial	Medial palmar septum	Intermediate palmar septum.
6. **Drainage :**	Incision in either the 3rd or 4th web space.	In first web space posteriorly.

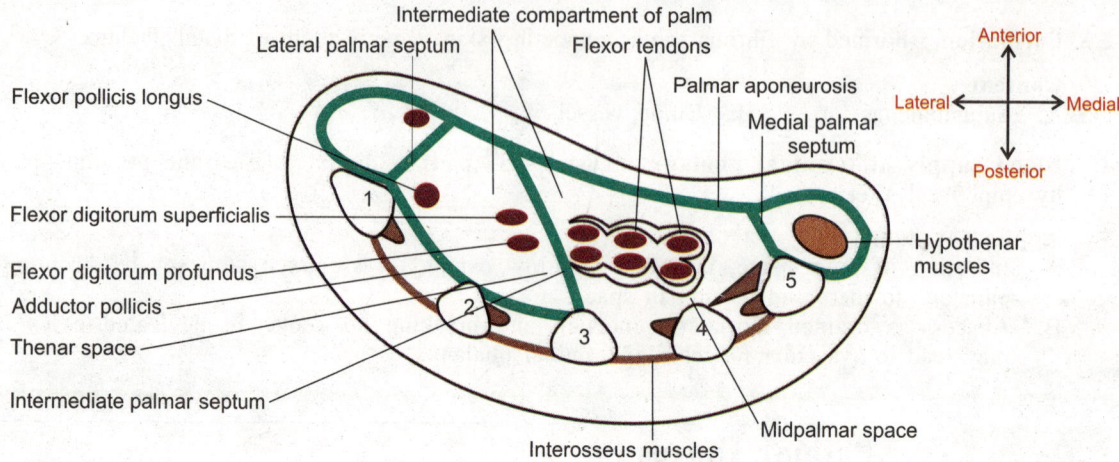

Fig. 1.56 : Thenar and midpalmar spaces.

SN-27   # Movements of the scapula

1.   **Introduction :** Movement of the acromio clavicular and coraco clavicular joint is always associated with the movement of the scapula.

2.   **Movements :** The movements of the scapula may or may not be associated with the movements of the shoulder joint. The various movements are described as follows :
     A.   Elevation (shrugging the shoulders) : It is associated with the raising of the acromio clavicular joint and depression of sternoclavicular joint.
          Muscles bringing the movements
          a.   Upper fibers of trapezius and
          b.   Levator scapulae.
     B.   Depression (drooping of the shoulder) : It is associated with depression of acromio clavicular joint and elevation of sternoclavicular joint.
          Factors bringing the movements
          a.   Gravity,
          b.   Muscles
               I.   Lower fibers of the serratus anterior and
               II.   Pectoralis minor.
     C.   Protraction (as in pushing and punching movement) : It is associated with the forward movement of lateral end and backward movement of the medial end of the clavicle.
          Muscles bringing the movements
          a.   Serratus anterior and
          b.   Pectoralis minor.
     D.   Retraction of the scapula (squaring of the shoulder) : It is associated with the backward movement of the lateral end and forward movement of the medial end of the clavicle.
          Muscles bringing the movements
          a.   Rhomboids major and minor.
          b.   Trapezius.

E. Forward rotation of the scapula round the chest wall takes place during overhead abduction of the arm. The scapula rotates round the coraco clavicular ligament.
Muscles bringing the movements
a. Upper fibers of trapezius.
b. Lower fibers of serratus anterior.
F. Backward rotation of the scapula occurs under the influence of gravity.
Muscles bringing the movements
a. Levator scapulae and
b. Rhomboids.

LAQ-16 Describe shoulder joint OR Glenohumeral joint under 1. Classification 2. Ligaments 3. Movements and muscles bringing movements 4. Relations 5. Blood supply 6. Nerve supply & 7. Applied anatomy.

1. **Classification :**
    A. Structural : Simple, ball and socket, multiaxial synovial joint.
    B. Functional : Diarthrosis.

2. **Ligaments :**
    A. Capsule
        a. Attachment :
            I. Humerus : It is attached to anatomical neck of humerus.
            II. Scapula : It is attached to peripheral margins of glenoid cavity including supraglenoid tubercle but excluding infraglenoid tubercle.
        b. Deficient : It is deficient in the region of bicipital groove for the passage of
            I. Tendon of long head of biceps,
            II. Synovial sheath,
            III. Ascending branch of anterior circumflex humeral artery.
        c. Laxity : It is lax on the inferior side, one cm below the surgical neck of humerus.
        d. Strengthened : It is strengthened by rotator cuff i.e.
            I. Supraspinatus,
            II. Infraspinatus,
            III. Teres minor &
            IV. Subscapularis.
        e. Capsule has two openings
            I. For long head of biceps muscle and
            II. For subscapular bursa.
    B. Synovial membrane : It lines inner surface of capsule and extends on long head of biceps, as tubular extension. It communicates with synovial membrane of subscapular bursa.
    C. Glenoid labrum : Structurally it is fibrocartilage in nature and triangular in cross section. It is attached to peripheral margin of glenoid cavity.
        a. It deepens the cavity of shoulder joint.
        b. It protects the edges of the articulating surfaces.
        c. It provides the cushion to head of humerus to roll as ball bearing.

    D. Glenohumeral ligament (It is condensation of anterior part of capsule). It extends superiorly from supero-medial margin of glenoid cavity. Inferiorly it is divided into 3 parts :

        a.   Superior band is attached to   ⟶ Upper end of lesser tubercle.
        b.   Middle band is attached to   ⟶ Lower end of lesser tubercle.
        c.   Inferior band is attached to   ⟶ Lower part of anatomical neck.

    E. Coracohumeral ligament : It is thick band in the upper part of fibrous capsule. It extends from the root of coracoid process to neck of humerus.

    F. Transverse humeral ligament : Bridges greater and lesser tubercle.

3. Movements :

    A. Flexion
        a.   Anterior fibres of deltoid &
        b.   Clavicular fibres of pectoralis major.

    B. Extension
        a.   Posterior fibres of deltoid with
        b.   Latissimus dorsi.

    C. Abduction
        a.   For every 15° of abduction 10° occurs at shoulder joint and 5° at shoulder girdle
        b. $1\text{-}15^o$ - Supraspinatus
        c. $15\text{-}90^o$ - Middle fibres of deltoid (acromial)
        d. $90^o\text{-}120^o$ by fibres of serratus anterior attached to inferior angle of scapula.
        e. 120° - 180° is by serratus anterior through shoulder girdle.

    D. Adduction
        a.   Sternal fibres of pectoralis major and
        b.   Latissimus dorsi

    E. Medial rotation   ☛   *Lady, soldier and majors* are medial rotators i.e. Muscles forming posterior boundaries of axilla, namely
        a.   Latissimus dorsi,
        b.   Subscapularis,
        c.   Two majors (pectoralis major and teres major) and
        d.   Anterior fibres of deltoid.

    F. Lateral rotation   ☛   **TIP**

        a.   **T**eres minor
        b.   **I**nfraspinatus
        c.   **P**osterior fibres of deltoid.

4. Relations :

    A. Superiorly :
        a.   Coracoacromial arch,
        b.   Sub-acromial bursa,
        c.   Supraspinatus and
        d.   Deltoid.

    B. Inferiorly : Long head of triceps.

    C. Anteriorly :
        a.   Subscapularis
        b.   Coracobrachialis   } These muscles are deep to deltoid.
        c.   Short head of biceps

D. Posteriorly :
    a. Deltoid,
    b. Infraspinatus,
    c. Teres minor and
    d. Intracapsular : Tendon of long head of biceps.

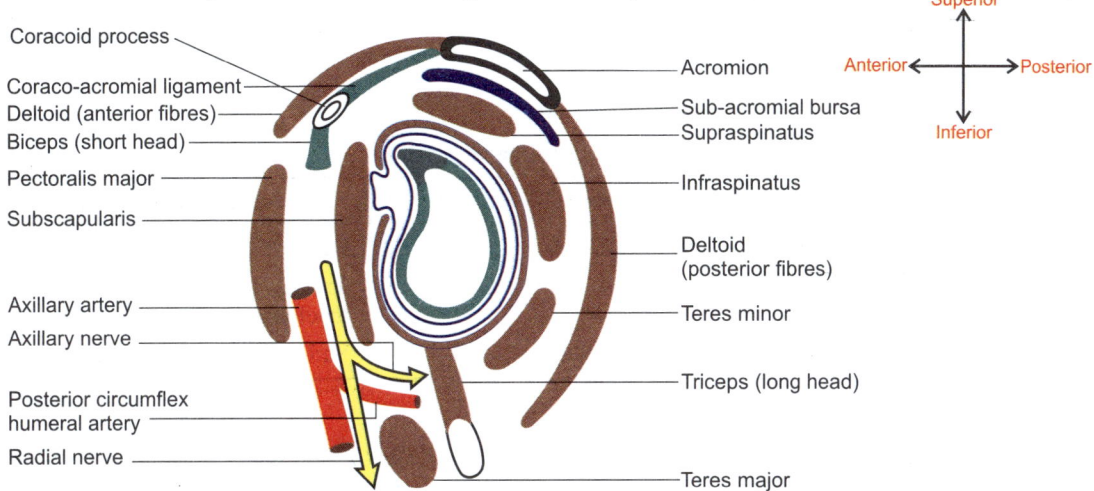

Fig. 1.57 : Relations of shoulder joint.

5. **Blood Supply :**
  A. Anterior circumflex humeral artery
  B. Posterior circumflex humeral artery } Branches of axillary artery
  C. Subscapular artery
  D. Suprascapular artery : Branch of thyrocervical trunk - branch of 1st part of subclavian artery.

6. **Nerve supply :** The shoulder joint obeys the Hilton's law, i.e. The nerve supplying muscles acting on the joint also supplies the joint and skin over the joint. Hence the nerves supplying joint are
  A. Axillary nerve,
  B. Musculocutaneous nerve and
  C. Suprascapular nerve.

7. **Applied anatomy :**
  A. Shoulder joint is the most frequently dislocating joint in the body. It is due to
    a. Disproportionate articular surfaces of head of humerus and glenoid cavity of scapula.
    b. Laxity of capsule : Capsule is lax inferiorly hence inferior dislocation is most common.
  B. It usually occurs when arm is forcefully abducted. Axillary nerve is usually injured.
  C. Frozen shoulder : It is common condition due to adhesion between rotator cuff and humeral head resulting into painful and restricted movements.
  D. Shoulder tip pain : Irritation of diaphragm causes referred pain to the shoulder tip. Since the root values of phrenic nerve supplying the diaphragm and supra clavicular nerve supplying shoulder joint are same, i.e. C_3 & C_4 spinal segment.

LAQ-17   **Describe elbow joint under**
1. **Classification**   2. **Ligaments**   3. **Movements**
4. **Relations**   5. **Blood supply**   6. **Nerve supply**
7. **Applied anatomy.**

1. **Classification :**
   A. Structural : Compound, uniaxial, hinge type of synovial joint.
   B. Functional : Diarthrosis.
   C. Cubital articulation : Consist of 3 joints.

Table 1.24 : The table showing bones forming the elbow joint.

Particulars	Humero radial joint	Humero ulnar joint
a. Bones	Humerus and radius	Humerus and ulna
b. Articular Surface	Head of radius with capitulum of humerus	Trochlear notch of ulna with trochlear surface of humerus
C. Type	Ball and socket type of synovial joint	Saddle type of synovial joint

2. **Ligaments :**
   A. Fibrous capsule : It is attached to peripheral margin of articular surface of humerus, radius and ulna
      a. It is thick medially, and laterally,
        Thin anteriorly, and posteriorly.
      b. Excludes medial and lateral epicondyles,
      c. Includes three fossae : Coronoid, radial and olecranon and
      d. Merges with the annular ligament of superior radioulnar joint.
   B. Synovial membrane - lines inner surface of capsule
   C. Anterior and
   D. Posterior ligaments } are formed by thickening of capsule of elbow joint and is thin.
   E. Ulnar collateral ligament is triangular in shape.
      It extends superiorly from lower part of medial epicondyle.
      Inferiorly it divides into 3 bands
      a. Anterior band is attached to medial margin of coronoid process.
      b. Inferior band is attached between olecranon and coronoid process.
      c. Posterior band is attached to medial margin of olecranon process.
   F. Radial collateral ligament : It extends from lateral epicondyle of humerus to annular ligament.

3. **Movements :**

Table 1.25 : The table showing movements and the muscles bringing the movements.

Movements	Muscles producing movement	Other muscles
A. Flexion	a. Brachialis b. Biceps c. Brachioradialis	Pronator teres, palmaris longus, flexor digitorum superficialis, flexor carpi radialis, flexor carpi ulnaris.
B. Extension	a. Triceps b. Anconeus	Extensor carpi radialis longus and brevis. Extensor carpi ulnaris, extensor digitorum

4. **Relations :**
   A. Anteriorly
      a. Brachialis
      b. Tendon of biceps
      c. Median nerve
      d. Brachial artery
      } Structures are contents of cubital fossa.
   B. Posterior : Triceps, anconeus.
   C. Medially :
      a. Ulnar nerve,
      b. Flexor carpi ulnaris and
      c. The common flexors of forearm.
   D. Laterally :
      a. Supinator,
      b. Extensor carpi radialis brevis and
      c. Common extensors.

5. **Blood supply :**
   A. Superior ulnar collateral artery
   B. Inferior ulnar collateral artery
   } Branches of brachial artery

   C. Anterior descending artery
   D. Posterior descending artery
   } Branches of profunda brachii artery

   E. Radial recurrent artery — Branch of radial artery
   F. Interosseous recurrent artery — Branch of common interosseous artery

   G. Anterior ulnar recurrent artery
   H. Posterior ulnar recurrent artery
   } Branches of ulnar artery

6. **Nerve supply :**
   A. Musculocutaneous nerve,
   B. Radial nerve,
   C. Median nerve and
   D. Ulnar nerve.

7. **Applied anatomy :**
   A. Supracondylar fractures results into Volkman's ischemic contracture. Which is due to injury to brachial artery.
   B. Usually the elbow dislocates posteriorly. It is associated with fracture of coronoid process.
   C. Effusion of joint occurs posteriorly because capsule is weak posteriorly.
   D. Tennis elbow : Pain and tenderness over lateral epicondyle due to
      a. Sprain of radial collateral ligament.
      b. Tearing of the fibers of extensor carpi radialis brevis.
      c. Inflammation of bursa over the extensor carpi radialis brevis.

SAQ-5   Carrying angle

1. **introduction** : It is an angle formed by arm with forearm when elbow is fully extended and forearm supinated, which opens laterally.

2. **Cause :** There are two reasons
    A. Medial flange of trochlea is 6 mm which is lower than lateral flange of trochlea.
    B. Obliquity of superior articular surface.

3. **Sex difference :** There is no much difference in the carrying angle in male and female.

4. **Function :** Carrying angle is helpful in holding the object.

5. **Degree of angle :**
    A. It is 163° in fully extended elbow and supinated forearm.
    B. It is 0° in full flexion and pronation of forearm.

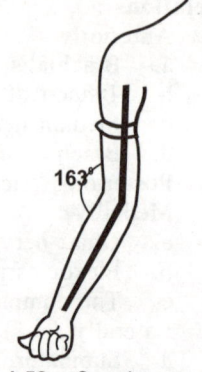

163°

Fig. 1.58 : Carrying angle.

LAQ-18   Describe supination and pronation

1. **Introduction :** Supination and pronation movements are mainly evolved for picking up the food and keeping into mouth.

Table 1.26 : The table showing comparison between supination and pronation.

	Supination	Pronation
A. Introduction :		
a. In anatomical position	a. Palm faces forward & thumb faces laterally.	Palm faces backwards and thumb faces medially.
b. In mid flexion of elbow joint	b. Palm faces upwards & thumb faces laterally.	Palm faces downwards and thumb faces medially.
B. Position of		
a. Bone	Radius is laterally, ulna is medially and both are kept parallel to each other.	Position of radius & ulna remains same. Radius is anteromedially, ulna is laterally in upper half, while it is reverse in lower half.
b. Interosseous membrane	Not spiralled.	Spirally twisted.
C. Movement of bone	Radius plays active role and ulna remains more or less fixed.	a. Head of radius rotates in the fibrosseous ring, a pivot joint. b. Lower end of radius and articular disc swing around ulnar head.
D. Strength	Strength is greater.	Strength is less.
E. Position of axis	Displaced medially.	Displaced laterally.
F. Situations in which these movements are used	Tightening of nuts picking the food.	Loosening of nuts.
G. Relation to gravity	Antigravity action.	Towards gravity.

2. **Mechanism of Action :**
   A. Position of forearm is semiflexed.
   B. Type of movement is rotatory.
   C. Evolved for picking up food and putting into mouth.
   D. Range of movements :
      a. In flexed elbow : 140° - 150°
      b. In extended elbow : 360°. It includes rotation of shoulder.
   E. Axis :
      a. Plane : Transverse.
      b. Representation : It is represented as axis passing through centre of head of radius and apex of articular disc to little finger.
   F. Homologous movements in lower limb : inversion and eversion
   G. Joints : Superior & inferior radio ulnar joints.

3. **Applied anatomy :**
   A. In children, head of radius is not developed as compared to annular ligament. Hence, subluxation of superior radioulnar joint is common under age of 6 years.
   B. Pronation and supination movements are used in mechanical jobs.
      e.g. tightening screw with screw driver.

LAQ-19 **Describe wrist joint (radio carpal) under**
1. Bones taking part   2. Classification   3. Ligaments
4. Relations   5. Movements   6. Blood supply
7. Nerve supply   8. Applied anatomy.

1. **Bones taking part :**
   A. Proximally :
      a. Distal articular surface of the radius and
      b. Articular disc of inferior radio-ulnar joint.
   B. Distally :
      a. Scaphoid, lunate, triquetral bone and
      b. Interosseous ligament.

2. **Classification :**
   A. Structural : Compound, biaxial, ellipsoid, type of synovial joint.
   B. Functional : Diarthrosis.

3. **Ligaments :**
   A. Capsule :
      a. Attachments : It is attached close to the peripheral margin of proximal and distal articular surfaces of bones including articular disc.
         Head of ulna is excluded.
      b. Variation of thickness : It is thin anteriorly and posteriorly
                                   thick laterally and medially.
      c. It blends with the palmar and dorsal radio carpal ligaments.
   B. Radial collateral ligament : It is thickening of lateral part of capsule and extends from styloid process of radius to the scaphoid and trapezium.
   C. Ulnar collateral ligament : It extends from styloid process of ulna to the triquetral and pisiform bone.

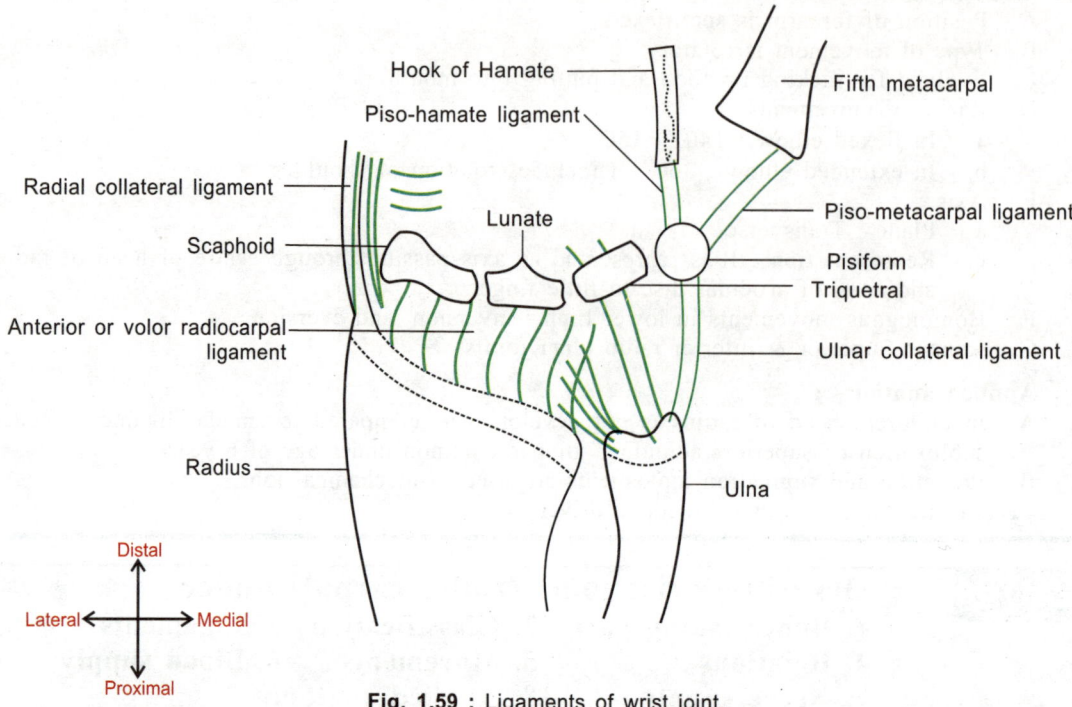

Fig. 1.59 : Ligaments of wrist joint.

4. **Relations :**
   A. In front : The tendons are arranged in three groups (from lateral to medial), they are
      a. Superficial :
         I.   Flexor carpi radialis,
         II. Palmaris longus and
         III. Flexor carpi ulnaris.
      b. Intermediate :
         I.   Radial artery,
         II. Median nerve,
         III. Flexor digitorum superficialis 🔑 **MR.**
              (tendons of middle and ring fingers are arranged superficially and tendons of
              index and little fingers are arranged deeply).
      c. Deep : Flexor pollicis longus, anterior interosseous vessels and nerve, flexor
         digitorum profundus.
   B. Behind : Beneath extensor retinaculum there are six osseofibrous compartments.
      These are arranged from lateral to medial as
      a. Abductor pollicis longus, extensor pollicis brevis,
      b. Extensor carpi radialis longus, extensor carpi radialis brevis,
      c. Extensor pollicis longus, tubercle of Lister,
      d. Extensor digitorum and extensor indicis,
      e. Extensor digiti minimi and
      f. Extensor carpi ulnaris.

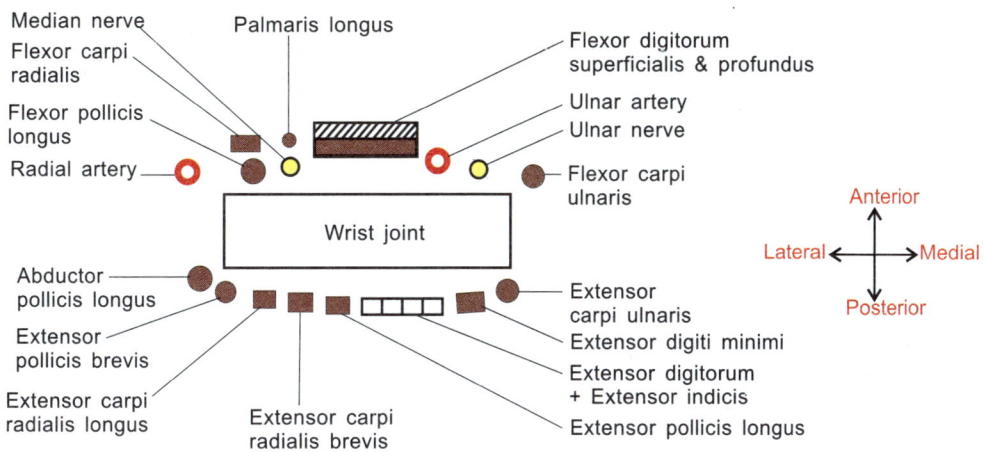

Fig. 1.60 : Relations of wrist joint.

5. **Movements :**

   A. Movements of wrist joint are associated with movements of midcarpal joint because they are produced by same group of muscle.

   B. Combination of wrist and midcarpal joint is called as link joint.

   Joint   Movements   🔑 READ

   a. Radiocarpal : Extension & Adduction.

   b. Midcarpal : Flexion and abduction.

Table 1.27 : The table showing muscles bringing different movements.

Movements	Range of move- ments	Main joint at which movements take place	Muscles bringing movements	Accessory muscles
A. Flexion	85°	Mid carpal	Flexor carpi radialis and flexor carpi ulnaris	Flexor digitorum superficialis, Flexor digitorum profundus, Flexor pollicis longus.
B. Extension	60°	Radiocarpal (wrist)	Extensor carpi radialis longus and brevis, Extensor carpi ulnaris	Extensor digitorum, Extensor indicis, Extensor pollicis longus, Extensor digiti minimi.
C. Abduction (Abduction is restricted than the adduction)	15°	Midcarpal	Abductor pollicis longus	Flexor carpi radialis, Extensor carpi radialis longus and brevis
D. Adduction	45°	Radio carpal	Flexor carpi ulnaris and Extensor carpi ulnaris	
E. Circumduction	Combination of flexion, extension, adduction and abduction			

6. **Blood supply :**
    A. Palmar carpal arch and
    B. Dorsal carpal arch which is derived from
        a.   Anterior interosseous artery.
        b.   Posterior interosseous artery.
        c.   Anterior carpal (branch of radial and ulnar arteries).
        d.   Posterior carpal (branch of radial and ulnar arteries).
        e.   Recurrent branches of deep palmar arch.

7. **Nerve supply :**
    A. Anterior interosseous nerve (branch of median nerve).
    B. Posterior interosseous nerve (branch of radial nerve).

8. **Applied anatomy :**
    A. Colles fracture (Dinner fork deformity)
        a.   It is due to fall on outstretched hand,
        b.   It involves distal end of radius,
        c.   Here fracture is transverse,
        d.   Force displaces the lower segment upwards and backwards and
        e.   Distal articular surface is inclined posteriorly.

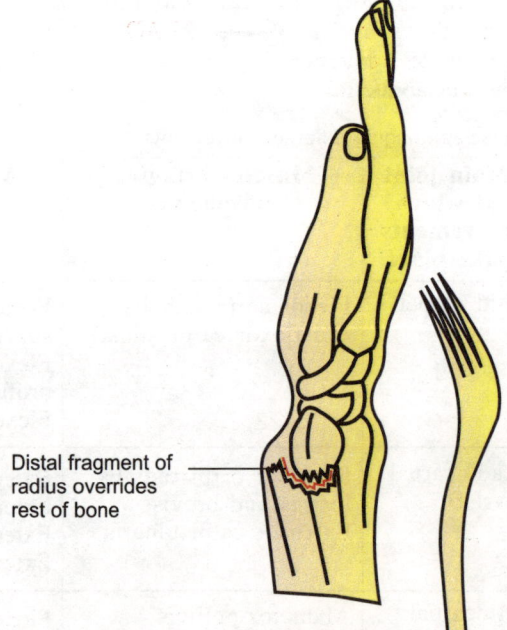

Distal fragment of
radius overrides
rest of bone

Fig. 1.61 : Colles fracture of distal radius.

B. Smiths fracture; it is reverse of Colles fracture :
    a.   It is produced by fall on the back of hand.
    b.   Here distal fragment is displaced forward and upward.

SN-28   First carpo metacarpal joint

1. **Classification :**
   A. Structurally : Biaxial, saddle variety of synovial joint.
   B. Functionally : Diarthrosis.

2. **Articular surfaces :**
   A. Distal surface of trapezium.
   B. Proximal surface of base of first metacarpal.

3. **Ligament :**
   A. Capsular ligament : Surrounds the joint. It is thickest, dorsally and laterally.
   B. Lateral ligament : Broad band, which thickens capsule.
   C. Anterior ligament.
   D. Posterior ligament.

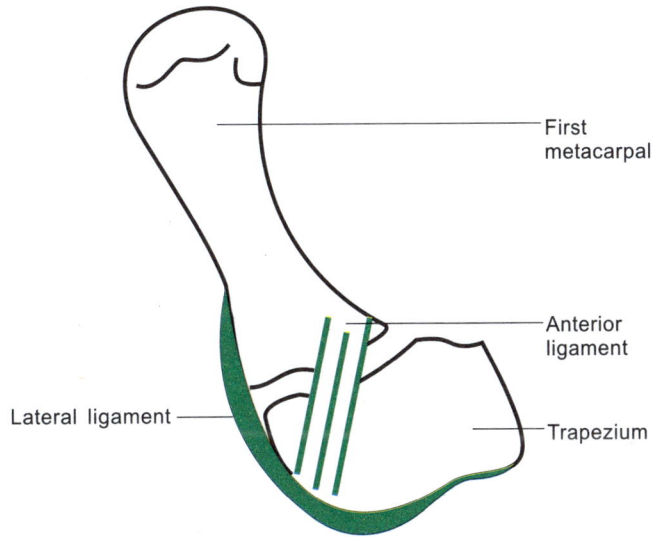

First
metacarpal

Anterior
ligament

Lateral ligament

Trapezium

Fig. 1.62 : Carpo-metacarpal joint of thumb.

4. **Relations :**
   A. Anterior : Muscles of thenar eminence.
   B. Dorsally : Long and short extensor of thumb.
   C. Medially : First dorsal interossei muscle.
   D. Laterally : Abductor pollicis longus.

5. **Nerve supply :** Median Nerve.

6. **Movements :** Flexion and extension are parallel to the plane of palm. Abduction and adduction movements are perpendicular to the plane of palm. Opposition is adduction with medial rotation.
   A. Flexion : Flexor pollicis brevis.
   B. Extension : Abductor pollicis longus. Extensor pollicis brevis.
   C. Abduction : Abductor pollicis brevis. Abductor pollicis longus.
   D. Adduction : Adductor pollicis.
   E. Opposition : Opponens pollicis.

First carpo-metacarpal joint

A. Classification
   A. Structurally : Biaxial, synovial joint of saddle variety.
   B. Functionally : Diarthrosis.

B. Articular surfaces
   A. Distal : trapezium (greater multangular).
   B. Proximal : saddle of base of first metacarpal.

C. Bonds
   A. Capsular ligament : surrounds the joint. Inner surface lined by synovial membrane.
   B. Lateral ligament.
   C. Anterior ligament.
   D. Posterior ligament.

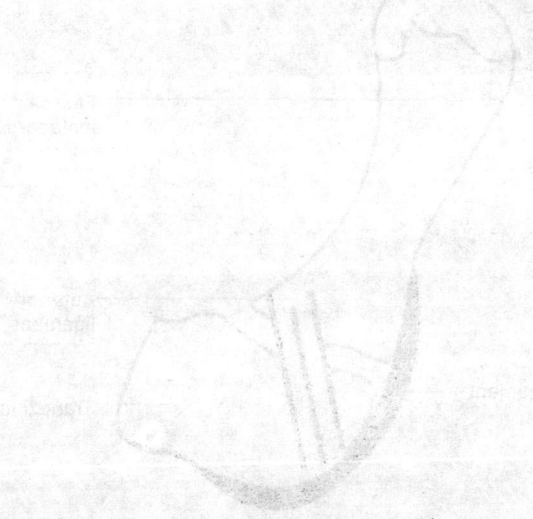

Fig. 4.32 : Carpo-metacarpal joint of thumb

D. Movements
   A. Flexion : flexor pollicis longus, flexor pollicis brevis.
   B. Extension : extensor pollicis longus, extensor pollicis brevis.
   C. Abduction : abductor pollicis longus, abductor pollicis brevis.
   D. Adduction : adductor pollicis.
   E. Opposition : opponens pollicis.

E. Nerve supply : Median nerve.

F. Movements : Flexion and extension are possible in the plane of palm. Abduction and adduction movements are perpendicular to plane of palm. Opposition is adduction with medial rotation.

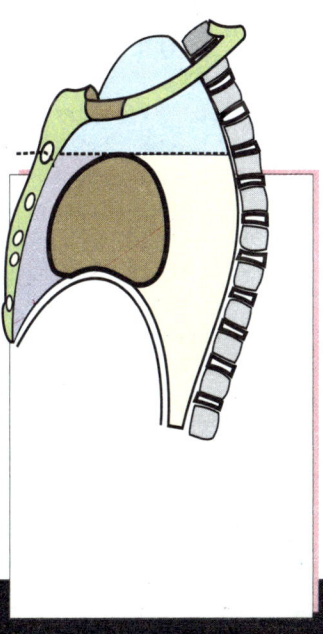

Index

SN-1   Angle of Louis / Sternal angle

1. **Introduction :** It is a bony angulation formed at the junction of manubrium and body of sternum.

2. **Situation :** It is situated five centimeters below the suprasternal notch.

3. **Events :**
   A. A plane which separates the superior and inferior mediastinum. It passes through angle of Louis to the intervertebral disc between fourth and fifth thoracic vertebra.
   B. Formation of cardiac plexus.
   C. Upper limit of the base of heart.
   D. Ascending aorta ends and arch of aorta begins.
   E. Arch of the aorta ends and descending aorta begins.
   F. Pulmonary trunk divides into two pulmonary arteries.
   G. Trachea divides into two principle bronchi.
   H. Azygos vein opens into superior vena cava.
   I. Thoracic duct crosses from right to left.

4. **Applied :** It is an important land mark for counting the ribs.

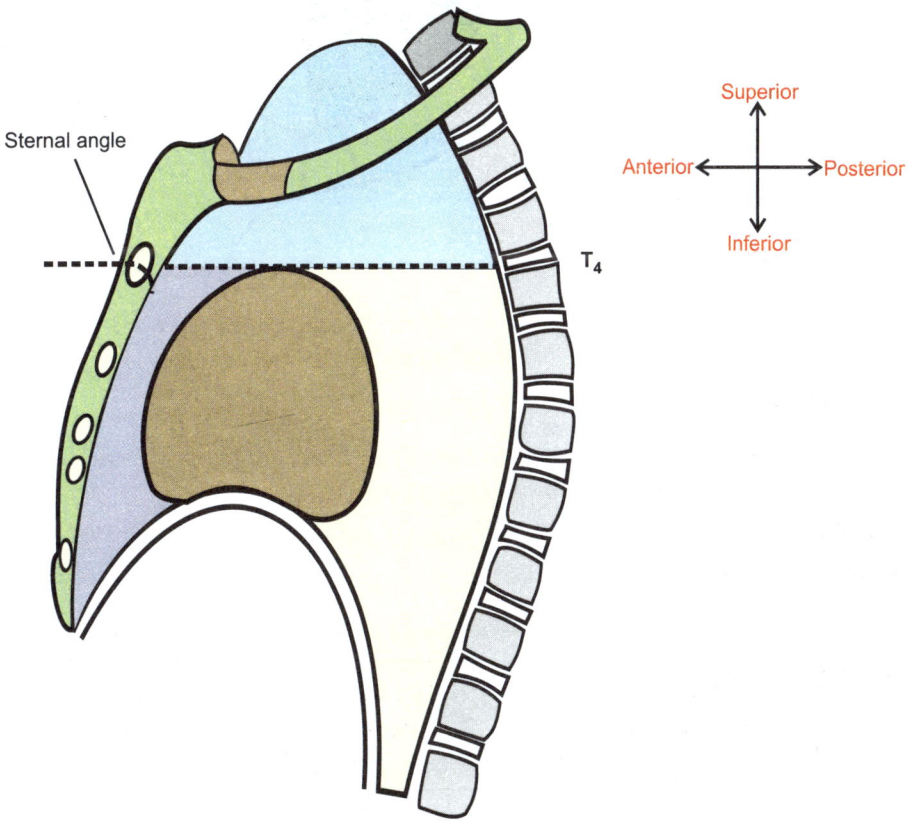

Fig. 2.1 : Angle of Louis / Sternal angle.

SN-2   Supra pleural membrane (Sibson's fascia)

1. **Fascia :** It is the dome shaped musculo facial membrane which roofs thoracic cavity.

2. **Formation :** It has
   A. Muscular part : It is formed occasionally by scalenus minimus muscle.
   B. Fascial part : It is formed from endothoracic fascia.

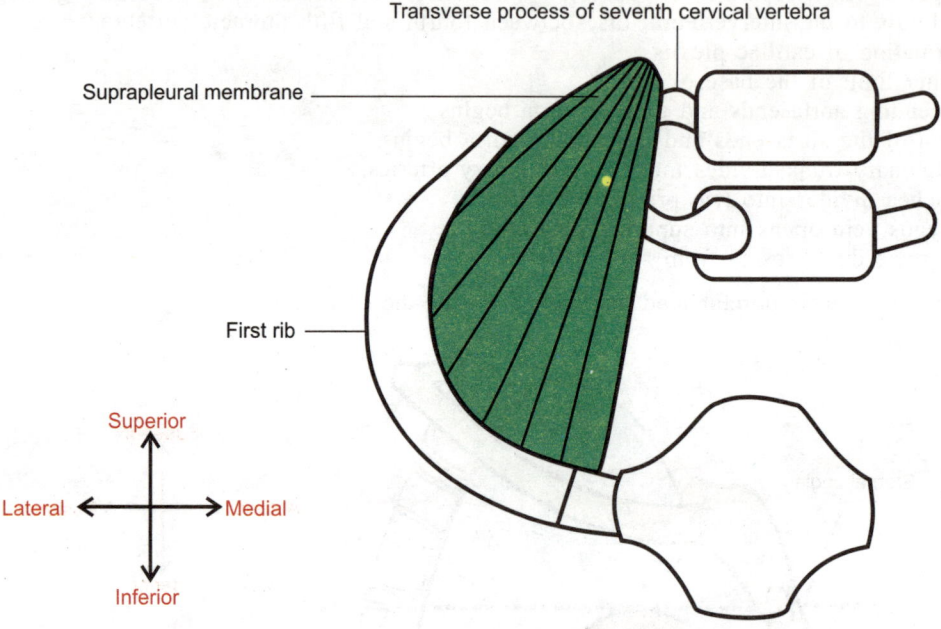

Transverse process of seventh cervical vertebra

Suprapleural membrane

First rib

Superior
Lateral ←→ Medial
Inferior

Fig. 2.2 : The suprapleural membrane.

3. **Attachments :**
   A. Anteriorly : Inner border of first rib.
   B. Posteriorly : Tip of the transverse process of seventh cervical vertebra.
   C. Medially : Continuous with the pretracheal fascia.

4. **Functions :** Protects the apex of the lung and cervical pleura during respiratory movements.

5. **Applied anatomy :** Herniation of cervical pleura is a result of rupture of supra pleural membrane.

LAQ-1   Describe intercostal space under following heads
1. Introduction   2. Intercostal muscles   3. Blood supply
4. Nerve supply & 5. Applied anatomy.

1. **Introduction :** It is the space between the two consecutive typical ribs on the same side.

2. Intercostal muscle :

Table 2.1 : The table shows origin, insertion and actions of intercostal muscles.

Muscle	Origin	Insertion	Actions
A. External intercostal	Lower border of the upper rib	Outer lip of the upper border of the rib below	Elevates 2nd to 12th ribs
B. Internal intercostal	Floor of the costal groove of the upper rib	Inner lip of the upper border of the rib below	
C. Transverse thoracis a. Subcostalis	Inner surface of the rib near the angle	Inner surface of the 2nd or 3rd rib below.	Depresses 2nd to 6th ribs
b. Intercostalis intimi	Inner surface of the upper rib	Inner surface of the rib below	
c. Sternocostalis	I. Lower $1/3^{rd}$ of the posterior surface of the body of the sternum. II. Posterior surface of the xiphoid process. III. Posterior surface of the costal cartilages of the lower 3 or 4 true ribs near the sternum.	Costal cartilages of the 2nd to 6th ribs.	

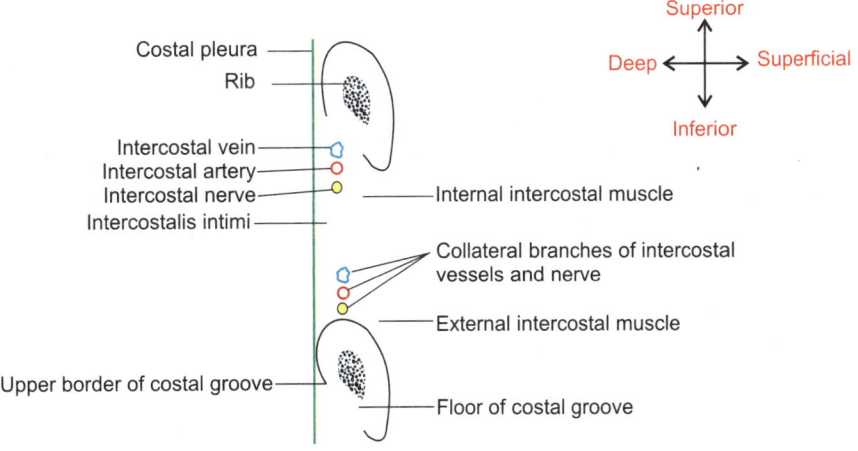

Fig. 2.3 : Longitudinal section through an intercostal space.

3. **Blood supply :**
   A. Arterial supply : The arteries in each intercostal space are arranged in two groups
      a. Anterior intercostal arteries : They are present in all spaces except the last two intercostal spaces. In each space there are two anterior intercostal arteries. One follows the lower margin of the upper rib and the other follows the upper margin of the lower rib.

      In the upper six spaces, the anterior intercostal arteries are the branches of the internal thoracic arteries.

      In the succeeding three spaces these are derived from musculophrenic arteries.

      b. Posterior intercostal artery : There is a posterior intercostal artery in each space. First and second posterior intercostal arteries are the branches of superior intercostal artery which is a branch of costo cervical trunk, a branch of subclavian artery.

      In the lower nine spaces the posterior intercostal arteries are the branches of descending thoracic aorta.

   B. Venous drainage : Each intercostal space is drained by anterior and posterior intercostal vein.
      a. Anterior intercostal veins : There are two anterior intercostal veins in each of the upper nine spaces.

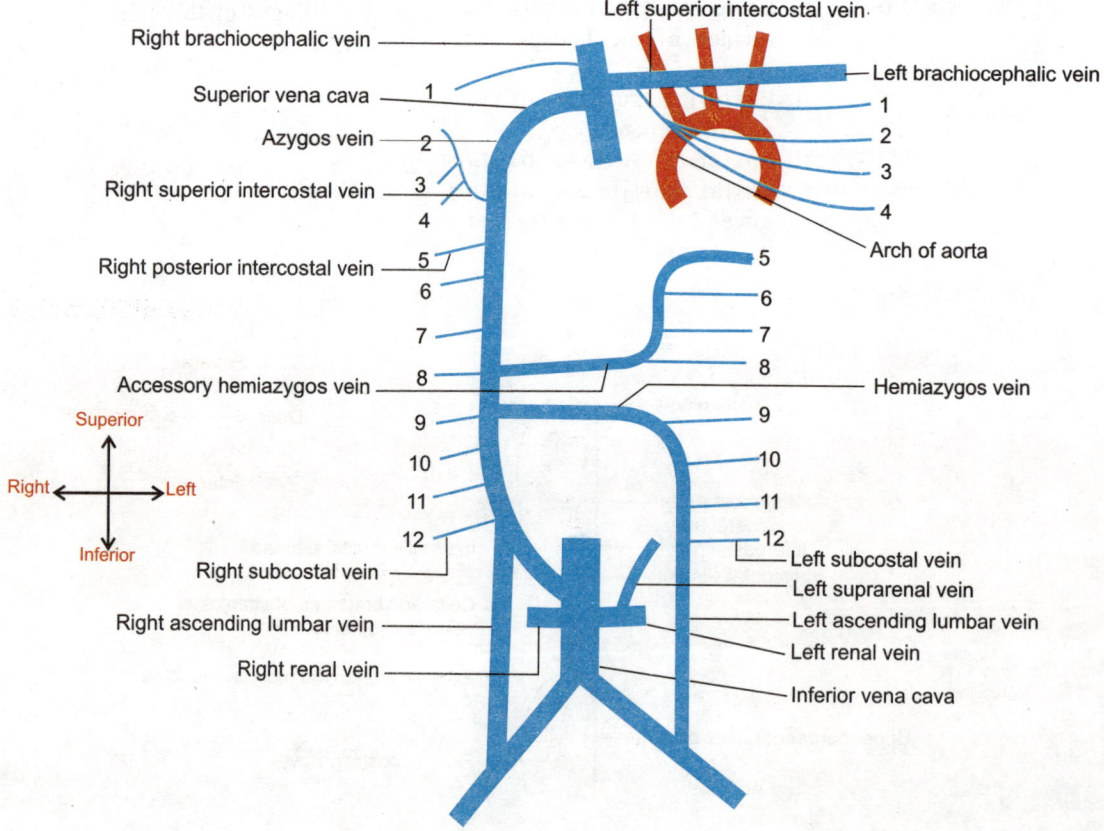

Fig. 2.4 : Venous drainage of posterior intercostal space.

      I.   Upper six intercostal veins drain into internal thoracic vein which drains into subclavian vein.

     II.   Lower six intercostal veins drain into musculophrenic vein.

    b.   Posterior intercostal veins :

Table 2.2 : The table showing venous drainage of intercostal space.

Veins	On right side they drain into	On left side they drain into
1st intercostal vein	Right brachiocephalic or Vertebral vein	Left brachiocephalic vein
2nd, 3rd & 4th intercostal vein	Join to form right 4th superior intercostal vein which drains into the azygos vein	Join to form left superior intercostal vein which drains into the left brachiocephalic vein
5th to 8th intercostal vein	Azygos vein	Accessory hemiazygos vein
9th to 11th and subcostal	Azygos vein	Hemiazygos vein

4. **Nerve Supply :** The intercostal muscles are supplied by intercostal nerves. They are anterior primary rami of spinal nerves T_1 to T_{11}. The anterior primary ramus of the 12th thoracic nerve forms the subcostal nerve. T_4, T_5 and T_6 supply only thoracic wall hence they are called typical intercostal nerves.

5. **Applied anatomy :**
    A.   Irritation of the intercostal nerve causes severe pain and is referred to the front of the chest or the abdomen. This is known as a root pain or girdle pain.
    B.   During tapping of the pleural effusion, the needle is inserted to the lower part of the intercostal space at the upper border of the rib to avoid injury to the intercostal nerve and vessels.
    C.   'Paracentesis thoracis' is usually done in the mid-axillary line because the level of pleural fluid is highest in the mid-axillary line.
    D.   'Paracentesis thoracis' is done in the lower part of the intercostal space to avoid the injury to the neurovascular bundle.
    E.   The tapping of pleural fluid should never be done medial to the angles of the ribs because the posterior intercostal arteries cross intercostal space obliquely from below upwards.
    F.   The pus from the vertebral column tends to track along the course of the neurovascular bundle and may point out any one of the three exit points.

SN-3   Azygos vein

1. **Meaning :** The word "azygos" means unpaired.

2. **Introduction :** It drains the thoracic wall and upper lumbar region. It is a link between superior and inferior vena cava.

3. **Situation :** It is situated in the posterior abdominal wall and posterior mediastinum.

4. **Formation :** It is formed by the union of
    A. The lumbar azygos vein,

    B.   Right subcostal vein and

    C.   Right ascending lumbar vein.

5.   **Course :**

    A.   It enters the thorax by passing through the right crus of diaphragm or by passing through the aortic opening of the diaphragm along with the abdominal aorta and thoracic duct. The abdominal aorta is on the left side and thoracic duct is on the right side of azygos vein.

    B.   It ascends up to the fourth thoracic vertebra, where it arches forward over the root of right lung.

6.   **Relations :**

    A.   Anteriorly : Oesophagus.

    B.   Posteriorly :

        I.   Lower eight thoracic vertebrae and

        II. Right posterior intercostal arteries.

    C.   To the right :

        I.   Right lung and pleura,

        II. Greater splanchnic nerve.

    D.   To the left :

        I.   Thoracic duct and aorta in the lower part,

        II. Oesophagus, trachea and right vagus in the upper part.

7.   **Tributaries :**

    A.   Right superior intercostal vein, formed by union of the 2nd and 3rd posterior intercostal vein (occasionally 4th posterior intercostal vein).

    B. 4th to 11th right posterior intercostal veins.

    C.   Hemiazygos vein (at the level of vertebra T_7 or T_8)

    D.   Accessory hemiazygos vein (at the level of vertebra T_8 or T_9)

    E.   Right bronchial vein, near the termination of the azygos vein.

    F.   Several oesophageal, mediastinal and pericardial veins.

    G.   The common trunk of azygos vein is formed by the union of the right ascending lumbar vein and the right subcostal vein.

8.   **Applied anatomy :** In obstruction of the superior or the inferior vena cava, the azygos vein acts as an important channel to establish collateral circulation.

SN-4   Typical spinal nerve

Each typical spinal nerve is formed by dorsal and ventral roots. Each spinal nerve divides into ventral and dorsal ramus.

Dorsal ramus goes posteriorly and divides into medial and lateral branch.

1.   The medial and lateral branches give muscular branches which supply muscles of the back and neck.

2.   Lateral branch of the dorsal ramus in the lower half and medial branch of the dorsal ramus in the upper half is cutaneous.   ⚷ L for L, L = lateral and lower

3.   Ventral rami in cervical, lumbar and sacral region unites together to form plexus.

SN-5 Typical intercostal nerve

1. **Introduction :** Anterior primary rami of 3rd to 6th thoracic spinal nerves are called typical intercostal nerves. They are confined only to thoracic wall.

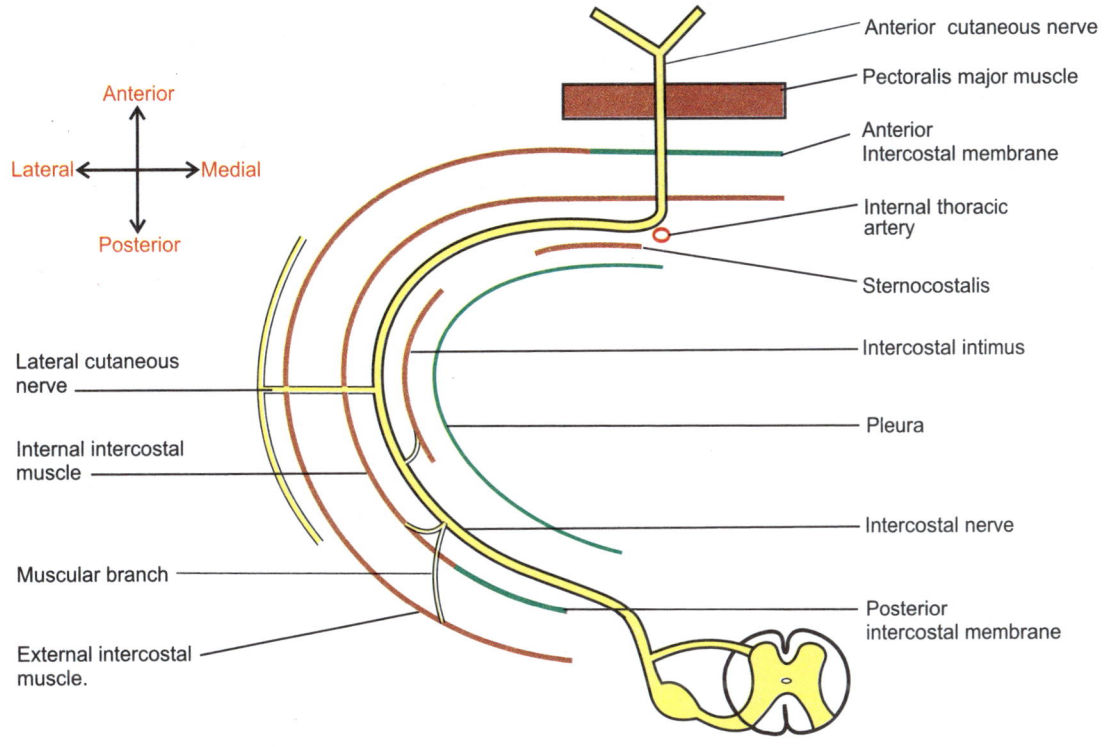

Fig. 2.5 : Course of typical inter-costal nerve.

2. **Course of typical intercostal nerve :**
   A. It emerges from the respective intervertebral foramen and passes between posterior intercostal membrane and the pleura. In major part of the space, the nerve lies between intercostalis intimi and the internal intercostal muscle.
   B. At the anterior edge of intercostalis intimus, it runs medially on the pleura and crosses in front of internal mammary artery.
   C. It turns forward and pierces the anterior intercostal membrane.
3. **Branches :** Each intercostal nerve gives
   A. Lateral cutaneous branch which appears at mid-axillary line and divides into anterior and posterior branches and
   B. Anterior intercostal nerve which comes anteriorly and crosses the sternum in front of the internal thoracic vessel and the sternocostalis muscle. It pierces
      a. Internal intercostal muscle,
      b. Anterior intercostal membrane,
      c. Pectoralis major muscle to supply the skin.

LAQ-2 — Describe parietal pleura under
1. Subdivisions of the pleura & 2. Applied anatomy.

1. **Subdivisions of the pleura :** Depending upon the structure it lines, it is called costal, diaphragmatic, cervical and mediastinal.

    A. Costal pleura : It lines the inner surface of the sternum, costal cartilage, ribs, intercostal spaces and sides of vertebral bodies but the costal layer is separated by endothoracic fascia.

    Tracing :

    a. It can be traced from back of the sternum - mediastinal pleura - sternoclavicular joint middle of the sternal angle - vertically upto the 4th costal cartilage.

        I. On the right side : It reflects vertically behind the xiphisternal joint - right costoxiphoid angle - 7th costal cartilage - costodiaphragmatic line of pleura.

        II. On the left side : It descends close to sternum - and deviates laterally from the sternum to 4th costal cartilage - costodiaphragmatic line.

    b. Behind : It continues with mediastinal pleura by the side of vertebral column along a line known as the costo vertebral reflection.

    c. Above : It continues as cervical pleura along the inner border of first rib.

    d. Below : It continues as the diaphragmatic pleura.

    B. Diaphragmatic pleura : It covers the thoracic surface of the corresponding part of diaphragm and laterally it continues as the costal pleura. It continues medially as mediastinal pleura.

    C. Cervical pleura : It extends from the inner border of first rib to the apex of the lung. It continues medially with mediastinal pleura. The summit of the cervical pleura is 3 to 4 cms above first costal cartilage. It does not extend above upper border of neck of first rib.

    D. Mediastinal pleura : It forms the lateral boundary of the mediastinum and is divided into three parts,

    a. Above the root of the lung : It extends from the sternum to vertebral column.

    b. At the root of the lung : The mediastinal pleura passes laterally in the form of a tube enclosing the structures of the root of lung and continues with pulmonary pleura.

    c. Below the root of the lung : The mediastinal pleura forms a bilaminar fold known as pulmonary ligament which extends from

        I. Oesophagus to corresponding lung below its hilum. At the hilum, the two layers are continuous with pulmonary pleura.

        II. Contents of pulmonary ligament : No important structures pass except

            i. Loose areolar tissue,

            ii. Lymphatics and

            iii. Sometimes accessory bronchial artery.

2. **Applied Anatomy :**

    A. Pleuritis : Inflammation of pleurae is known as pleurisy or pleuritis. It may be dry or wet pleurisy.

    B. Paracentesis : It is the tapping of the fluid from the pleural cavity. It is performed posterior to mid - axillary line.

    C. Pneumothorax : Presence of the air in the pleural cavity is called pneumothorax.

SN-6   Mediastinal surfaces of the right and left lung

1. Right side (venous)

A. Right atrium and auricle.
B. A small part of the right ventricle.
C. Superior vena cava.
D. Lower part of the right brachiocephalic vein.
E. Azygos vein.
F. Oesophagus.
G. Inferior vena cava.
H. Trachea.
I. Right vagus nerve.
J. Right phrenic nerve.

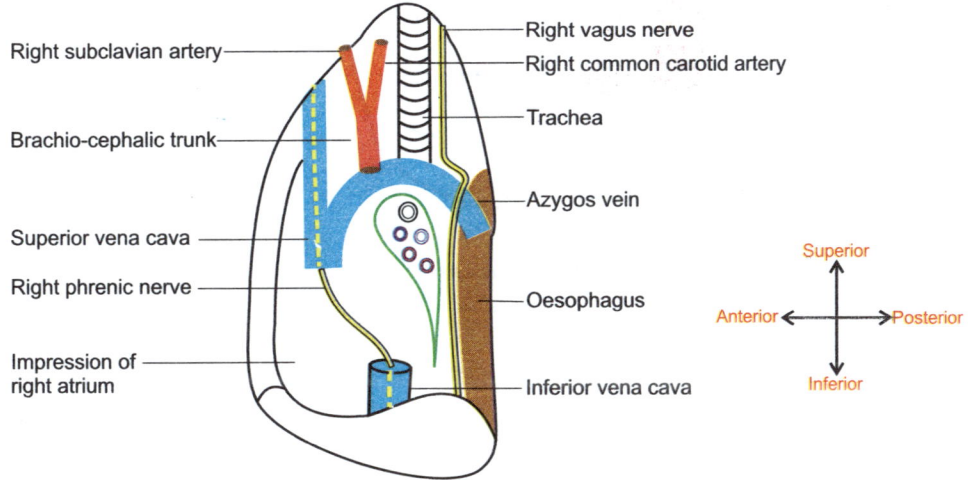

Fig. 2.6 : Mediastinal surface of right lung.

2. Left side (arterial)

A. Left ventricle and left auricle.
B. Infundibulum and adjoining part of the right ventricle.
C. Pulmonary trunk.
D. Arch of aorta.
E. Descending thoracic aorta.
F. Left subclavian artery.
G. Thoracic duct.
H. Oesophagus.
I. Left brachiocephalic vein.
J. Left vagus nerve.
K. Left phrenic nerve.
L. Left recurrent laryngeal nerve.

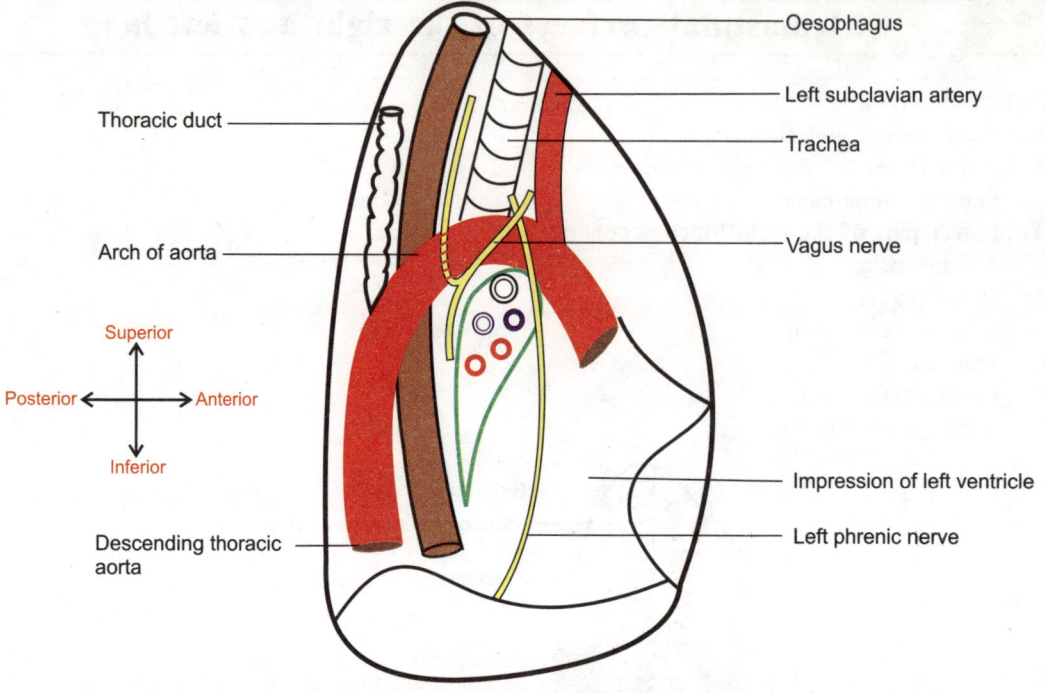

Fig. 2.7 : Mediastinal surface of left lung.

| SN-7 | **Draw and label structure of the roots of the right and left lung.** |

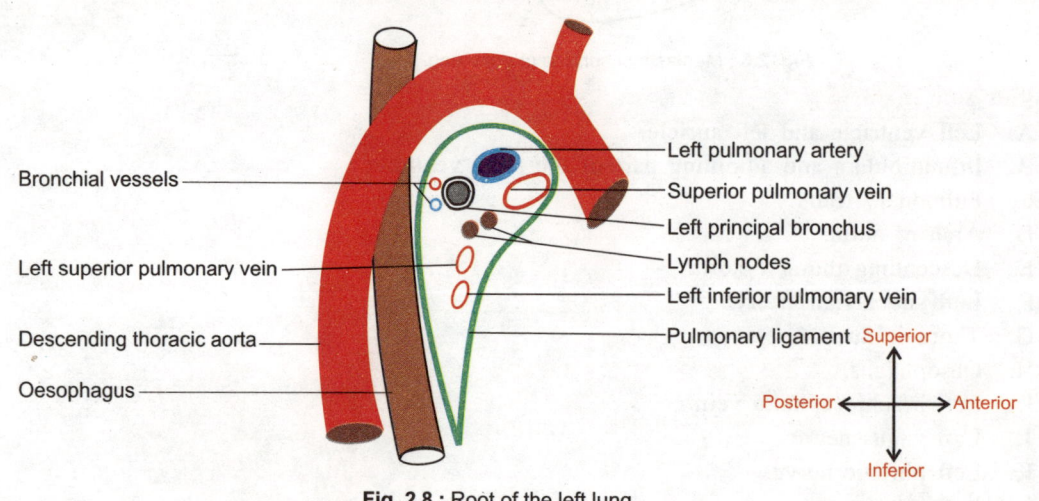

Fig. 2.8 : Root of the left lung.

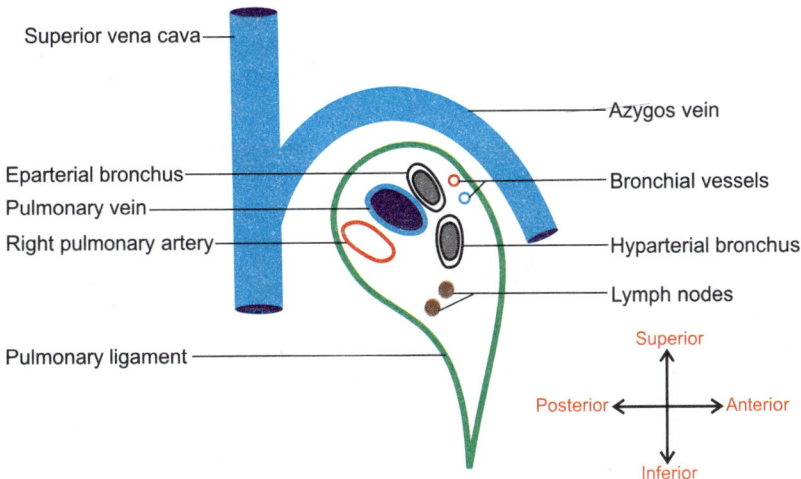

Fig. 2.9 : Root of the right lung.

| SN-8 | Azygos lobe (*A* not; *zygos* paired) |

1. **Types :** Accessory or supernumerary lobes of lungs are called as azygos lobe. They are of three types
   A. Upper azygos lobe.
   B. Lower azygos lobe.
   C. Lobe of azygos vein.
   The formal two types have little practical importance. And these are described in reference to hilum of the lung.
   The lobe of the azygos vein is present in 1% of population. It affects the upper lobe of the right lung, where the apex of the lung splits into medial and lateral parts of the fissure, the bottom of which contains the arch of the azygos vein suspended by a pleural septum, the meso-azygos. The medial part of the split apex forms the lobe of the azygos vein.

2. **Development :** It is because of the upward development of apical bronchus. It develops medial to the arch of azygos vein instead lateral to it.

3. **Applied anatomy :**
   A. The plane x-ray of the chest shows a small dense shadow close to the right sternal angle.
   B. It is one of the differential diagnosis of enlarged lymph node in the chest.

| SN-9 | Blood supply of lung |

1. **Arterial supply :**
   A. The nutrition of the lungs is by bronchial arteries.
      a. These are small arteries varying in origin, size and number.

    b.   On the right side there is one bronchial artery which is a branch of third posterior intercostal artery or from the upper left bronchial artery.

    c.   On the left side there are two bronchial arteries which arise from descending thoracic aorta.

B.   De-oxygenated blood to the lungs is brought by the pulmonary arteries.

C.   Oxygenated blood is returned to the heart by pulmonary veins.

2. Venous drainage :

A.   Bronchial veins drain the lungs. They are usually two in number on each side. The right bronchial veins drain into the azygos vein. The left bronchial vein either drain into left superior intercostal vein or azygos vein.

B.   The greater part of the blood from the lung is drained by the pulmonary veins.

LAQ-3   Draw and describe bronchopulmonary segment under
1. Definition   2. Gross anatomy
3. Lymphatic drainage   &   4. Applied anatomy.

1. Definition : It is the independent respiratory, surgical segment or unit of lung aerated by tertiary or segmental bronchus.

2. Gross anatomy :

A.   Shape : Pyramidal

    a.   Apex : Directed towards the root of lung

    b.   Base : Towards the surface of lung

B.   Segment : There are 10 segments in each lung. They are described in the following table.

Table 2.3 : The table shows bronchopulmonary segments of right and left lung.

Right lung		Left lung	
Ten		Ten	
Lobes	**Segment**	**Lobes**	**Segment**
a. Upper	1. Apical 2. Anterior 3. Posterior	a. Upper I. Upper division	1. ⎫ 2. ⎬ Apicoposterior 3. Anterior
b. Middle	4. Medial 5. Lateral	II. Lingular lobe	4. Superior 5. Inferior
c. Lower	6. Superior (Apical or dorsal) 7. Anterior basal 8. Posterior basal 9. Lateral basal 10. Medial basal	b. Lower	6. Apical (Superior) 7. ⎫ 8. ⎬ Anteromedial basal 9. Lateral basal 10. Posterior basal

C.   Intersegmental plane : It is the connective tissue septa between two adjacent lobes. It is continuous on the surface with pulmonary subpleural connective tissue.

D. Relations : 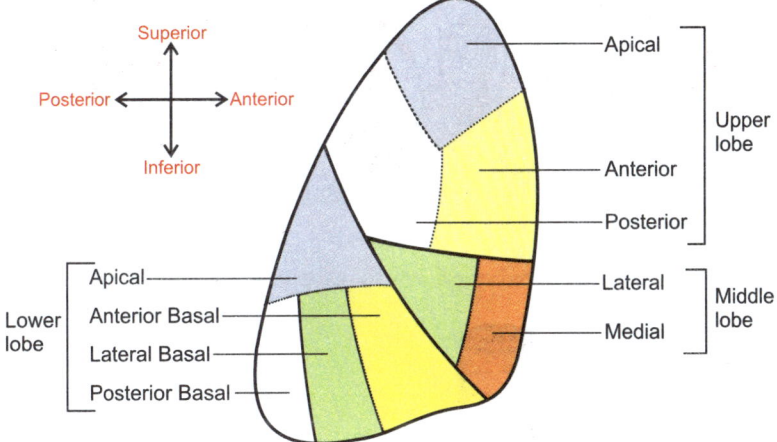 **PAD**
  a. <u>P</u>ulmonary <u>a</u>rteries lie <u>d</u>orsolateral to bronchus.
  b. Pulmonary veins do not accompany the bronchial or pulmonary arteries. Near the hilum of the lung, the pulmonary veins lie ventro medial to the bronchus.

3. **Lymphatic drainage :** There are two sets of lymphatics both of which drain into bronchopulmonary nodes
  A. Superficial lymphatics drain into peripheral lung tissue lying beneath the pulmonary pleura. The vessels pass round the borders of lung and margins of fissure to reach the hilum.
  B. Deep lymphatics drain into bronchial tree, the pulmonary vessels and the connective tissue septa. They run towards the hilum where they drain into bronchopulmonary nodes.

Fig. 2.10 : Bronchopulmonary segment of right lung.

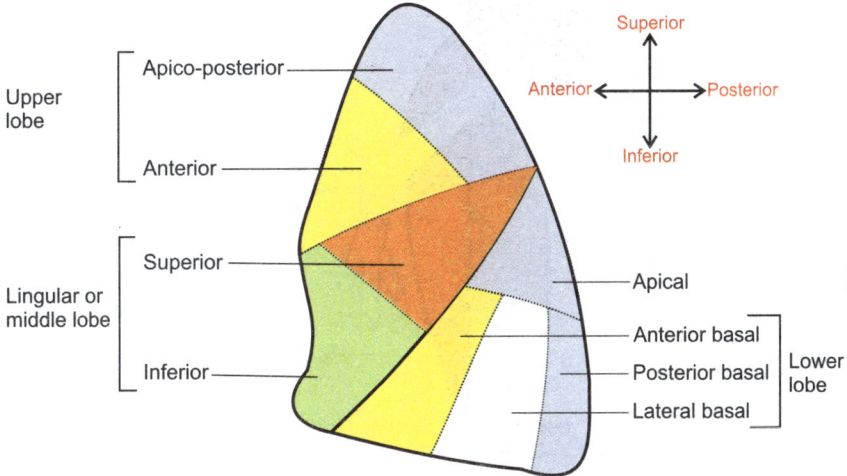

Fig. 2.11 : Bronchopulmonary segment of left lung.

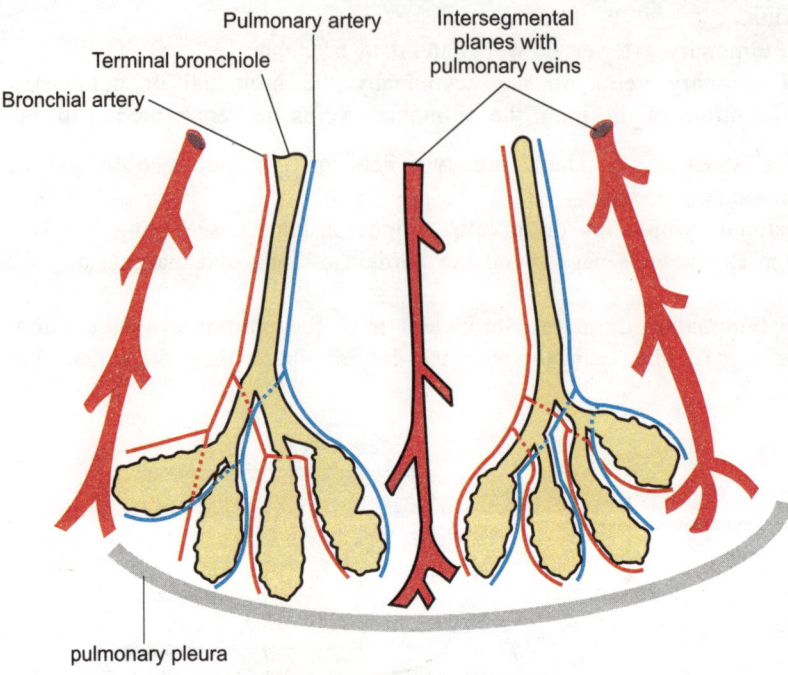

Fig. 2.12 : Relations of the bronchiole with the bronchial artery and pulmonary vessels.

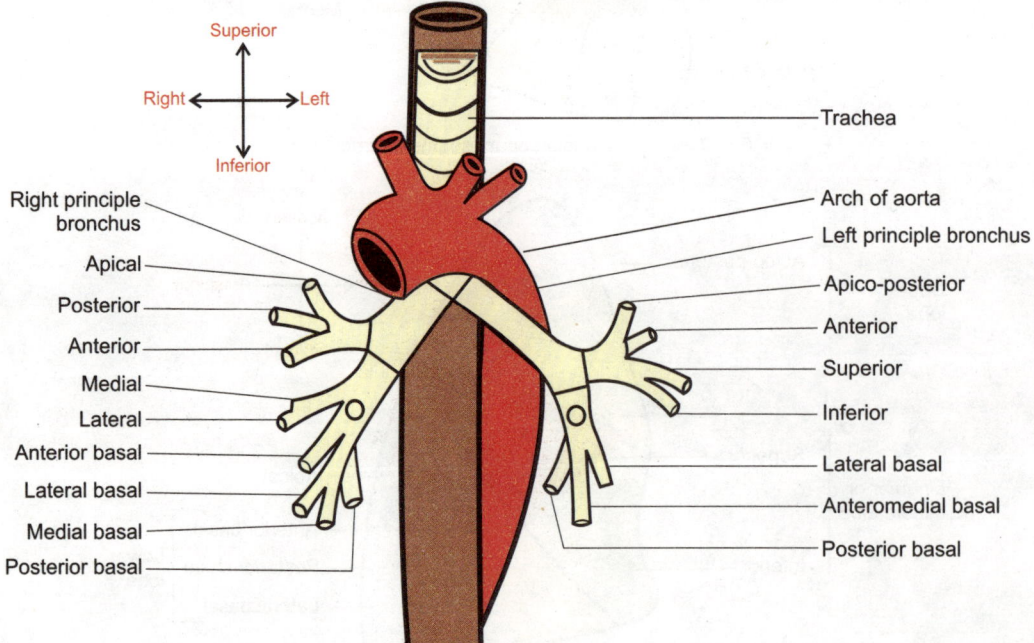

Fig. 2.13 : The bronchial tree.

4.   **Applied Anatomy :**
   A.   Bronchography : It is the study of bronchopulmonary segments radiologically by instillation of radiopaque dye. Study of bronchopulmonary segments helps to localize the affected segment of the lung and helps in postural drainage.
   B.   Lung abscess is more common in,

   PUL ALL   P = posterior, UL = upper   lobe
   A = apical   LL = lower lobe

   a.   **P**osterior segment of **u**pper **l**obe
   b.   **A**pical segment of **l**ower **l**obe
        (Mendelson's Syndrome - the aspiration pneumonia is common in posterior segment of upper lobe and apical segment of lower lobe. Because these segments are most dependent in recumbent position).
   c.   Each bronchopulmonary segment acts as an independent unit hence infection is restricted only to respective segment, except in tuberculosis.
   d.   The benign neoplasm is restricted to each segment. However malignant growths are not restricted to the respective segment.
   e.   Posterior segment of right upper lobe is frequent site for tuberculosis infection.
   f.   Anterior segment of upper lobe shows cancerous changes.

SN-10   Mediastinum (Partition)

1.   **Introduction :** Thoracic mediastinum is the space between right and left pleural sacs and limited on each side by mediastinal pleura.

2.   **Extent :** It extends vertically from thoracic inlet to diaphragm.

3.   **Division :** The mediastinum is divided by an imaginary horizontal plane extending from sternal angle to lower border of fourth thoracic vertebra.
   A.   Superior mediastinum and

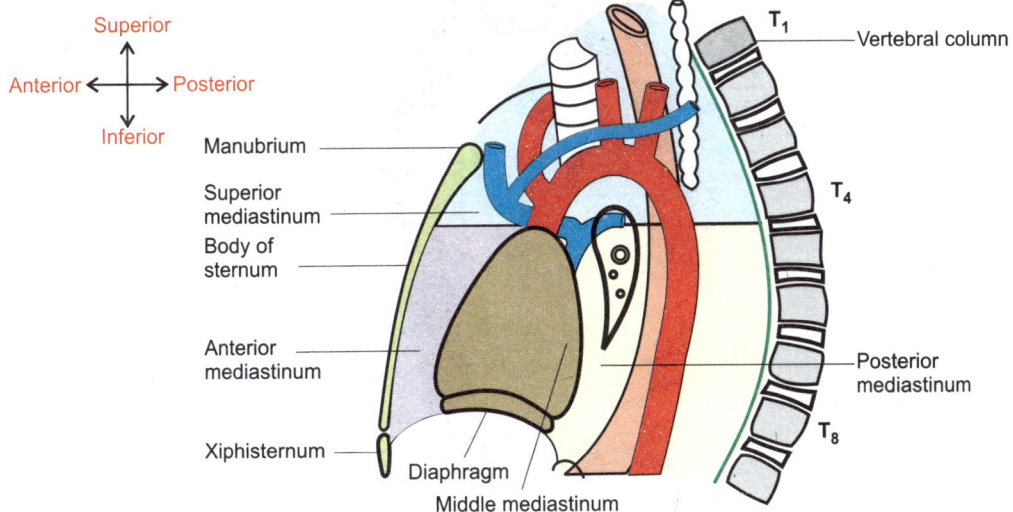

Fig. 2.14 : Subdivisions of the mediastinum.

B.   Inferior mediastinum : It is subdivided by pericardium and heart into
  a.   Anterior mediastinum,
  b.   Middle mediastinum and
  c.   Posterior mediastinum.
      Anterior mediastinum is narrowest; middle mediastinum is widest; while posterior mediastinum is longest.

4.   **Development :** It develops from primitive ventral and dorsal meso oesophagus.

SN-11   Superior mediastinum

1.   **Definition :** It is the area of the thoracic cavity above the imaginary plane extending from sternal angle to the lower border of body of the fourth thoracic vertebra.

2.   **Boundaries :**
  A.   Anteriorly : Manubrium sternum.
  B.   Posteriorly :
    a.   Upper four thoracic vertebrae,

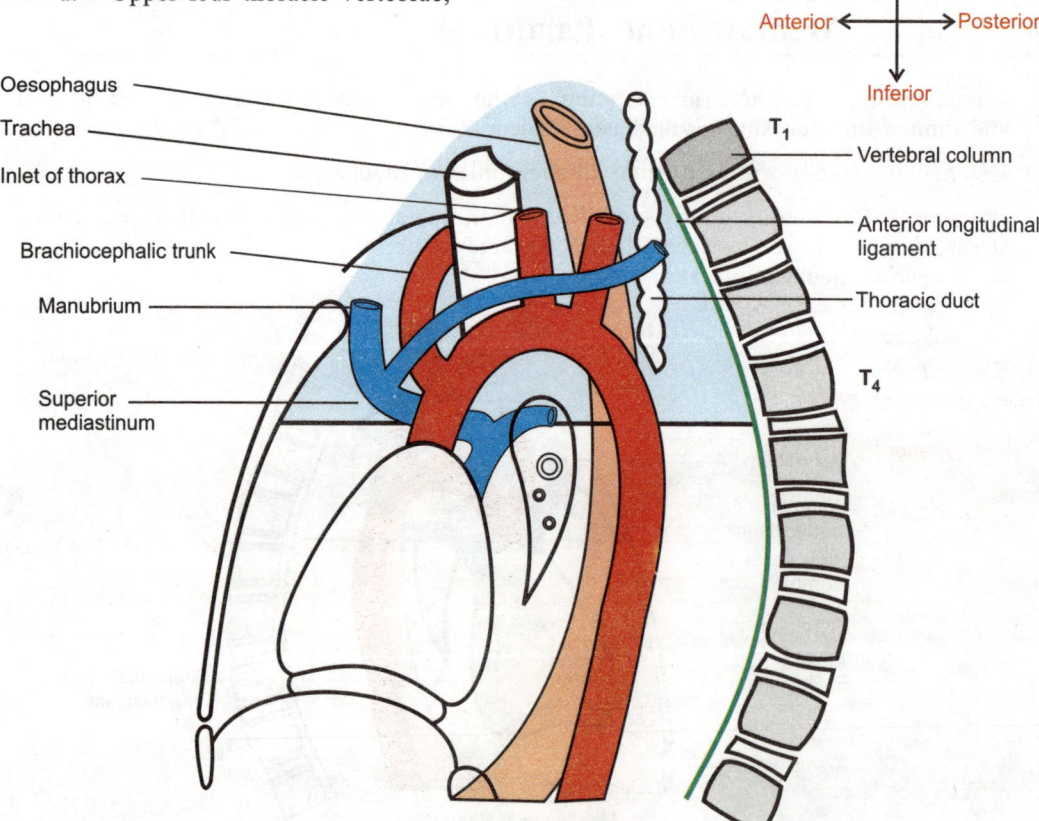

Fig. 2.15 : Superior mediastinum.

b. Intervertebral discs and

c. Anterior longitudinal ligament.

C. Above : Thoracic inlet

D. Below : Horizontal plane extending from sternal angle to lower border of fourth thoracic vertebra.

E. On each side : Mediastinal pleura.

3. **Contents :**

A. Retro sternal structures

a. Superior vena cava

b. Veins opening into superior vena cava

I. Right and left brachiocephalic vein

II. Left superior intercostal vein

c. Thymus gland

d. Muscles : Sterno thyroid, sterno hyoid

B. Intermediate structures (aorta)

a. Arch of aorta and its branches from right to left.

I. Brachiocephalic trunk.

II. Left common carotid.

III. Left subclavian.

b. Nerve :

I. Phrenic nerve,

II. Vagus nerve and

III. Cardiac plexus.

C. Prevertebral structures (Trachea and oesophagus)

a. Trachea,

b. Oesophagus,

c. Left recurrent laryngeal nerve,

d. Thoracic duct

e. Muscle - longus colli and

f. Paratracheal and tracheo bronchial lymph node.

4. **Applied :**

A. Abscess (caries of cervical vertebra) or bleeding behind prevertebral fascia enters superior mediastinum.

B. Obstruction to superior vena cava gives rise to engorgement of veins in the upper half of the body.

C. Pressure over trachea causes dyspnoea, and cough.

D. Pressure on the oesophagus causes dysphagia.

E. Pressure on the left recurrent laryngeal nerve gives rise to hoarseness of voice.

F. Pressure over sympathetic chain causes Horners syndrome.

Horner's syndrome : It is due to involvement of the sympathetic nerve, which is contributed by T_1 segment of the spinal cord. There is injury to the root of brachial plexus.

SN-12   Anterior mediastinum

1. **Introduction :** It is a potential space present in the anterior part of inferior mediastinum.

2. **Boundaries :**
   A. Superiorly : Imaginary line extending from sternal angle to lower border of fourth thoracic vertebra.
   B. Inferiorly : The diaphragm.
   C. Anteriorly : Posterior surface of body of sternum.
   D. Posteriorly : Fibrous pericardium.

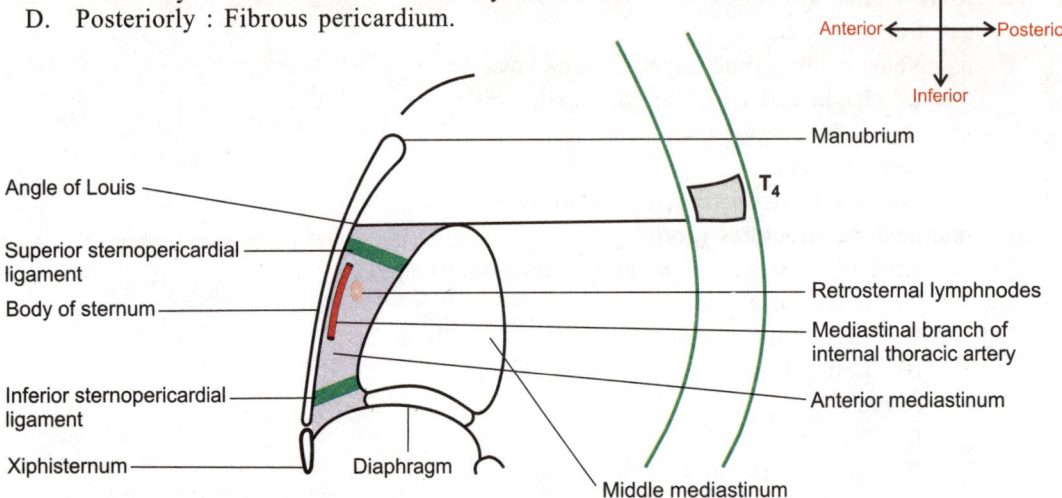

Fig. 2.16 : Boundaries and contents of anterior mediastinum.

3. **Contents :**
   A. Thymus gland is the principal content of the anterior mediastinum
   B. Mediastinal artery, branch of internal thoracic artery.
   C. Ligaments : Superior and inferior sterno pericardial.
   D. Retro-sternal lymph node.
   E. Loose areolar tissue.

4. **Applied anatomy :** Abscess or bleeding or growth in front of the pretracheal fascia of the superior mediastinum enters the anterior mediastinum.

SN-13   Middle mediastinum

1. **Introduction :** It is a widest of all the mediastinum and is occupied by the heart and the pericardium.

2. **Boundaries :**
   A. Superiorly : Horizontal plane from sternal angle to lower border of fourth thoracic vertebra.
   B. Inferiorly : By the diaphragm.
   C. Anterior :
   D. Posteriorly :   } By fibrous pericardium

3. **Contents :**
    A. Heart and the related structures
        a. Pericardium.
        b. Deep cardiac plexus.
        c. Structures entering pericardium
            I.   Four pulmonary veins and
            II. Arch of azygos vein.
        d. Structures leaving the pericardium
            I.   Ascending aorta and
            II. Pulmonary trunk.
    B. Trachea and related structures
        a. Right bronchus and
        b. Left bronchus.
        c. Inferior tracheobronchial lymph node.
    C. Other structures
        a. Phrenic nerve and
        b. Pericardiacophrenic vessels.

SN-14 Posterior mediastinum (longest)

1. **Introduction :** It is a longest part of the inferior mediastinum.

2. **Boundaries :**
    A. Superiorly : By the plane extending from sternal angle to lower border of fourth vertebra.
    B. Inferiorly : The diaphragm.
    C. Anteriorly : From above downward
        a. Bifurcation of trachea.
        b. Pulmonary vessels.
        c. Fibrous pericardium.
        d. Posterior surface of the diaphragm.
    D. Posteriorly :
        a. Bodies of lower eight thoracic vertebrae.
        b. Intervertebral discs and
        c. Anterior longitudinal ligament.
    E. On each side : Mediastinal pleura.

3. **Contents :**
    A. Longitudinal structures
        a. Vagus nerve
        b. Descending thoracic aorta
        c. Thoracic duct
        d. Azygos vein
        e. Posterior mediastinal lymph nodes
        f. Oesophagus
        g. Splanchnic nerve
    B. Transverse structures
        a. Superior and inferior hemiazygos vein.
        b. Posterior intercostal vein.
        c. Posterior intercostal artery.

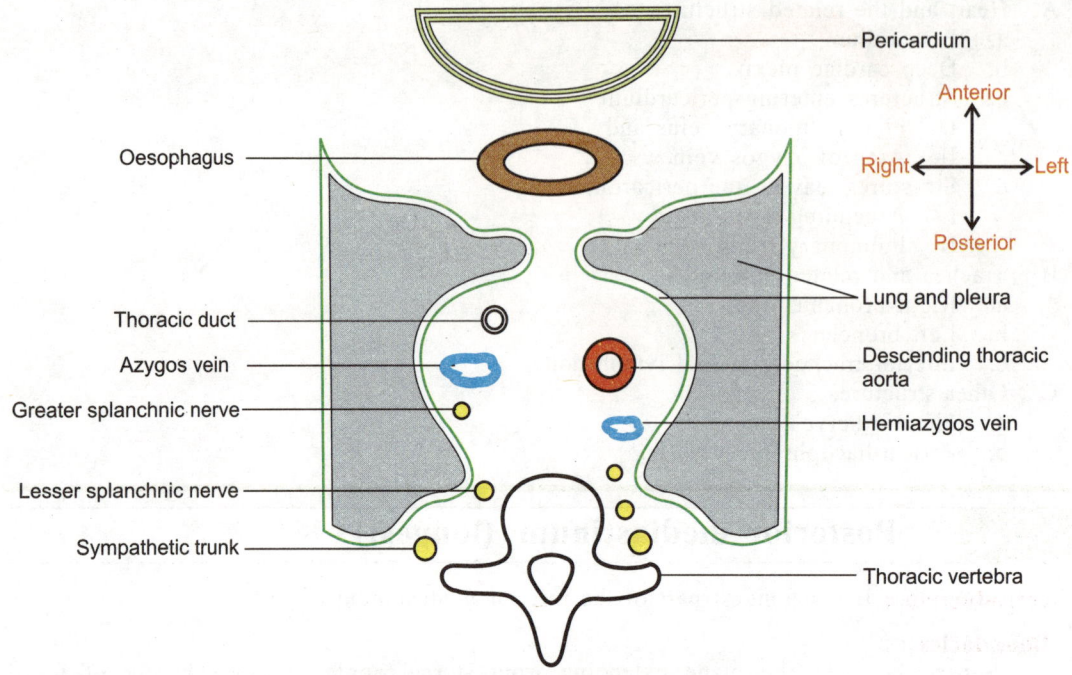

Fig. 2.17 : Posterior mediastinum.

4.   **Applied anatomy :** Abscess or bleeding between prevertebral and pretracheal fascia enters superior mediastinum and enters the posterior mediastinum.

LAQ-4	**Describe the fibrous pericardium under**

1. Gross anatomy   2. Relations   3. Blood supply
4. Nerve supply   5. Functions   6. Development

1.   Gross anatomy :
   A.   Synonymous : Outer layer of pericardium.
   B.   Introduction : It is a cone shaped open sac and has apex and base.
       a.   Apex : It merges with the tunica adventitia of (pulmonary trunk and ascending aorta) and pre tracheal layer of the deep cervical fascia.
       b.   Base : It fuses with the upper surface of central tendon and musculature of the left part of the diaphragm.
       c.   In front : It is attached to the upper and lower ends of the body of sternum by the superior and inferior sterno-pericardial ligaments respectively.
   C.   Structures piercing fibrous pericardium.
       a.   Ascending aorta,
       b.   Pulmonary trunk,
       c.   Two venae cavae and
       d.   Four pulmonary veins.

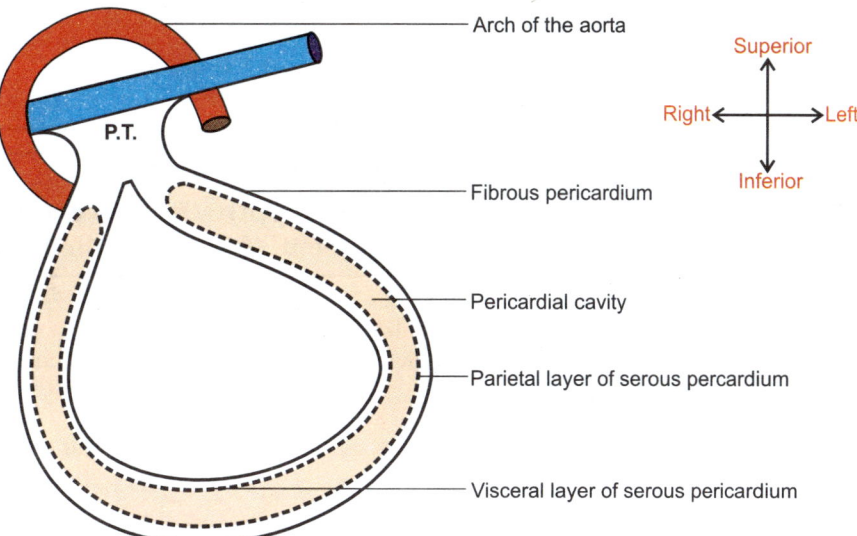

Fig. 2.18 : General arrangement of parietal and visceral layers of pericardium.

2. **Relations :**
    A. Anteriorly : Thoracic wall is separated by lung, pleura and occasionally by thymus.
    B. Posteriorly :
        a. Right and left bronchi
        b. Oesophagus
        c. Oesophageal plexus of nerves
        d. Descending thoracic aorta
        e. Thoracic duct
        f. Azygos vein
        g. Hemiazygos vein
        h. Posterior part of the mediastinal surface of both lungs.
    C. On each side :
        a. Cardiac impression of the corresponding lung
        b. Phrenic nerves
        c. Pericardiaco phrenic vessels.
    D. Below :
        a. Left lobe of the liver
        b. Fundus of the stomach.

3. **Blood supply :**
    A. Arterial supply
        a. Pericardiacophrenic artery (branch of internal thoracic artery)
        b. Musculophrenic artery (terminal branch of internal thoracic artery)
        c. Branches of descending thoracic aorta.
    B. Venous drainage :
        a. Azygos vein and
        b. Internal thoracic vein.

4. **Nerve supply :** Fibrous pericardium is pain sensitive and is supplied by phrenic nerve.

5. **Functions :**
   A. It keeps the heart in position.
   B. It prevents the over distention of the heart.

6. **Development :** It develops from septum transversum.

LAQ-5   **Describe the serous pericardium under**
         1. Gross anatomy   2. Blood supply   3. Nerve supply
         4. Functions   5. Development &   6. Applied anatomy.

1. **Gross anatomy :**
   A. Synonymous : Inner layer of pericardium.
   B. Introduction : It is a closed sac and lies within the fibrous pericardium. It consists of
      a. Visceral layer (epicardium) and
      b. Parietal layer.
   There is a potential sac present between fibrous and visceral layer. The maximum capacity of the sac is 300 ml.

2. **Blood supply :**
   A. Arterial supply : Coronary arteries branches of ascending aorta.
   B. Venous drainage : Coronary sinus.

3. **Nerve supply :** Cardiac plexus.

4. **Functions :**
   A. It allows the free movement of the heart within the fibrous pericardium.
   B. It keeps the surface moist and slippery.

5. **Development :**
   A. Parietal layer of the serous pericardium develops from somato pleuric layer of pericardial sac.
   B. Visceral layer of serous pericardium develops from splanchnopleuric layer of pericardial sac.

6. **Applied anatomy :**
   A. The accumulation of fluid in the pericardial sac is called pericardial effusion.
   B. Pericardial tamponade : Pericardial effusion compresses the heart and decreases the diastolic capacity of heart. This results in diminished cardiac output but increased pulse rate and increased venous pressure.
   C. Paracentesis : Aspiration of pericardial fluid is called paracentesis. It is done by
      a. Subcostal route and
      b. Parasternal route.

SN-15   **Transverse sinus** (Inter visceral space)

1. **Synonymous :** Inter visceral space.

2. **Introduction :** It is a horizontal gap present between arterial and venous ends of heart tube.
   A. Arterial end
      a. Ascending aorta and
      b. Pulmonary trunk.

    B. Venous end
      a. Superior vena cava,
      b. Inferior vena cava and
      c. Pulmonary vein.

3.   **Location :** It is present between two layers of serous pericardium and situated on the upper part of the posterior surface of the heart.

4.   **Boundaries :**
    A. Anteriorly :
      a. Ascending aorta and
      b. Pulmonary trunk
    B. Posteriorly :
      a. Superior vena cava,
      b. Upper margin of left atrium and
      c. Four pulmonary veins.

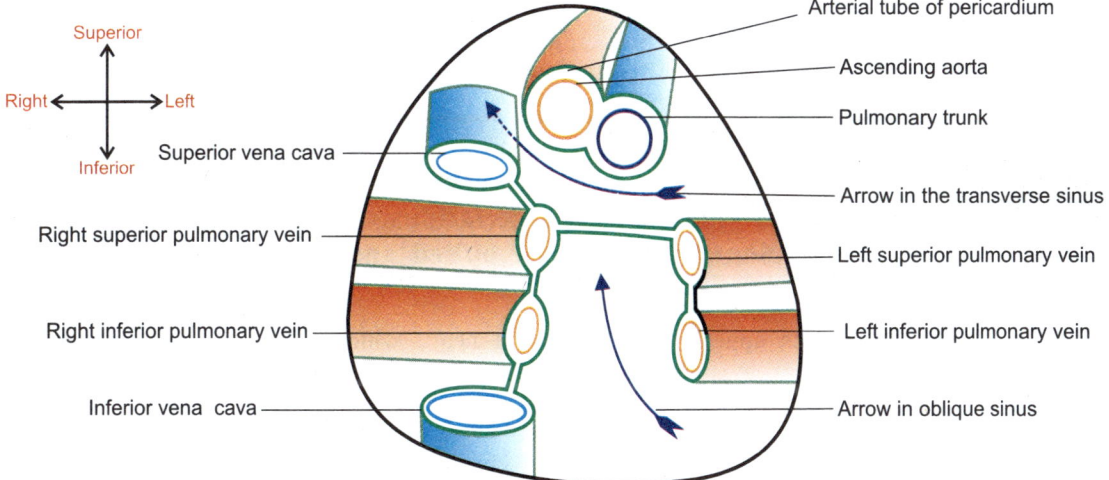

Fig. 2.19 : Oblique & transverse sinus.

    C. Superiorly : Bifurcation of pulmonary trunk.
    D. Inferiorly : Upper surface of left atrium.
    E. Each side : Pericardial cavity.

5.   **Development :** It develops from degeneration of the central cells of dorsal mesocardium.

6.   **Applied anatomy :** During cardiac surgery the ligature may be passed through the transverse sinus around the aorta and pulmonary trunk.

SN-16   Oblique Sinus

1.   **Synonymous :** Parieto visceral space

2.   **Introduction :** It is a cul-de-sac (blind alley) present behind left atrium or it is a space between four pulmonary veins. It is closed on all sides except inferiorly.

3. **Location** : It is located on the posterior surface of heart between parietal and visceral layer of pericardium.

4. **Formation** : It is formed by a reflected part of parietal pericardium.

5. **Boundaries** :
   A. Anteriorly : Posterior surface of left atrium.
   B. Posteriorly : Parietal pericardium.
   C. On right side : Right pair of pulmonary veins and inferior vena cava.
   D. On left side : Left pair of pulmonary veins.
   E. Above : Upper margin of left atrium.

6. **Functions** :
   A. It suspends heart in pericardial cavity.
   B. It permits free pulsations of left atrium.

7. **Development** : It is developed due to the rearrangement of the veins at venous end.

8. **Applied** :
   A. Pericarditis : Inflammation of pericardium.
   B. In pericarditis the pain is referred to epigastrium.

LAQ-6   **Describe right atrium under**
1. Gross anatomy   2. Relations   3. Blood supply
3. Development & 4. Applied anatomy.

1. **Gross anatomy :**
   A. Introduction : It is upper right chamber of heart, which receives venous blood from all parts of the body by following veins.
      a. Superior vena cava brings venous blood from upper half of the body.
      b. Inferior vena cava brings venous blood from lower half of the body.
      c. Coronary sinus brings venous blood from the substance of heart.
   B. Right atrium forms
      a. Right and upper border of the heart,
      b. Sternocostal surface and base of the heart.
   C. Extent : It extends from the opening of superior vena cava to the opening of inferior vena cava. It corresponds to right third costal cartilage to right sixth costal cartilage.
   D. External features : It is elongated chamber and presents following features:
      a. Right auricle :
         I. It is an ear like projection arising from right atrium. It covers
            i. Ascending aorta and
            ii. Infundibulum of right ventricle
         II. Its margins are notched and interior surface is sponge like.
         III. It prevents free flow of blood but favours thrombosis. It causes pulmonary embolism in auricular fibrillation.
      b. Sulcus terminalis : It extends
         I. From the angle made by superior vena cava and the right margin of right auricle
         II. To right border of inferior vena cava.

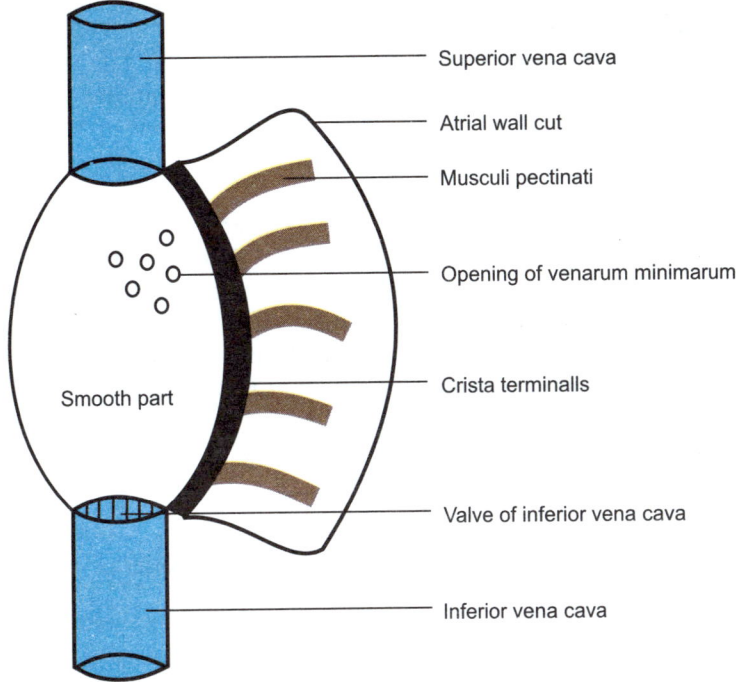

Fig. 2.20 : Interior of right atrium.

E.   Interior of the right atrium : It is divided into three parts

    a.   Anterior part (it is also called as pectinate part or rough part). It shows following features :

        I.   Crista terminalis is produced by internal muscular ridge.

        II. Transverse muscular ridges called musculi pectinati. They give the appearance of teeth of comb. They arise from crista terminalis and inserts on atrioventricular orifice. They are connected to each other and form reticular network.

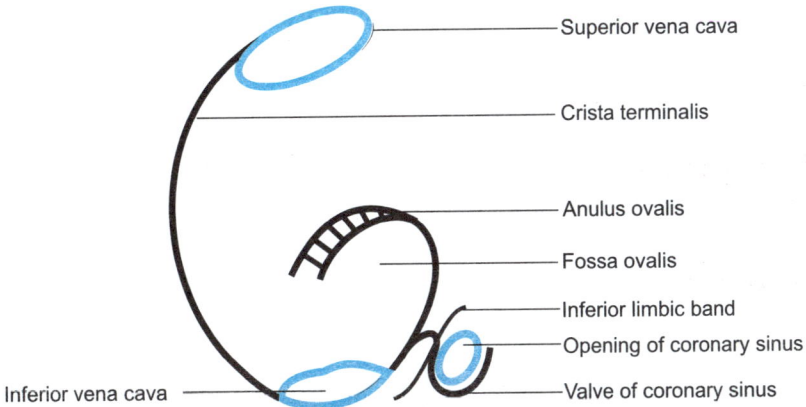

Fig. 2.21 : Interior of right atrium.

    b.   Posterior part : It is also called sinus venorum or smooth part. It demonstrates following features :

        I.   Intervenous tubercle of Lower,

            i.   Site : It is present between superior and inferior vena cava.

            ii.   Function : In foetal life it directs the flow of blood from superior vena cava to right ventricle.

        II.   Opening of superior vena cava

        III.   Opening of inferior vena cava : It is guarded by Eustachian valve which is formed by duplication of the endocardium. It contains few muscle fibers. In foetal life the valve regulates the flow of blood from the inferior vena cava to the left atrium through the foramen ovale.

        IV.   Coronary sinus : It is guarded by valve of coronary sinus.

        V.   Openings of the vanae cordis minimi (Thebesian vein).

    c.   Septal wall (It is also called central part of posterior wall).

        I.   Fossa ovalis a shallow saucer shaped depression, derived from septum primum.

        II.   Limbus fossa ovalis : It is a prominent margin of fossa ovalis. Its anterior edge is continuous with left end of valve of inferior vena cava.

2. Relations :

A.   Anterior :

    a.   Pericardium

    b.   Pleura.

    c.   Anterior part of the mediastinul surface of the right lung.

B.   Posterior

    a.   Right : Pair of pulmonary veins.

    b.   Left : Interatrial septum.

C.   Laterally :

    a.   Right phrenic nerve and pericardiaco phrenic vessels.

    b.   Mediastinal pleura.

    c.   Cardiac impression of right lung.

D.   Medially :

    a.   Root of ascending aorta and

    b.   Root of pulmonary trunk.

3. Blood supply :

A.   Arterial : Right coronary artery, branch of ascending aorta.

B.   Venous : Drains into coronary sinus.

4. Development :

A.   Chronological age : It develops at the end of fourth week of intrauterine life (IUL).

B.   Germ layer : Mesoderm

    a.   The endocardium develops from angioblastic tissue.

    b.   The myocardium develops from splanchnopleuric mesoderm.

    c.   The pericardium develops from somatopleuric intraembryonic mesoder

C. Site : Primitive atrial chamber.

D. Sources : It is divided into

    a. Posterior smooth part (sinus vena'rum) develops from the absorption of the right horn of sinus venosus.

    b. Crista terminalis develops from

        I. Upper part of right venous valve.

        II. Septum spurium.

    c. Valves of the inferior vena cava and coronary sinus develop from lower part of the right venous valve.

    d. Rough trabeculated part (atrium proper) and right auricle develops from right half of the primitive atrium.

    e. Most ventral smooth part is derived from right half of the atrio ventricular canal.

    f. Upper part of interatrial septum develops from septum secundum and lower part develops from septum primum.

F. Anomalies :

    a. Atrial septal defect : It is due to the failure of fusion of the septum primum and the septum secundum. This results into admixture of arterial and venous blood.

    b. Patent foramen ovale.

    c. Persistence of foramen primum.

    d. Persistence of foramen secundum.

5. **Applied anatomy :**

A. Pressure in the right atrium can be measured by recording venous pressure in external jugular vein.

B. For the repair of the atrial septal defect the right atrium is incised along the right border avoiding the region of SA node.

SN-16   Peculiarities of coronary arteries

The following are the peculiarities of coronary arteries. They can be memorized by the word

    Functional end arteries   **FEA**

    F = **f**illed in diastole,

    E = **e**lastic lamina is absent,

    A = **a**rtery of artery.

1. Functional end artery : The coronary arteries reveal communications i.e. they do anastomose. Hence structurally they are not end arteries. But in case of blockage of coronary artery, the blood received through anastomosing channel is so less that they do not meet the required demand. Therefore they are called end functional end arteries.

2. Filled in diastole :   All the blood vessels in the body are filled in systole. However coronary arteries are filled in diastole.

3. Elastic lamina is absent : Coronary arteries are highly muscular vessels and internal elastic lamina is discontinuous and poorly developed.

4. Coronary arteries demonstrate the longitudinal oriented muscles in the outer part of intima or inner part of media.

LAQ-7 **Describe right coronary artery under**
1. **Origin**   2. **Course**   3. **Branches**
4. **Distribution** & 5. **Applied anatomy.**

1. **Origin :** It arises from anterior aortic sinus of ascending aorta.

2. **Course :**
   A. It passes between right auricular appendage and the infundibulum of the right ventricle.
   B. It passes vertically downwards in the atrio-ventricular groove.
   C. The artery turns backwards at the inferior border of the heart and runs posteriorly. The terminal part of the right coronary artery is small and anastomoses with the circumflex branch of left coronary artery.
   D. Peculiarity : Right coronary artery has a characteristic loop at the point where the posterior inter ventricular artery and AV nodal artery arises.

3. **Branches :**
   A. Right conus artery :
      a. The word 'conus' means infundibulum of right ventricle. It is a first branch of right coronary artery.
      b. It is meant for the nutrition of the conus arteriosus.
      c. It may arise as the third **coronary artery.**
      d. It anastomoses with the left conus artery, a branch of the anterior inter-ventricular branch of the left coronary artery to form an anastomotic necklace around the infundibulum or the commencement of the pulmonary trunk.

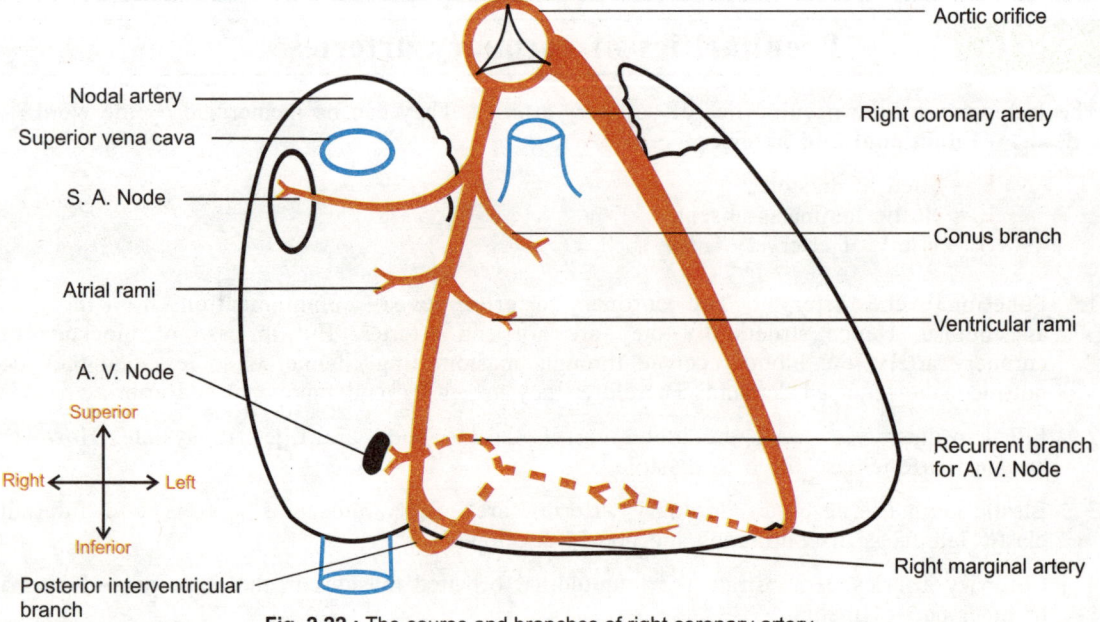

Fig. 2.22 : The course and branches of right coronary artery.

B. SA nodal artery : It forms vascular ring around the termination of superior vena cava. It supplies SA node in 60% of the hearts.

C. Right anterior ventricular branches : They are three to four in number. They pass along the sterno-costal surface and as the name suggests they supply anterior surface of right ventricle. One of the branch is longest and is known as right marginal artery. It runs along the inferior border of the heart.

D. Posterior inter-ventricular branch : It passes along the inter-ventricular groove towards the apex of the heart to supply the diaphragmatic surface of right ventricle.

E. AV nodal artery : This supplies AV node.

4. **Distribution :**
   A. Right atrium,
   B. SA node,
   C. Superior parts of the right ventricle,
   D. Posterior $1/3^{rd}$ of inter-ventricular septum,
   E. AV node and
   F. Right AV bundle.

5. **Applied anatomy :**
   A. The right coronary artery is a second commonest occluded artery in causing myocardial infarction.
   B. In 20% to 25% of population, the right coronary artery also supplies diaphragmatic surface (substantial) of left ventricle. This is called 'right dominant' coronary surface.

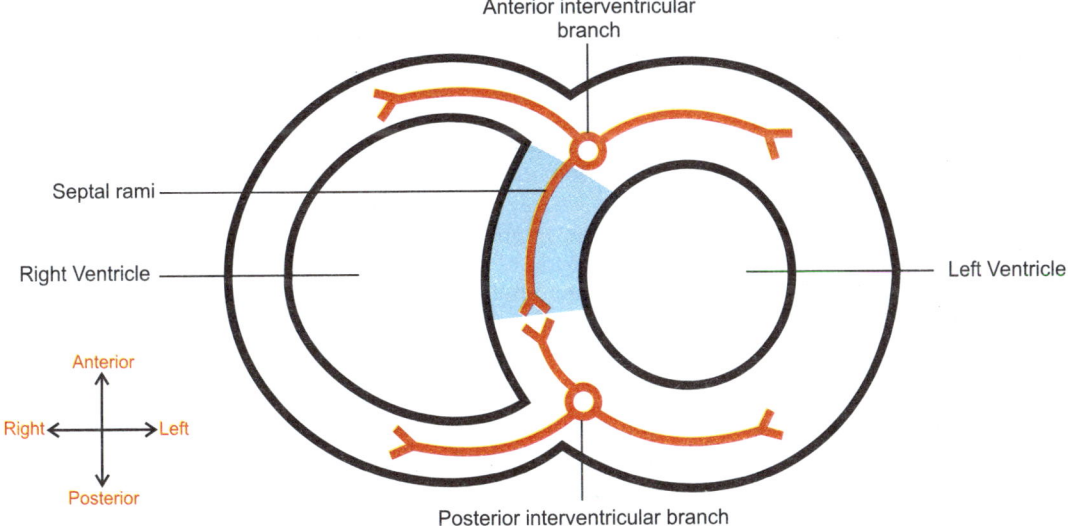

Fig. 2.23 : Arterial supply of the interventricular septum.

C. Although the coronary arteries have numerous anastomoses at the arteriolar level, they are essentially 'functional end arteries' i.e. when a coronary artery is blocked the blood received by collateral channels is inadequate to meet the required demand in required time.

D. The cardiac pain (due to angina pectoris or myocardial infarction) is usually referred to the left precordium and inner aspects of left arm and forearm.

The heart is supplied by upper 4 thoracic (i.e. T_1, $_2$, $_3$ & $_4$) spinal segment. The skin over precordium is supplied by T_4, T_3 and T_2 spinal segments. The inner aspect of arm is innervated by T_2 spinal segment. And the inner aspect of forearm and hand is innervated by T_1 spinal segment.

The cardiac pain is therefore referred to the precordium and inner aspects of the arm and forearm because of the same segmental innervation.

The cardiac pain is usually referred to the left side because:

Cardiac lesions mostly occur in the left half of the heart, but if the lesion is in right half of the heart, the pain will be referred on the right side. Hence it is wrong notion that cardiac pain is always referred to the left side 'the left arm myth'.

E. The coronary disease in old age is less fatal than in young age because anastomoses increase and collateral channels develop with the advancement of age.

F. The slow gradual blocking coronary artery is less dangerous than sudden blockage because the arteries taking part in extra pericardiac anastomosis will dilate and provide blood supply to the heart.

LAQ-8   Describe left coronary artery under
1. Origin   2. Course   3. Branches
4. Distribution & 5. Applied anatomy.

1. **Origin :** It is shorter but wider than the right coronary artery and supplies the greater mass of myocardium. It arises from left posterior aortic sinus of ascending aorta.

2. **Course :**
   A. It passes between left auricle and the infundibulum of the right ventricle.
   B. After the short course it divides into two terminal branches (circumflex and anterior inter-ventricular branch).
   C. The circumflex branch is one of the terminal branch of left coronary artery, runs from the left border of the heart to the back of the heart in the Antrio-ventricular groove.
   D. It gives various branches to atrium and ventricle and anastomosis with the right coronary artery.

3. **Branches :**
   A. Anterior inter-ventricular artery : It is downward continuation of the main trunk along the anterior inter-ventricular groove. It winds round the inferior border of the heart to anastomose with the posterior inter-ventricular artery i.e. junction of anterior $1/3^{rd}$ and posterior $2/3^{rd}$ of the posterior inter-ventricular groove. It has following branches
      a. Anterior ventricular branches for the sternocostal surfaces of both left and right ventricles. One of the right anterior ventricular branch gives the left conus artery which supplies the conus arteriosus of the right ventricle and forms anastomotic necklace with the right conus artery, branch of right coronary artery.
      b. Septal branches : To supply anterior $2/3^{rd}$ of the inter-ventricular septum.
   B. Circumflex artery : It passes along the left part of the posterior atrio-ventricular groove. The branches are as follows,

a.   Atrial branches : They are in three groups - Anterior, lateral and posterior for each corresponding three surfaces of the left atrium.
b.   Ventricular branches : They are 1 to 5 in number. One of these branches is larger and descends along the left border of the heart to the apex and is called left marginal artery.
c.   Nodal artery for the SA node in 35% of cases.

4.   **Distribution :**
   A.   Anterior aspects of both right and left ventricles,
   B.   Anterior $2/3^{rd}$ of the ventricular septum,
   C.   Left branch of the AV bundle,
   D.   Left surface of the left ventricle &
   E.   Posterior aspect of the left atrium.

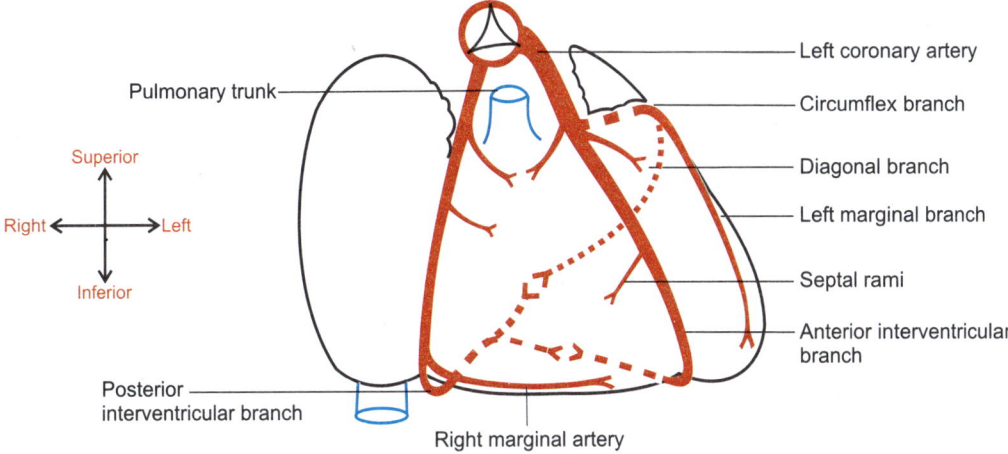

Fig. 2.24 : The course and branches of left coronary artery.

5.   **Applied anatomy :**
   A.   Anterior inter-ventricular branch of left coronary artery is the most commonly occluded vessel in the myocardial infarction. The circumflex branch of left coronary artery is a third commonly occluded vessel in myocardial infarction.
   B.   The left coronary artery in addition to the usual distribution, supplies blood to the entire inter-ventricular septum and atrioventricular node. In such cases it is called left dominant coronary artery.

> **Note :** Please write the points of C, D, E and F of applied anatomy of right coronary artery.

| LAQ-9 | **Venous drainage of the heart** |

The veins draining the heart are divided in two groups
1.   Veins draining into coronary sinus : This is a wide vessel that lies in the posterior part of atrio-ventricular groove. It is covered by thin layer of myocardium and opens in the posterior wall of right atrium left to the opening of inferior vena cava.

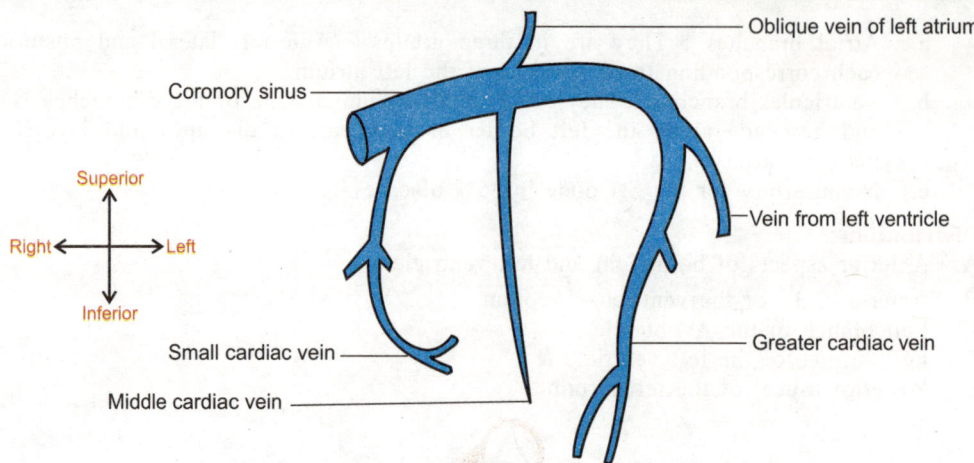

Fig. 2.25 : The figure showing veins draining the heart.

The tributaries of the coronary sinus and their details is described in the following table.

Table 2.4 : The table showing the veins draining into coronary sinus.

Particulars	Situation	Draining area	Artery accompanying the vein
A. Great cardiac	Anterior inter ventricular groove	a. Anterior part of inter ventricular septum b. Anterior part of both ventricles	Anterior interventricular artery (left coronary)
B. Middle cardiac	Posterior inter ventricular groove	a. Posterior part of inter ventricular septum b. Posterior part of both ventricles	Posterior ventricular (right coronary artery)
C. Small cardiac	Coronary sulcus	Margins of right ventricle	-
D. Oblique vein of the left atrium (vein of Marshal)	Posterior part of left atrium	-	-

2. Veins directly opening into the right atrium are described in the following table.

Table 2.5 : The table showing veins directly draining into right atrium.

Particulars	Situation	Draining area	Termination
Anterior cardiac vein.	Atrioventricular groove	Anterior surface of right ventricule	Right atrium
Venae cordae minimi (Thebesian vein)	-	Endocardium	Right atrium

LAQ-10 Describe superior vena cava under
1. Gross anatomy   2. Relations   3. Tributaries
4. Development & 5. Applied anatomy.

1. **Gross anatomy :**
   A. Introduction : This is the large venous channel which collects the blood from the upper half of the body and drains into the right atrium.
   B. Formation : It is formed by the union of right and left brachiocephalic veins.
   C. Site : It is formed behind the lower border of first right costal cartilage.
   D. Length : 7 cms.
   E. Termination : It terminates by opening into the upper part of the right atrium behind the third costal cartilage.

2. **Relations :**
   A. Anterior :
      a. Chest wall.
      b. Internal thoracic vessels.
      c. Anterior margin of the right lung and pleura.
      d. The vessel is covered by pericardium in its lower half.
   B. Posterior :
      a. Trachea and right vagus (posteromedial to the upper part of the vena cava).
      b. Root of right lung (posterior to the lower part).
   C. Medial :
      a. Ascending aorta.
      b. Brachiocephalic artery.
   D. Lateral :
      a. Phrenic nerve (with accompanying vessels).
      b. Right pleura and lung.

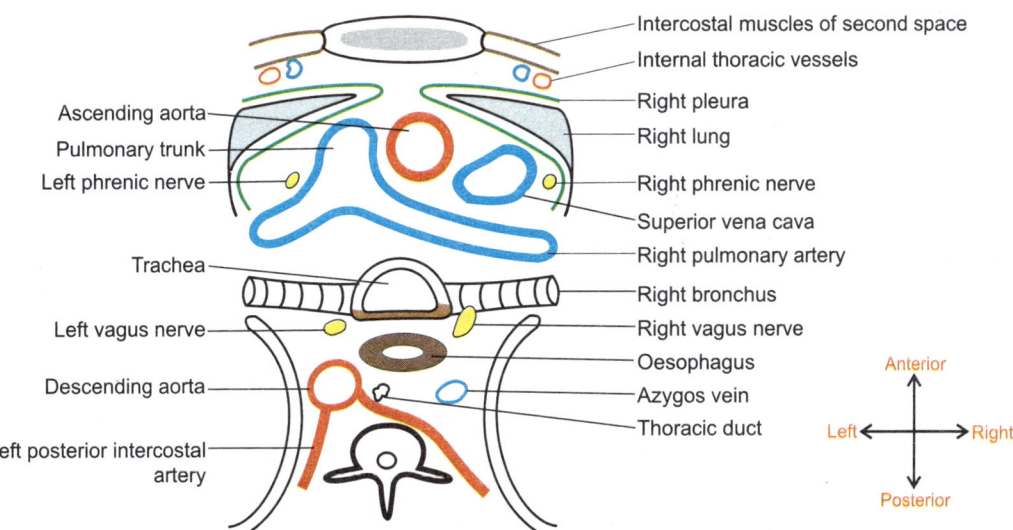

Fig. 2.26 : Relations of superior vena-cava at fifth thoracic vertebra.

3. **Tributaries :**
   A. Azygos vein : It opens into the superior vena cava at the level of second costal cartilage just before it enters the pericardium.
   B. Small mediastinal veins.
   C. Pericardial veins.

4. **Development :**
   A. Upper half develops from right anterior cardinal vein.
   B. Lower half develops from right common cardinal vein.

5. **Applied anatomy :**
   A. In the obstruction of the superior vena cava above the opening of azygos vein, the venous blood of the upper half of the body is returned through the azygos vein and the superficial veins are dilated on the chest upto the costal margin.
   B. In the obstruction of the superior vena cava below the opening of the azygos vein, the blood is returned through the inferior vena cava via the femoral vein.
   C. Here the superficial veins are dilated on both the chest and abdomen.
   D. In cases of the mediastinal syndrome, the signs of the superior vena caval obstruction are first to appear.

LAQ-11 **Describe the arch of the aorta under**
1. Origin   2. Course   3. Relations
4. Branches 5. Development & 6. Applied anatomy.

1. **Origin :** It is the continuation of the ascending aorta behind the manubrium sternum. It is situated in the superior mediastinum.

2. **Course :**
   A. It begins behind the upper border of the second right sternochondral joint.
   B. It runs upwards, backwards and to the left, across the left side of the bifurcation of the trachea. Then it passes downwards behind the left bronchus and on the left side of the body of the fourth thoracic vertebra. It thus arches over the root of the left lung.
   C. It ends at the lower border of the body of the fourth thoracic vertebra by becoming continuous with the descending aorta.
   Thus the origin and termination of the aortic arch is at the same level, although it begins anteriorly and terminates posteriorly.

3. **Relations :**
   A. Anteriorly and to the left :
      a. Nerves (from before backwards)
         I.   Left phrenic
         II. Lower cervical cardiac branch of the left vagus,
         III. Upper cervical cardiac branch of left sympathetic chain,
         IV. Left vagus.
      b. Left superior intercostal vein, deep to the phrenic nerve and superficial to the vagus nerve.
      c. Left pleura and lung.
      d. Remains of thymus.

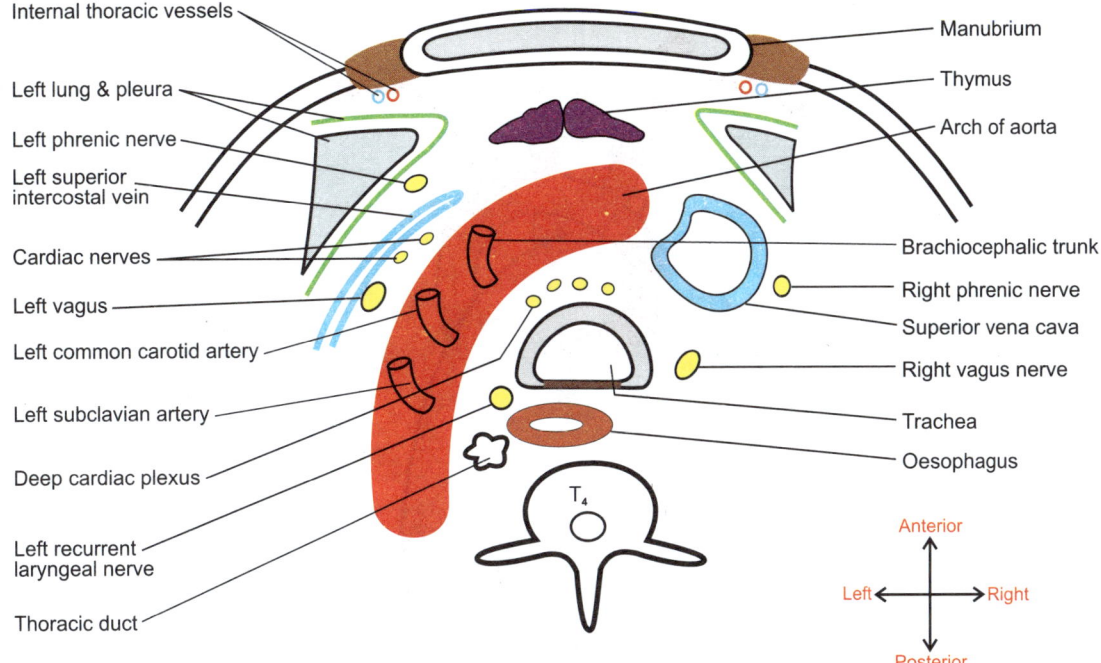

Fig. 2.27 : Relations of arch of aorta at T$_4$ level.

    B.   Posterior and to the right :
        a.   Trachea, with the deep cardiac plexus and the tracheobronchial lymph nodes.
        b.   Oesophagus.
        c.   Left recurrent laryngeal nerve.
        d.   Thoracic duct.
        e.   Vertebral column.
    C.   Superior :
        a.   Three branches of the arch of the aorta
            I.   Brachiocephalic
            II. Left common carotid and
            III. Left subclavian artery.
        b.   All these arteries are crossed, close to their origin by the left brachiocephalic
           vein.
    D.   Inferior :
        a.   Bifurcation of the pulmonary trunk.
        b.   Left bronchus.
        c.   Ligamentum arteriosum with superficial cardiac plexus on it.
        d.   Left recurrent laryngeal nerve.

4.   Branches :
    A.   Brachiocephalic artery which divides into the right common carotid and right
        subclavian artery.
    B.   Left common carotid artery.
    C.   Left subclavian artery.

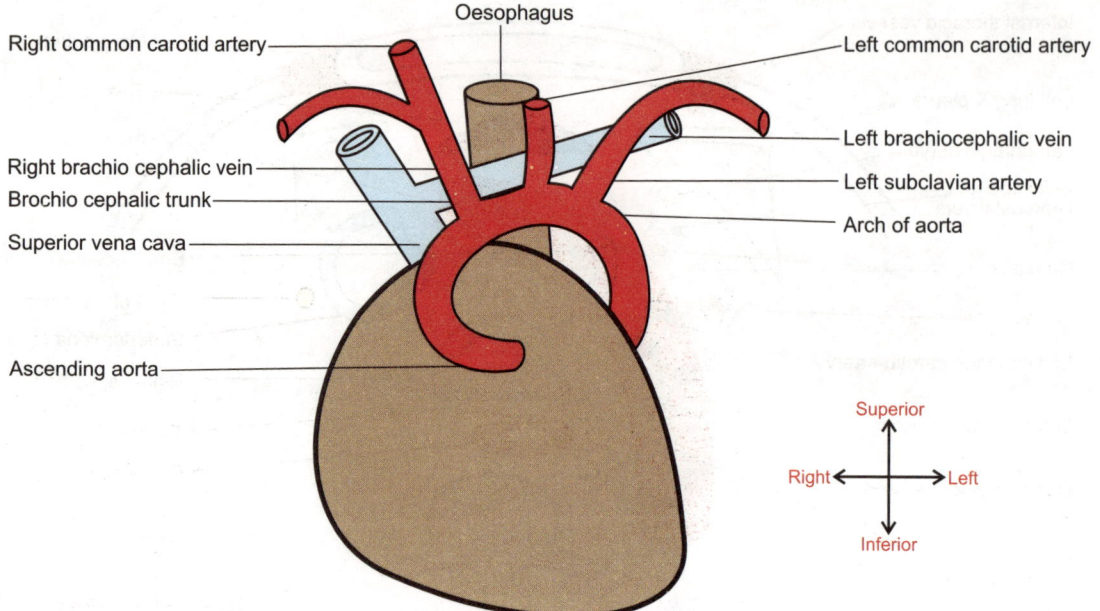

Fig. 2.28 : Branches of the arch of the aorta.

5. Development :

A. **Chronological age :** It develops at the end of fourth week of intrauterine life (IUL).

B. **Germ layer :** Mesoderm.

C. **Site :** Ventral to the foregut.

D. **Sources :** The arch of the aorta is developed from three sources (from before backward)

    a. **Left horn of aortic sac (truncus arteriosus) :** It forms the part of arch of the aorta between brachiocephalic trunk and left common carotid artery.

    b. **Left fourth aortic arch :** It forms the part between left common carotid artery and ductus arteriosus.

    c. **Left dorsal aorta :** It forms the rest of the arch upto the descending aorta.

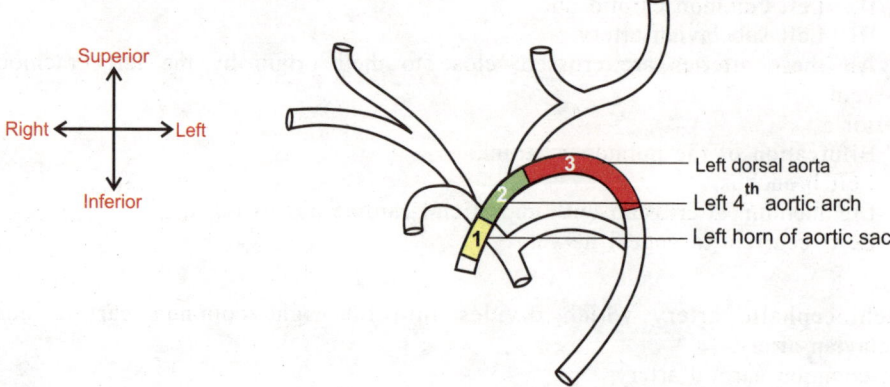

Fig. 2.29 : Development of arch of the aorta.

E. Anomalies :
  a. Coarctation of aorta : It takes place due to the congenital stenosis or atresia of the arch of the aorta distal to the origin of left subclavian artery. The stenosis is due to defect of the tunica media which may be
    I. Preductal &
    II. Postductal.
  b. Right sided aortic arch : This is common in birds. It is due to the persistence of the right dorsal aorta below the seventh intersegmental artery.
  c. Double aortic arch : It is common in frogs. It is due to the persistence of left dorsal aortae.
  d. Patent ductus arteriosus.

6. **Applied anatomy :**
  A. Aortic knuckle : A convex bulging known as aortic knuckle is found on the left side of the sternal angle in a plain X-ray chest. It is formed by the distal part of the arch of the aorta.
  B. Aortic aneurysm.

LAQ-12 Describe oesophagus under
1. Gross anatomy 2. Blood supply 3. Lymphatic drainage
4. Nerve supply 5. Histology & 6. Applied anatomy.

1. **Gross anatomy :**
  A. Introduction : It is the longest muscular tube of gastrointestinal tract extending from pharynx to stomach.
  B. Extent : It extends from lower border of cricoid cartilage (sixth cervical vertebra) to cardiac orifice of stomach (tenth thoracic vertebra).
  C. Constriction : Normally the oesophagus shows four constrictions at the following levels 🔑   **ABCD**
    a. Where it is crossed by the **a**ortic **a**rch.
    b. Where it is crossed by the left **b**ronchus.
    c. At its **c**ommencement (caused by **c**ricopharyngeus sphincter).
    d. Where it pierces the **d**iaphragm.

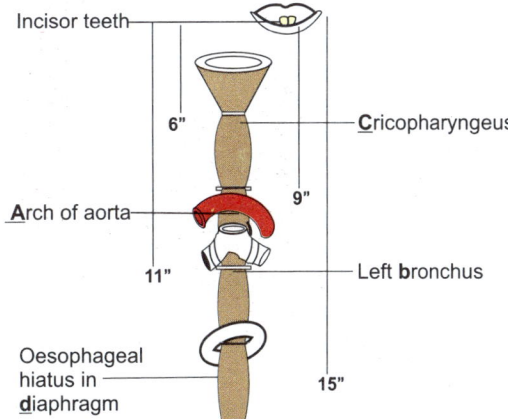

Fig. 2.30 : Constrictions of oesophagus.

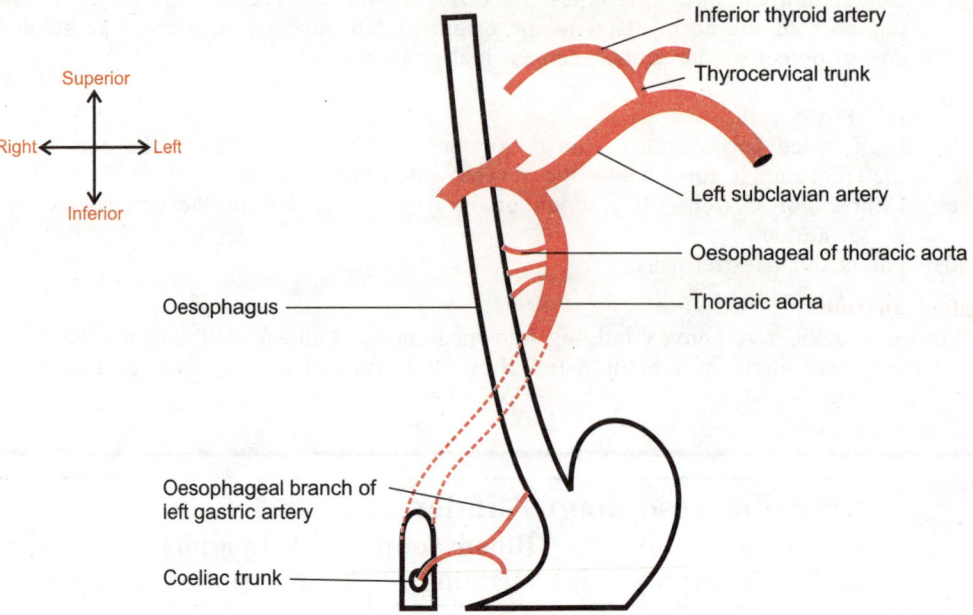

Fig. 2.31 : Arterial supply of oesophagus.

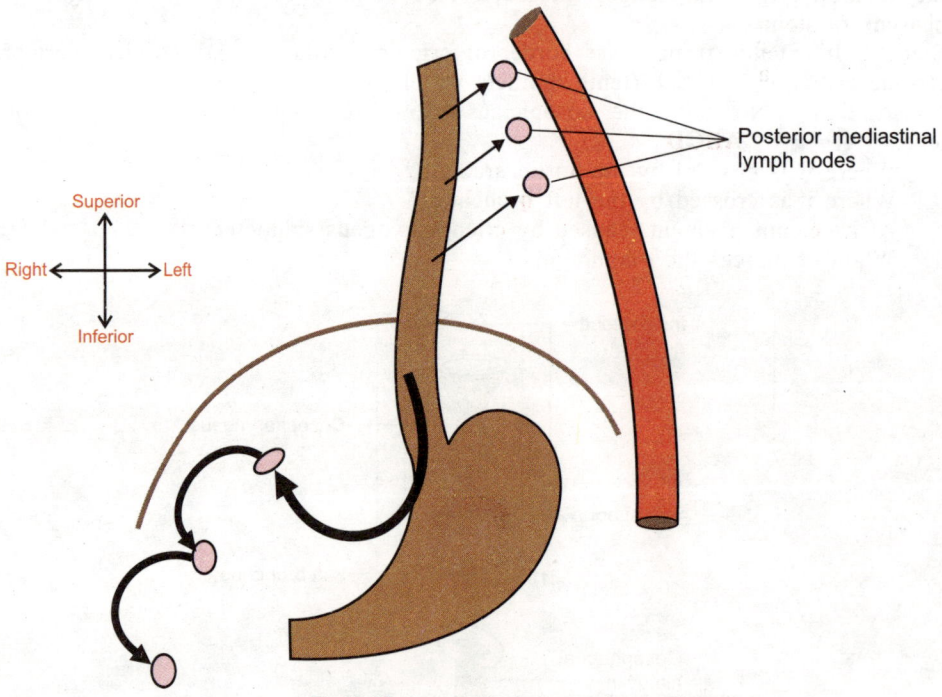

Fig. 2.32 : Lymphatic drainage of oesophagus.

Table 2.6 : The table showing blood supply and lymphatic drainage of oesophagus.

Particulars	Upper (cervical)	Middle (thoracic)	Lower (abdominal)
2. Blood supply A. Arterial supply	Oesophageal branches of inferior thyroid arteries (subclavian artery)	a. Oesophageal branches of thoracic aorta b. Oesophageal branches of bronchial arteries	Oesophageal branches of left gastric artery.
B. Venous drainage	Oesophageal veins drain into brachiocephalic vein which drains into superior vena cava	Oesophageal veins drain into azygos vein which drains into superior vena cava	Oesophageal vein drains into left gastric veins which drains into portal vein
3. Lymphatic drainage *Lymphatics of oesophagus follows arteries*	Deep cervical lymph nodes	Tracheobronchial lymph nodes and posterior mediastinal nodes.	Left gastric nodes & coeliac lymph nodes

4. **Nerve supply :**
   A. Sympathetic fibers : These arise from T_5 - T_9 segments of the spinal cord and form the oesophageal plexus.
   B. Parasympathetic fibers : These are derived from vagi and recurrent laryngeal nerves. The nerve cells in the myenteric and submucous plexuses act as postganglionic neurons for parasympathetic fibers only.
   The congenital absence of these nerve cells produces disturbance in peristalsis and the condition is known as cardio-spasm or achalasia (*a* not ; *chalasis* relaxation).

5. **Histology :** It is formed by four layers from inside out.
   A. Mucosa : It is thick and is in the collapsed state thrown into longitudinal folds. It consists of

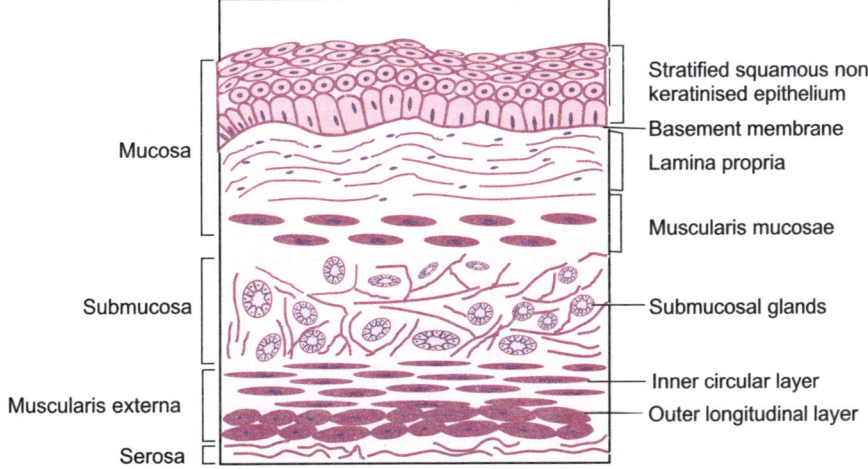

Fig. 2.33 : Oesophagus.

a.   Surface epithelium of stratified squamous non-keratinised. It is replaced by columnar epithelium at the gastro oesophageal junction.
b.   Lamina propria.
c.   Thick muscularis mucosa which shows an internal circular layer and an external longitudinal layer. A nerve plexus may be found among the muscle fibers.

B.   *Submucosa : It contains mucous glands which are sparse and are found in the upper and lower ends.*
C.   Muscularis externa : It consists of inner circular and outer longitudinal, which are of skeletal muscle in the upper part and smooth muscle in the lower part. *It is the longest smooth muscle cells of the body.*
D.   Serosa is lined by thick fibrous coat.

6.   **Applied anatomy :**

A.   Oesophageal varices : The lower end of oesophagus is one of the main sites of porto caval anastomosis. Here the tributaries of left gastric vein anastomose profusely with the tributaries of azygos and hemiazygos veins.
     In portal hypertension there is shunting of the blood from portal to caval system.
     There is dilatation and tortuosity of these collateral channels which is called oesophageal varices. Rupture of these veins results into haematemesis (i.e. vomiting of frank red colored blood). This differentiates haematemesis arising from perforation of gastric ulcers which is black-red in colour.
B.   Dysphagia : Obstruction to oesophagus results into painful swallowing or difficult swallowing which is called as dysphagia. This can be diagnosed by barium swallow.
C.   Achalasia cardia : It is due to neuromuscular in-coordination of muscles of the lower end of oesophagus. This results into loss of peristalsis & there is a failure of relaxation of the lower end of oesophagus. Consequently the food accumulates in the oesophagus causing regurgitation. The regurgitant does not include gastric contents and is not sour tasting. The achalasia is the most common oesophageal motility disorder, with an incidence of 6 per 100,000 individuals.

LAQ-13 Describe thoracic duct under
1. Gross anatomy   2. Course and relations 3. Tributaries
4. Histology   5. Development &   6. Applied anatomy.

1.   **Gross anatomy :**

A.   Introduction : It is a lymphatic channel present in the thoracic region draining the lymph from lower half and left upper half of the body.
B.   Appearance : Beaded.
C.   Measurement : Length x width (cm) 45 x 0.5
D.   Extent : Lower border of T_{12} vertebra to 7th cervical vertebra.
E.   Commencement : It commences from the cranial end of cisterna chyli.
F.   Termination : It terminates in the left brachiocephalic vein at the junction of left subclavian and left internal jugular vein.

2.   **Course and relations :**

A.   It passes through the aortic opening of diaphragm which is present at 12th thoracic vertebra.

B. Here it accompanies on the left side by descending thoracic aorta and on the right side by azygos vein.

C. It lies posterior to oesophagus upto 5th thoracic vertebra.

D. It ascends upward and at level of 5th thoracic vertebrae it takes left turn and enters the superior mediastinum.

E. At the level of 7th cervical vertebra, it arches laterally, which is 3 cms to 4 cms above the left clavicle.

3. **Tributaries :**

A. At commencement it receives confluence of lymph trunk.

B. In thorax it receives lymph trunk from
   a. Upper lumbar region
   b. Posterior mediastinum and
   c. Upper six intercostal space.

C. In the neck it receives two tributaries
   a. Left subclavian lymph trunk &
   b. Left jugular lymph trunk.

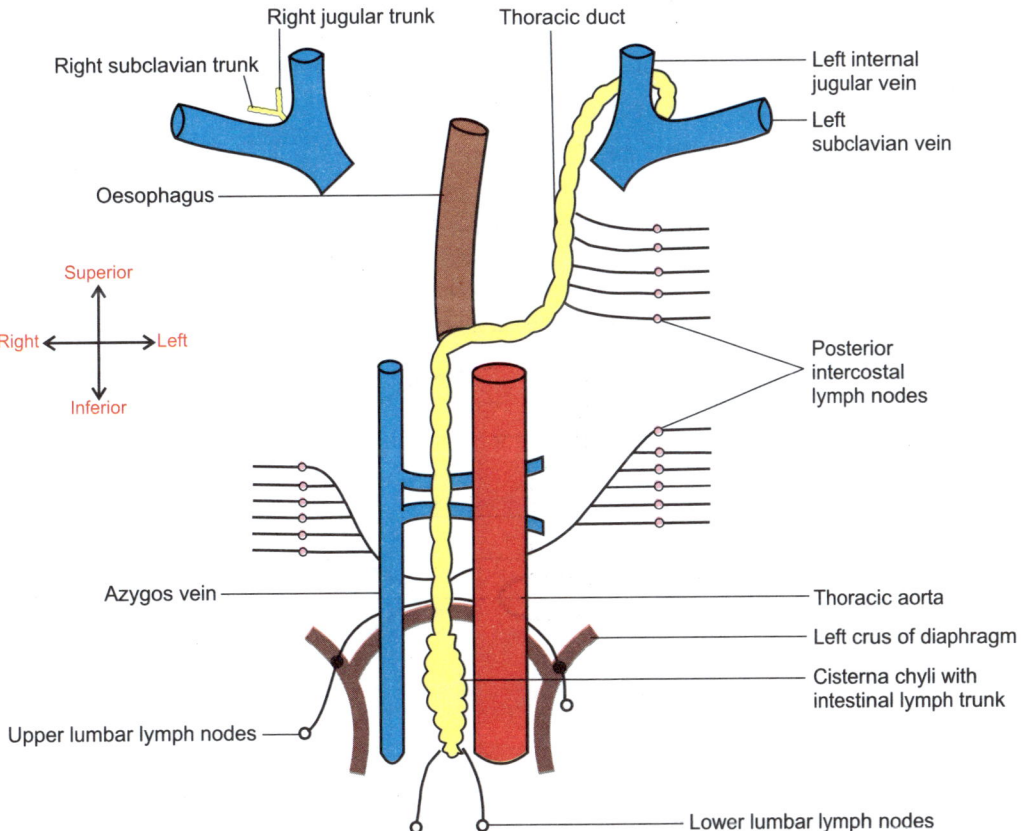

Fig. 2.34 : The course & relations of the thoracic duct.

4. **Histology :** It has three layers
   A. Tunica externa
   B. Tunica media : It shows connective tissue fibers arranged along long axis of the vessels.
   C. Tunica intima : It shows well defined sub-endothelial layer.
5. **Development :** It develops from
   A. Two longitudinal channels which are present by the side of primitive vertebral column.
   B. They are connected by transverse channels at the level of 5th thoracic vertebra.
   C. Right upper and left lower limbs of the original longitudinal channel disappears and the remaining part gives to thoracic duct.
6. **Applied anatomy :**
   A. Obstruction of duct is caused by
      a. Surrounding tumours or by
      b. Microfilaria.
   B. Rupture of duct leads to leakage of chyle and the condition is called chylothorax.

SN-17   Development of inter-atrial septum

1. **Chronological age :** It develops in the fourth week of intrauterine life (IUL).

2. **Germ layer :** Splanchnic layer of lateral plate mesoderm.

3. **Site :** From the roof of primitive atrial chamber.

4. **Sources :**
   A. Septum primum : A thin crescent shaped membrane grows from the roof of primitive common atrial chamber. It grows downward in the direction of septum intermedium (fused atrio ventricular cushion). This septum is called septum primum.

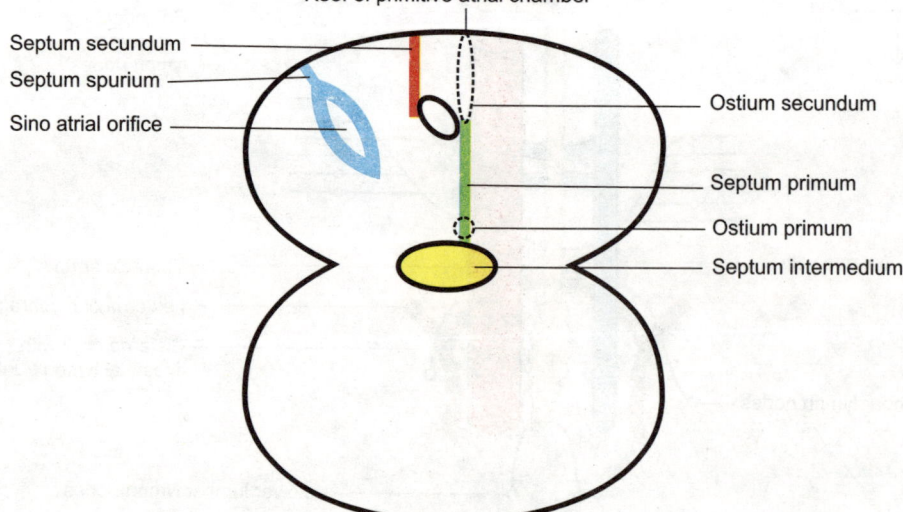

Fig. 2.35 : Development of inter-atrial septum.

There is a gap between lower end of septum primum and septum intermedium called as ostium primum. Before lower end of septum primum fuses with septum intermedium, upper part breaks open and the gap is formed which is called ostium secundum.

B. Septum secundum : Another crescentic membrane arises on right side of septum primum and on left side of valve of septum spurium (false). There is a gap between septum primum and septum secundum which is oval in shape and is called as foramen ovale. The blood coming from right atrium passes to left atrium through foramen ovale.

C. At birth the left atrium receives blood from lungs by four pulmonary veins. Due to the increase in the volume of blood the pressure is increased in left atrium. The septum secundum and septum primum approximates and interatrial septum is developed.

5. **Anomalies :** Atrial septal defect is common anomaly.
   A. Incidence : 0.07%
   B. Prevalence : 2 to 1 in female versus male infant.
   C. Types : It is of three types
      a. Cor triloculare biventriculare : This is the most serious abnormality of atrial septal defect. There is complete absence of the atrial septum. It is always associated with serious defects elsewhere in the heart.
      b. Osteum primum defect is caused by
         I. Defective formation of atrio-ventricular (endocardial) cushion or
         II. Failure of the septum primum to reach the atrioventricular cushion.
      c. Osteum secundum defect : It is a most significant defect. It is caused by
         I. Failure of development of septum secundum.
         II. Excessive resorption of septum primum.
      d. Patent foramen ovale is caused by failure of approximation of septum primum and septum secundum after birth. It is clinically not significant as it does not allow shunting of blood.

SN-18 — Development of inter ventricular septum

1. **Chronological age :** It develops in the seventh week of intrauterine life (IUL).

2. **Germ layer :** Splanchnic layer of lateral plate mesoderm.

3. **Site :** From the floor of the common ventricular chamber (bulboventricular cavity).

4. **Sources :** It has two parts : muscular and membranous part
   A. Muscular part forms the major part of the interventricular septum. It arises as a muscular ridge or fold, the interventricular septum from the primitive ventricular chamber.
   B. Membranous part : It is also called interventricular foramen. It exists between the free age of interventricular septum and the fused endocardial cusion. It permits communication between right and left ventricles upto the end of seventh week. It has two parts

a. Anterior membranous part which develops from atrioventricular endocardial cushion. It is also called intermediate septum (septum between right atrium and left ventricle). The atrioventricular canal is formed between the primitive atrium and primitive ventricle. Initially the canal is round and changes to oval. Two elevations develop on the anterior and posterior wall of this canal, which gets fused and forms septum intermedium. This communicates with right and left side of atrium to right and left side of ventricle.

b. Posterior membranous part is formed by right and left bulbar septum.

5. **Anomalies :**

A. Ventricular septal defect (VSD) : This is the most common congenital anomaly of the heart. It is because of failure of fusion of endocardial cushion or the atrioventricular canal.

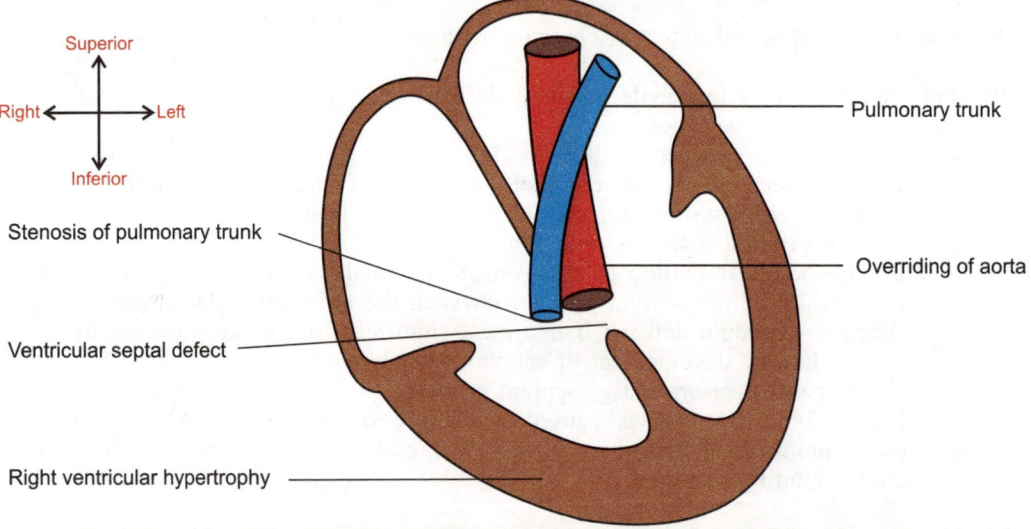

Fig. 2.36 : Fallot's tetrology.

B. Fallot's tetralogy : (Tetralogy means four defects) It is most common congenital cyanotic heart disease. The main defect is an unequal division of the conus leading to narrow pulmonary and wide ascending aorta. It is characterized by

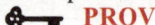 **PROV**

A. **P**ulmonary stenosis
b. **R**ight ventricular hypertrophy.
c. **O**verriding of the aorta.
d. **V**entricular septal defect.

The clinical manifestations are breathlessness on exertion. The child suddenly ceases his activity and lies in the knee chest position "squatting posture", by doing so he gets relief probably because squatting reduces the venous return by compressing the abdominal veins and increases the systemic vascular resistance by kinking the femoral and popliteal arteries. Both these mechanisms tend to decrease the right to left shunt through ventricular septal defect and improves the pulmonary circulation.

SN-19 Development of left atrium

1. **Chronological age :** It develops in the fifth to seventh week of intrauterine life (IUL).

2. **Germ layer :** Mesoderm.

3. **Site :** Primitive atrial chamber.

4. **Sources :**
   A. The posterior smooth part (between the openings of the pulmonary veins) develops from the incorporation of the endocardial cushions of the four pulmonary veins.
   B. The anterior part which is somewhat trabeculated including the left auricle develops from the left half of the primitive atrium.
   C. The most ventral part develops from the left half of the atrio-ventricular canal.

SN-20 Development of portal vein

1. **Chronological age :** It develops in the fifth to seventh week of intrauterine life (IUL).

2. **Germ layer :** Mesoderm.

3. **Site :** Around the duodenum.

4. **Sources :**

Table 2.7 : The table showing sources of different part of the portal vein.

Part	Develops from
A. Infra duodenal part	Part of left vitelline vein from joining of splenic vein to dorsal inter vitelline anastomosis.
B. Retro duodenal part	Dorsal anastomoses between right and left vitelline veins.
C. Supra duodenal part	Right vitelline vein between dorsal anastomosis and cephalic ventral anastomosis.
D. Right branch	Cephalic part of right vitelline vein cranial to cephalic inter vitelline anastomosis.
E. Left branch	Cephalic ventral anastomosis and left vitelline cranial to cephalic ventral inter vitelline anastomosis.

SN-21 Development of inferior vena cava

1. **Chronological age :** It develops in the fifth to seventh week of intrauterine life (IUL).

2. **Germ layer :** Splanchnic layer of lateral plate mesoderm.

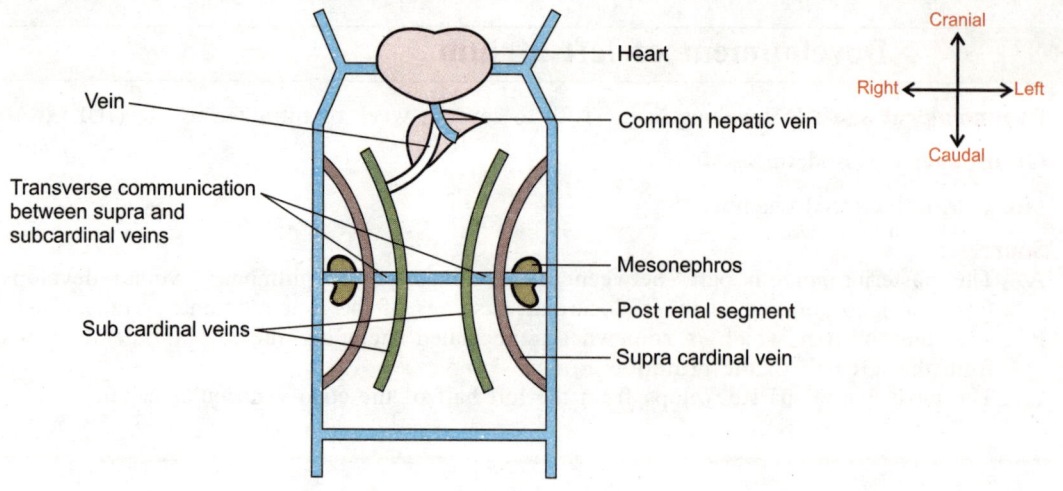

Fig. 2.37 : Development of inferior vena-cava.

3. **Site :** Posterior abdominal wall.

4. **Sources :**
   A. Right posterior cardinal vein caudal to joining of right supracardinal vein.
   B. Right supracardinal vein caudal to right supra subcardinal anastomosis.
   C. Right supracardinal - subcardinal anastomoses.
   D. Right subcardinal vein caudal to right subcardino hepatocardiac channel anastomoses.
   E. Right subcardinal hepatic cardiac channel anastomoses.
   F. Hepatocardiac channel.

5. **Anomalies :**
   A. Absence of inferior vena cava - results when the right subcardinal vein fails to establish connection with the liver.
   B Double inferior vena cava - (at lumbar level) - results from persistence of left supracardinal vein.

HEAD FACE NECK

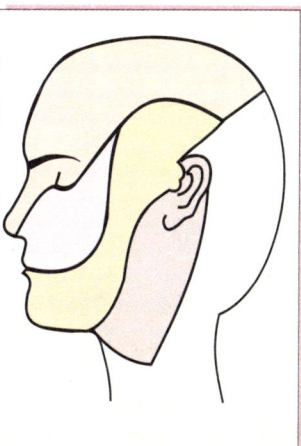

Index

SAQ-1   Pterion

It is a H shaped suture present on the lateral side of the skull.

1. **Formation :** It is formed by four bones.
   A. Frontal
   B. Parietal
   C. Sphenoid and
   D. Temporal

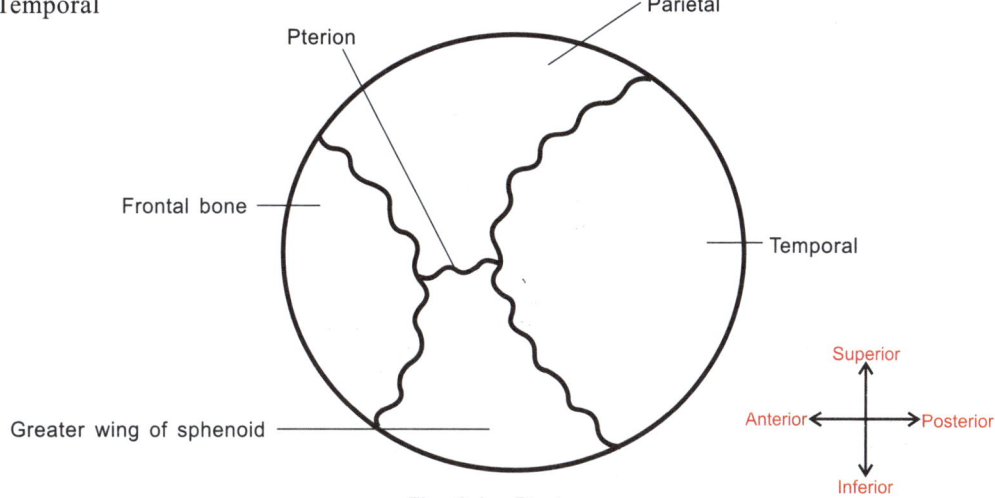

Fig. 3.1 : Pterion.

2. **Situation :** It is situated 4 cm. above the midpoint of zygomatic arch and 2.5 cm behind the fronto zygomatic suture.

3. **Relation :** Following structures are related deep to the pterion.
   A. Middle meningeal vessels.
   B. Stem of lateral sulcus of cerebral fissure (Sylvian point).

4. **Applied anatomy :**
   A. A blow at pterion may lead to an extradural haemorrhage. This may be due to rupture of middle meningeal artery.
   B. The extradural haematoma exerts a local pressure on the underlying motor area in the precentral gyrus.
   C. The center of the pterion is an important landmark to neurosurgeon. In case of increased intracranial tension, the Burr holes are placed at pterion.

SAQ-2   Suprameatal triangle (Mecewan's triangle)

It is a triangular depression, present behind the external acoustic meatus.

1. **Boundaries :** Margins of suprameatal triangle are **SET** 🔑
   A. Above by **s**upramastoid crest.
   B. Anteriorly by posterosuperior margin of **e**xternal acoustic meatus.
   C. Behind by **t**angential line drawn from posterior margin of external acoustic meatus.

2. **Applied anatomy :**

A. The suprameatal triangle corresponds with conchae of the auricle and the mastoid antrum.

B. At birth, mastoid antrum is situated at about 3 mm deep to the suprameatal triangle. In adult, it is situated at about 15 mm from the surface.

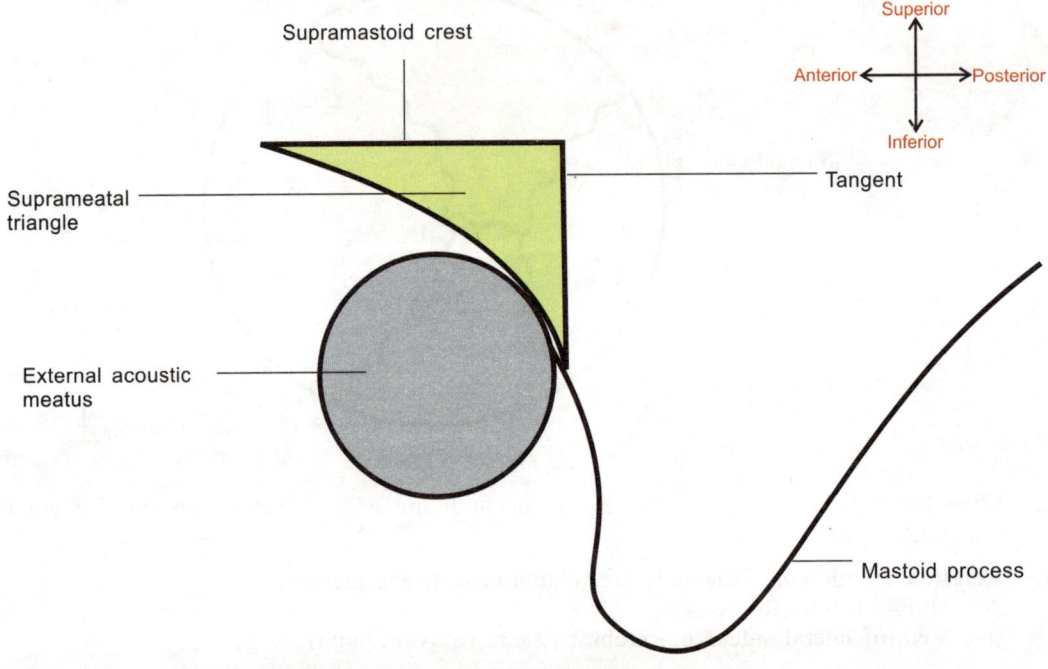

Fig 3.2 : Boundaries of suprameatal triangle.

LAQ-1   Mastoid process

(*Masts* breast, *oid* like)
It is a large projection from the lower part of mastoid part of temporal bone. It forms the lateral wall of the mastoid notch.

1. **Situation :** Posteroinferior part of external acoustic meatus.

2. **Development :** During second year and is usually better developed in men then in women.

3. **Attachments :** Following muscles are attached from before backwards.

    ⚷ SSC LC

A. Sternocleidomastoid,
B. Splenius capitis,
C. Longissimus capitis.

4. **Relations :**
   A. It is grooved on the deep aspect by digastric notch for the origin of posterior belly of digastric. Medial to the notch is a groove for the occipital artery.
   B. Stylomastoid foramen which transmits facial nerve and stylomastoid branch of posterior auricular artery.

5. **Applied anatomy :** Since mastoid process is not developed at birth and the external acoustic meatus is small, it results into exposure of facial nerve. This nerve is likely to get damaged during application of forceps at birth.

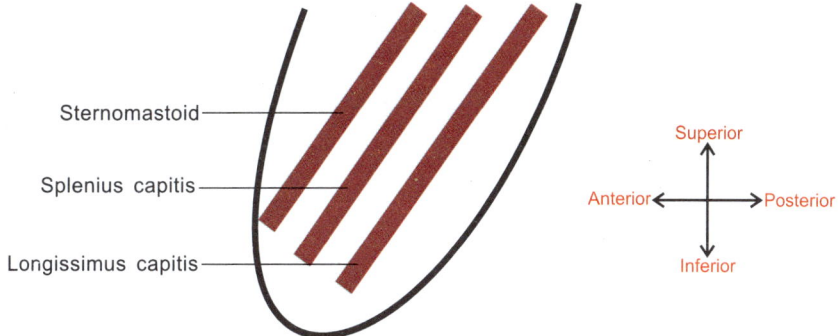

Fig. 3.3 : Muscles attached to the mastoid process.

SN-1   **Styloid process**   Imp

It is a long, slender and pointed bony process arises from temporal bone. It is directed downwards and forwards.

1. **Site :** It is present between external and internal carotid artery.

2. **Relations :**
   A. Medially - internal jugular vein.
   B. Laterally - parotid gland.

3. **Attachments :**

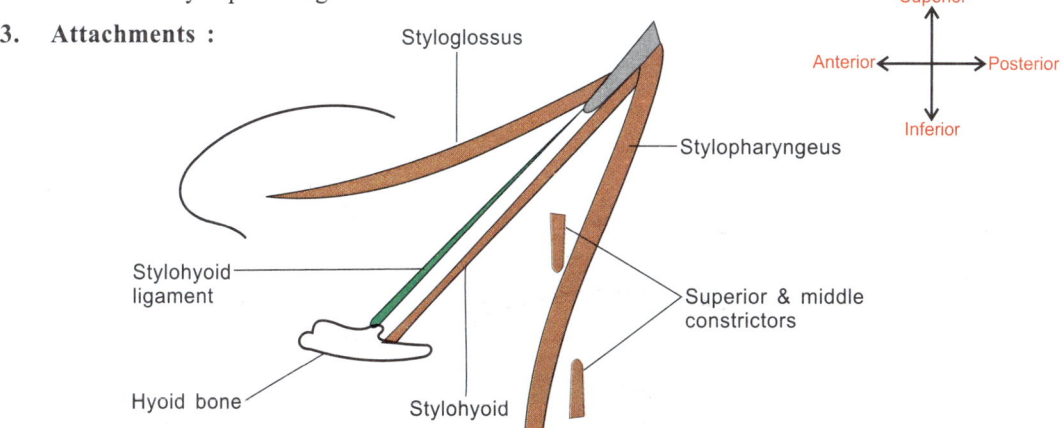

Fig. 3.4 : Attachments to styloid process.

Table 3.1 : Structures attached to styloid process and their nerve supply.

Parts of styloid process	Structure	Nerve supply
At the tip & anterior surface	Styloglossus muscle	Hypoglossal (XII)
Medial surface	Stylopharyngeus muscle	Glossopharyngeal (IX)
Posterior surface	Stylohyoid muscle	Facial nerve VII
Tip of styloid process & anterior surface	Stylomandibular ligament	------------
Tip of styloid process	Stylohyoid ligament	

LAQ-2   **Describe scalp under**
1. **Layers**   2. **Blood supply**
3. **Nerve supply &**   4. **Applied anatomy.**

1.   **Layers :** 🔑 **SCALP**

A.   **S**kin: Skin is hairy and contains plenty of sebaceous glands. It is adherent to the epicranial aponeurosis through the dense superficial fascia, as in the palms and soles.

B.   **C**onnective tissue (superficial fascia) : It is very dense and contains plenty of blood vessels and nerves. The cut vessels are not able to retract due to adherence of their wall with the dense connective tissue.

C.   **A**poneurosis (galea aponeurotica or epicranial aponeurosis) : This contains occipitofrontalis muscle. It has occipital and frontal belly. The occipital belly arises from external occipital protuberance and highest nuchal lines. The Frontal belly arises from epicranial aponeurosis and merges with the procerus, corrugator supercilli and orbicularis oculi. The direction of the fibers is antero posteriorly.

D.   **L**oose areolar tissue : It extends
   a.   Posteriorly from highest and superior nuchal lines,
   b.   Laterally from superior temporal lines and
   c.   Anteriorly into the eyelids.
   The fourth layer i.e. loose areolar tissue is called dangerous area of the scalp. The infection of this layer reaches dural venous sinuses through emissary veins.
   The bleeding in this layer results into black eye.

E.   **P**ericranium or periosteum : It is loosely attached to the surface of the bone and is firmly adherent to the sutures. Fluid collected in this layer takes the shape of underlying bone.

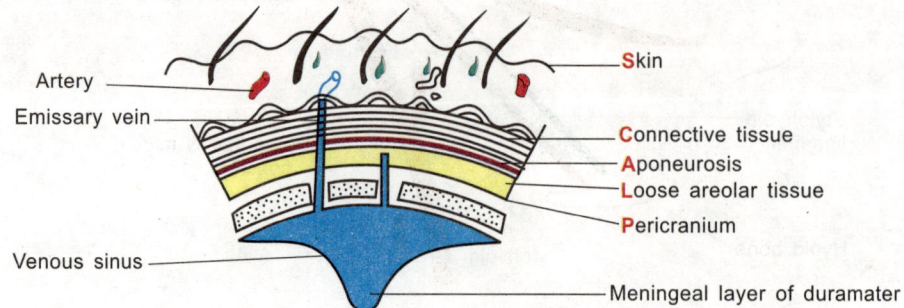

Fig. 3.5 : Layers of the scalp.

2. **Blood supply**
   A. Arterial supply:

Table 3.2 :

In front of auricle	Behind the auricle
a. Supratrochlear artery b. Supraorbital artery } Ophthalmic artery (internal carotid) c. Superficial temporal artery (External carotid artery)	a. Posterior auricular artery b. Occipital artery } External carotid artery

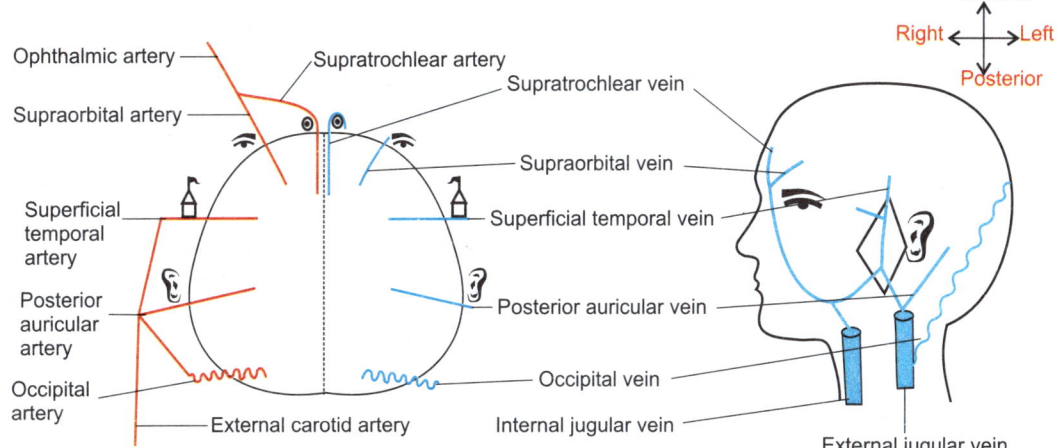

Fig. 3.6 : Arterial supply and venous drainage of scalp.

   B. Venous drainage :
      a. The supratrochlear vein joins with supraorbital vein and drains into angular vein. It continues as facial vein joins with anterior division of retromandibular vein and opens into common facial vein which drains into internal jugular vein.
      b. Superficial temporal vein joins with maxillary vein and drains into retromandibular vein. It divides into anterior and posterior divisions. The anterior division joins with the facial vein and drains into internal jugular vein and posterior division combines with the posterior auricular vein and drains into external jugular vein.
      c. Occipital vein drains into
         I. Suboccipital venous plexus which are connected by emissary veins or
         II. External jugular vein.

3. **Nerve supply :**
   A. Sensory :
      a. In front of auricle :
         I. Supraorbital and supra trochlear branches of ophthalmic division of trigeminal nerve.
         II. Zygomaticotemporal branch of zygomatic nerve which is a branch of maxillary division of trigeminal nerve.
         III. Auriculotemporal - mandibular division of trigeminal.

    b.   Behind the auricle   🔑   **GaLeO - Go To**
         I.   Posterior division of great auricular nerve. (Ventral rami of C_2 - C_3)
         II. **L**esser **O**ccipital nerve. Ventral rami of (C_2)
         III. **G**reater **O**ccipital nerve - dorsal ramus of C_2 nerve.
         IV. **T**hird **O**ccipital nerve - dorsal ramus C_3 nerve.

B. Motor
    a.   In front of the auricle : Temporal branch of facial nerve supplies frontal belly of occipito frontalis.
    b.   Behind the auricle : Posterior auricular branch of facial nerve supplies occipital belly of occipito frontalis.

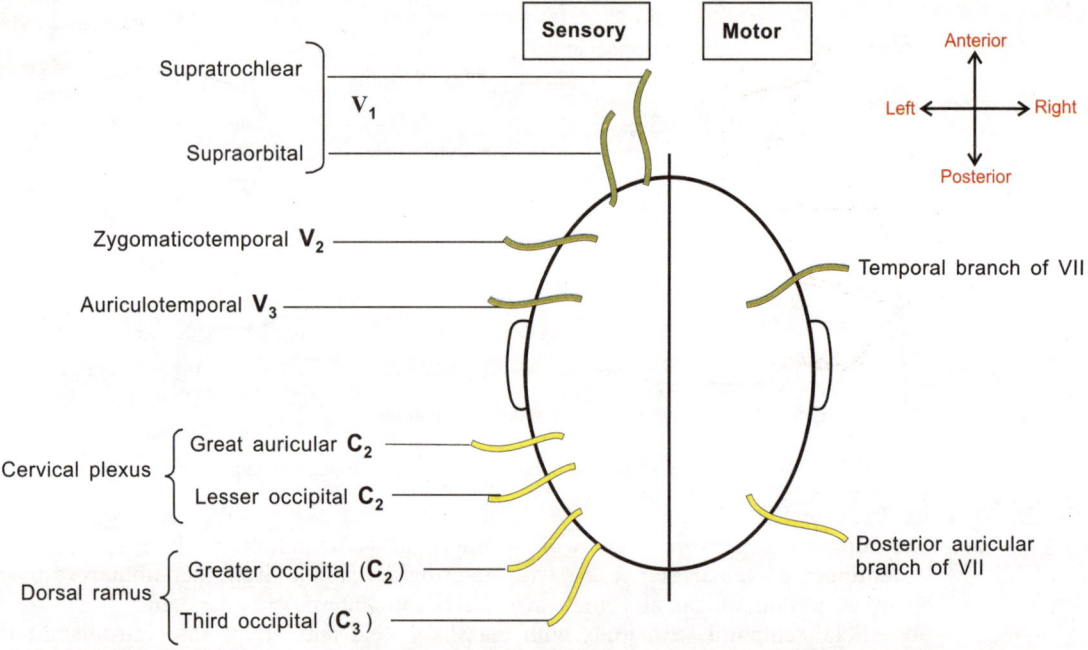

Fig. 3.7 : Sensory and motor supply of the scalp.

4. **Applied anatomy :**
    A. First layer : Skin is thick and hairy. It is the common site of sebaceous cyst.
    B. Second layer :
        a.   The bleeding in second layer is profuse. This is because of two reasons.
           I.   The scalp has rich blood supply (five arteries on each side),
           II. The torn vessels are prevented from constriction because the walls of the blood vessels are adherent to the dense connective tissue.
        b.   The bleeding can be immediately arrested by compressing against hard bone i.e. cranium.
    C. Third layer : The injury in anteroposterior direction heals fast. There is a delay in the healing of the transverse injury. Because the direction of the fibers of muscles is anteroposterior.

D. Fourth layer :
    a. *This is the dangerous area of scalp.* The infection from this layer spreads to the brain through emissary vein.
    b. Accumulation of blood and pus in this layer result in black eye.
E. Fifth layer : Bleeding in fifth layer takes the shape of underlying bone.

LAQ-3 Describe muscles of face under
1. Actions   2. Nerve supply &   3. Applied anatomy.

1. Actions : The muscles of facial expression can be grouped as
  A. Muscles acting on the orifice of the orbit : These are sub grouped as constrictor (sphincters) and dilators.
    a. The frontal belly of occipitofrontalis is responsible for elevation of eyebrows as in an expression of surprise and it also contracts in looking upwards. The action is antagonistic to the orbital part of orbicularis oculi.
    b. Corrugator supercilli drags the eyebrow medially and downward and protects the eye from bright sunlight. It produces vertical wrinkles of the forehead.
    c. Orbicularis oculi has three parts.
      I.   Palpebral part closes the eye gently as in sleep and blinking.
      II.   Orbital part closes the eye firmly as happens during a dust storm.
      III. Lacrimal part dilates the lacrimal sac.
  B. Muscle acting on the orifice of the nose, these are
    a. Procerus produces transverse wrinkles across bridge of nose as in frowning.
    b. Nasalis has two parts.
      I.   Transverse part called as compressor naris. It compresses nasal aperture.
      II.   Alar part called dilator naris. It dilates the anterior nasal aperture in deep inspiration.
      III. Depressor septa dilates anterior nasal aperture in anger.

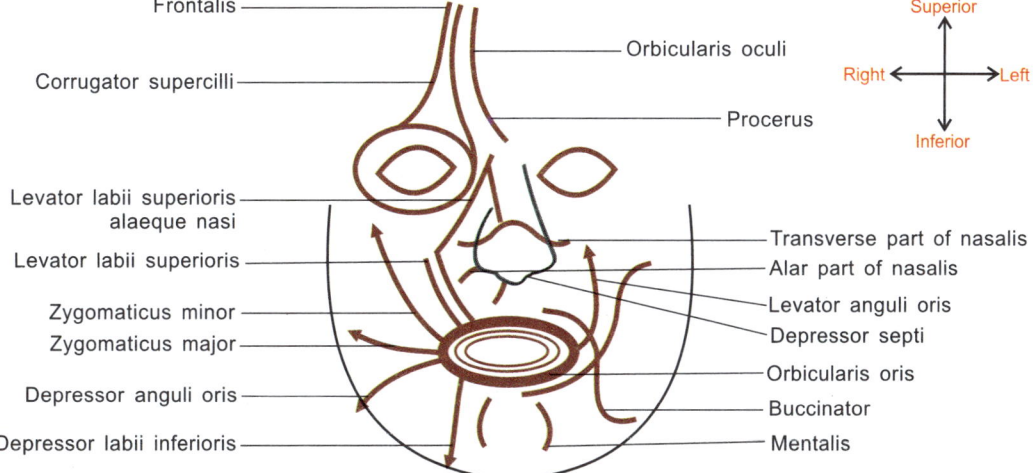

Fig. 3.8 : Muscles of the face.

Table 3.3 : The table shows muscles acting on openings of the face.

Openings	Constrictor (sphincter)	Dilator
A. Eyelid	a. Orbicularis oculi b. Corrugator supercilli	a. Levator palpebrae superioris b. Frontal belly of occipito Frontalis
B. Lacrimal sac	–	Lacrimal part of orbicularis oculi
C. Anterior nasal aperature	–	a. Alar part of nasalis. b. Depressor septi. c. Levator labii superioris alaeque nasi
D. Upper lip	Orbicularis oris	a. Levator labii superioris b. Levator labii superioris alaeque nasi c. Zygomaticus minor d. Levator anguli oris.
E. Angle of mouth	Depressor anguli oris	a. Zygomaticus major.

C.　Muscles acting on the orifice of the mouth can be grouped as
　　a.　Sphincter : Orbicularis oris closes the mouth
　　b.　Dilators :
　　　　I.　Subcutaneous layer : Risorius (risus, to laugh).
　　　　II.　Superficial layer :
　　　　　　i.　Zygomaticus major draws the angle of mouth upward and laterally as in laughing.
　　　　　　ii.　Zygomaticus minor elevates and everts upper lip.
　　　　　　iii.　Levator labii superioris alaeque nasi elevates and everts the upper lip & dilates the nostril.
　　　　III.　Middle layer
　　　　　　i.　Depressor anguli oris draws the angle of mouth downward.
　　　　　　ii.　Levator anguli oris
　　　　　　iii.　Depressor labii inferiors draws angle of mouth downward and somewhat laterally as in expression of irony.
　　　　　　iv.　Levator labii superioris elevates the lip.
　　　　IV.　Deeper layer
　　　　　　i.　Mentalis protrudes the lower lip.
　　　　　　ii.　Buccinator flattens the cheek and forcibly expels the air between the lips.

2.　**Nerve supply** : The muscles of the face are developed from second pharyngeal arch and the nerve of the second pharyngeal arch is facial nerve. Hence all the muscles are supplied by facial nerve.

3.   Applied anatomy :

Table 3.3 : The table shows difference between upper motor and lower motor neuron lesion

Particulars	Upper motor neuron lesion	Lower motor neuron lesion
A. Synonym	a. Supra nuclear facial palsy.	a. Infra nuclear facial palsy. e.g. Bell's palsy.
B. Site of lesion	b. Above the facial nerve nucleus i.e. corticonuclear fibers.	b. Below the facial nerve nucleus i.e. facial nerve.
C. Muscles paralysed	c. Contralateral muscles of lower half of face are paralysed.	c. Ipsilateral muscles of the whole face are paralysed.
D. Clinical features	d. Clinical features on the opposite side of lesion. I. Facial asymmetry II. Inability of angle of mouth to move upwards III. Loss of nasolabial fold IV. Accumulation of food in the vestibule of the mouth. V. Dribbling of saliva VI. Inability to inflate the cheek laterally.	d. Clinical features on the side of paralysis. I. Facial asymmetry. II. Loss of wrinkles on forehead. III. Inability to close eye. IV. Inability of angle of mouth to move upwards. V. Loss of nasolabial fold. VI. Accumulation of food in the vestibule of the mouth. VII. Dribbling of saliva. VIII. Inability to inflate the cheek laterally.

SN-2   # Sensory nerve supply of the face

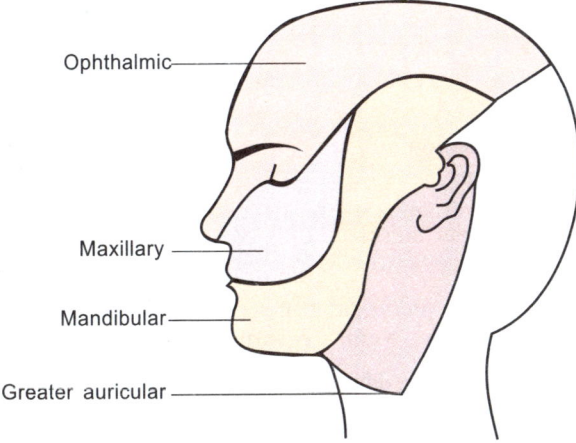

Ophthalmic

Maxillary

Mandibular

Greater auricular

Fig. 3.9 : Sensory nerve supply of the face.

Table 3.4 : The table shows cutaneous nerve supply of the face.

Source	Cutaneous nerve	Area of distribution
1. Ophthalmic division of Trigeminal nerve	A. Supratrochlear nerve B. Supraorbital nerve C. Lacrimal nerve D. Infratrochlear nerve E. External nasal nerve	Scalp up to vertex, Forehead; Upper eyelid; Conjunctiva; and Root, dorsum and tip of nose.
2. Maxillary division of trigeminal nerve	A. Infraorbital nerve B. Zygomaticofacial nerve C. Zygomaticotemporal nerve	Upper lip; Side and ala of nose; lower eyelid; upper part of cheek; and anterior part of temple.
3. Mandibular division of trigeminal nerve	A. Auriculotemporal nerve B. Buccal nerve C. Mental nerve	Lower lip; chin; lower part of cheek; Lower jaw except over the angle and Lower margin; upper $2/3^{rd}$ of lateral surface of auricle; and side of head.
4. Cervical plexus	A. Anterior division of great auricular nerve $(C_{2, 3})$. B. Upper division of transverse (anterior) cutaneous nerve of neck $(C_{2, 3})$.	Skin over the angle of the jaw and over the parotid gland. Lower margin of the lower jaw.

SN-3　　　Dangerous area of face

1. **Introduction :** The embolus arising from dangerous area of the face causes serious complication of muscles of eyeball.

2. **Site :** 🔑　　**USA**
   A. **U**pper lip.
   B. **S**eptum of nose.
   C. **A**djoining area of cheeks.

3. **Reasons** facilitating thrombus formation.
   A. Absence of deep fascia in face,
   B. Absence of valves in facial vein and
   C. Facial vein lies directly on facial muscles.

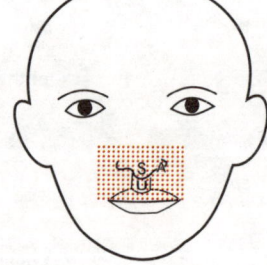

Fig. 3.10 : Dangerous area of the face.

4. **Communications :**
   A. Deep facial vein -- facial vein – pterygoid venous plexus -- cavernous sinus.
   B. Angular vein -- superior ophthalmic vein – cavernous sinus.

5. **Applied anatomy :** The infection of the dangerous area of the face leads to cavernous sinus thrombosis. The embolus compresses cranial nerves present in the cavernous sinus and results into paralysis of the muscles of the eyeball.

LAQ-4 Describe lacrimal apparatus under
1. Components 2. Blood supply
3. Nerve supply and 4. Applied anatomy.

1. **Components or parts :**
   A. Lacrimal gland with ducts

   Table 3.5 : The table shows details of orbital and palpebral part of lacrimal gland.

Particulars	a. Orbital	b. Palpebral
Situation	Medial surface of frontal process of zygomatic bone	Below levator palpebrae superioris
Shape	Almond	Flat
No. of ducts	4 - 5	8

   c. **Functions :** 🔑 **TEARS**
   I. Maintains **T**ransparency of cornea,
   II. **E**xpresses emotion,
   III. **A**cts as bactericidal,
   IV. **R**enders nourishment to cornea,
   V. Keeps the **s**urface moist.
   B. Conjunctiva :
   a. Gross features :
   It is transparent mucous membrane covering sclara and lining the inner surface of eyelid.
   Conjunctival sac : It is a potential space between eyelid & eyeball, consists of
   I. Orbital part which is in contact with the sclera.

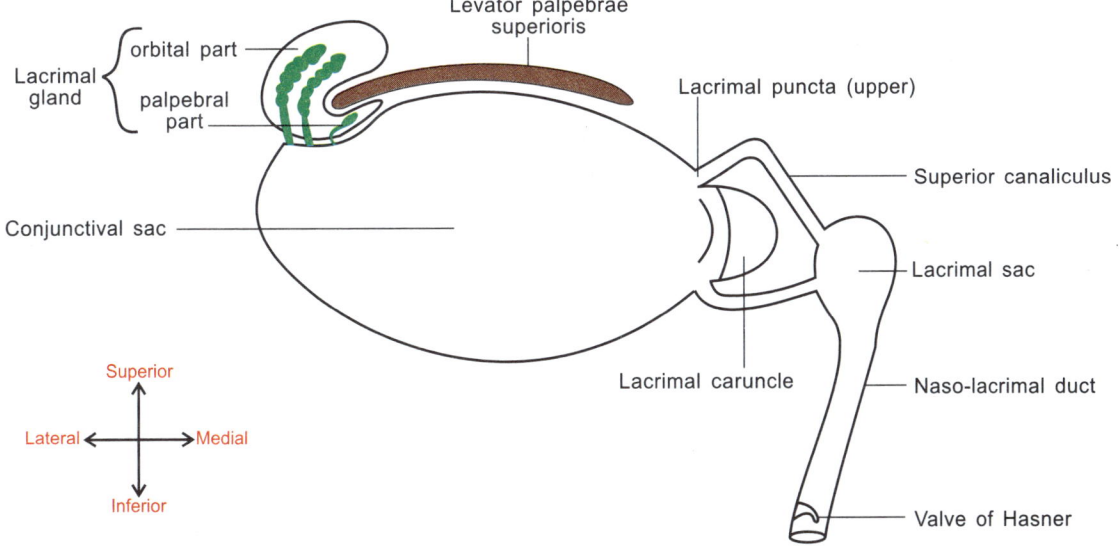

Fig. 3.11 : Lacrimal apparatus.

      II. Palpebral part : It is highly vascular, adherent to tarsal plate. It lines the eyelid.
- b. Nerve supply :
  - I. Ophthalmic division of trigeminal nerve.
  - II. Maxillary division of trigeminal nerve.
- c. Blood supply : Palpebral branch of ophthalmic artery.

C. Puncta with lacrimal canaliculi: Each lacrimal canaliculus begins with punctum.
- a. Length of canaliculus :   10 mm.
  - Vertical - 2 mm
  - Horizontal - 8 mm
- b. It is lined by stratified squamous non-keratinized epithelium.
  - It opens in the lateral wall of lacrimal sac behind medial palpebral ligament.

D. Lacrimal sac :   It is membranous part continues with nasolacrimal duct. It is blind pouch measuring 12 x 5mm.

Relations of lacrimal sac :
- a. Anterior :
  - I. Medial palpebral ligament.
  - II. Orbicularis oculi muscle.
- b. Medially: Lacrimal groove.
- c. Laterally: Lacrimal fascia and lacrimal part of orbicularis oculi.

E. Nasolacrimal duct : It is a membranous passage of 18 mm long. It runs from the lower end of lacrimal sac & opens in the inferior meatus of nose. The lower end of the duct is guarded by valve of Hasner. It prevents backward flow of fluid.

2. Blood supply : Lacrimal branch of ophthalmic artery.

3. Nerve supply :
A. Sensory : Lacrimal branch of ophthalmic division of trigeminal nerve.
B. Sympathetic :
- a. Preganglionic fibers arise from spinal cord (T_1 - T_5 segment) and goes to superior cervical sympathetic ganglion.
- b. Post ganglionic fibers are the plexus around internal carotid artery and around ophthalmic artery.

C. Parasympathetic nerve carries secretomotor fibers.
- a. Preganglionic fibers arise from lacrimatory nucleus present in the pons pass via facial nerve ⟶ greater petrosal nerve and joins with deep petrosal nerve to form nerve to pterygoid canal ⟶ **pterygopalatine ganglion** ⟶ relay ⟶
- b. Postganglionic fibers by maxillary nerve - (zygomatico temporal) – lacrimal nerve - lacrimal gland.

4. Applied anatomy :
A. Dacryoadenitis (*Dacryo* tear) - It is the inflammation of lacrimal gland.
B. Inflammation of lacrimal sac is known as dacryocystitis and presents with pain, oedema and redness.
C. Dacryocystectomy is removal of lacrimal sac.
D. Removal of palpebral part is equal to the removal of entire gland because the ducts of the orbital part passes through palpebral part.
E. Epiphora (*Epiphora* sudden burst) - overflow of tears.

| **LAQ-5** | **Describe investing layer of deep cervical fascia under**
1. Attachments 2. Features & 3. Applied anatomy. |

It is deep fascia of neck, lies deep to platysma and surrounds the neck like a collar.

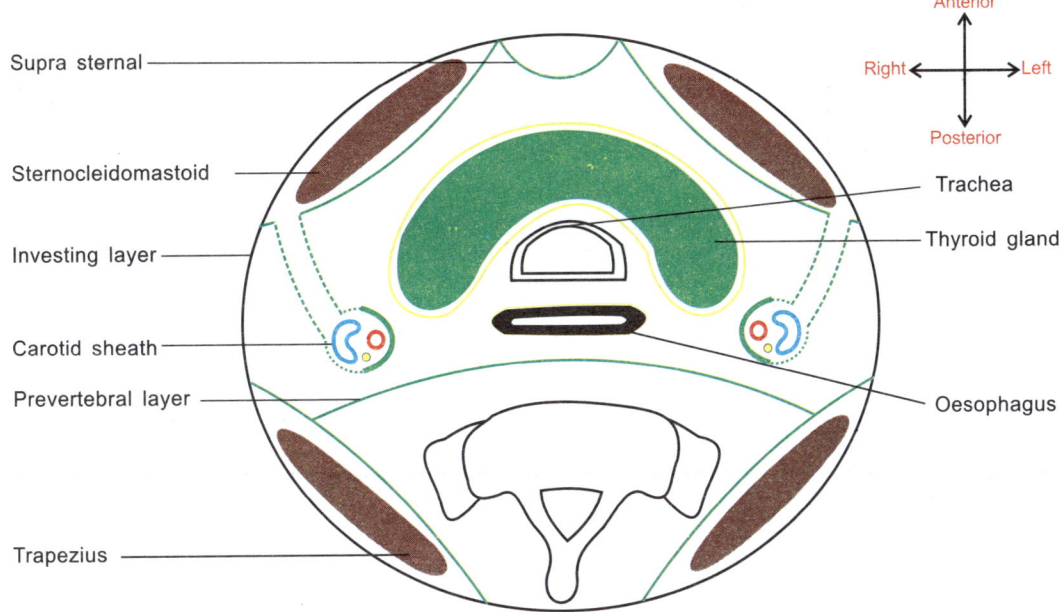

Fig. 3.12 : Investing layers of the deep cervical fascia.

1. **Attachments :**
   A. Superiorly
       a. External occipital protuberance.
       b. Superior nuchal line.
       c. Mastoid process.
       d. Base of mandible &
       e. It splits to enclose parotid between the angle of mandible and mastoid process.
   B. Inferiorly
       a. Spine of scapula.
       b. Acromion process.
       c. Clavicle.
       d. Manubrium.
   C. Anteriorly
       a. Symphysis menti.
       b. Hyoid bone.
       c. Oblique line of thyroid cartilage.

2. **Features**
   A. Thickness - varies
       a. Thick over parotid gland, called parotid fascia.
       b. Thick between styloid process and angle of mandible (stylomandibular ligament).
       c. Thin on styloid process, mandible & tympanic plate.

B. Magic of two. 🔑 "2"
   a. Encloses **2** muscles : Trapezius & sternocleidomastoid.
   b. Encloses **2** glands : Parotid & submandibular.
   c. Forms **2** laminae : Pretracheal & prevertebral.
   d. Forms roof of **2** triangles :
      I. Anterior &
      II. Posterior.
   e. Forms **2** spaces : Suprasternal and supraclavicular.
   f. Forms **2** structures : Stylomandibular ligament & parotidomassetric fascia.
   g. Forms **2** slings : Intermediate tendon of digastric & omohyoid.

3. **Applied anatomy :**
   A. Ludwigs angina : It is a triangular swelling due to infection in the submandibular region. It is limited laterally by two halves of mandible and posteriorly by hyoid bone. This is because of the attachments of investing layer of deep cervical fascia to the base of mandible and hyoid bone.
   B. Collar stud abscess : The deep cervical lymph nodes are the sites of tuberculous infection. The lymph node caseates and the abscess is formed. It penetrates the deep fascia and forms a swelling under the skin.
   C. Mumps : Infection of parotid gland is painful due to thick & strong fascia covering it.

SN-4   Pretracheal fascia

The condensed deep fascia in front of trachea is called pretracheal fascia.

1. **Attachments :**
   A. Superiorly :
      a. Hyoid bone in the median plane,
      b. Oblique line of thyroid cartilage and
      c. Cricoid cartilage, more laterally.
   B. Inferiorly :
      Below the thyroid gland it encloses the inferior thyroid veins, passes behind the brachiocephalic veins, and finally blends with the arch of the aorta.
   C. On either side it fuses with the front of the carotid sheath deep to the sternomastoid.

2. **Other features :**
   A. On either side it sends a septa which connects the thyroid gland and forms a supensory ligament of the thyroid gland and is called ligament of Berry.
   B. The ligaments are attached chiefly to the cricoid cartilage and may extend to the thyroid cartilage.
   C. It supports the thyroid gland and do not let it sink into the mediastinum.
   D. The capsule of the thyroid gland is very weak along the posterior borders of the lateral lobes. Hence the thyroid gland can enlarge posteriorly and compress oesophagus and produces dysphagia.

3. **Functions :**
   A. The fascia provides a slippery surface for free movements of the trachea during swallowing.
   B. It forms neurovascular sheath to carotid vessels.

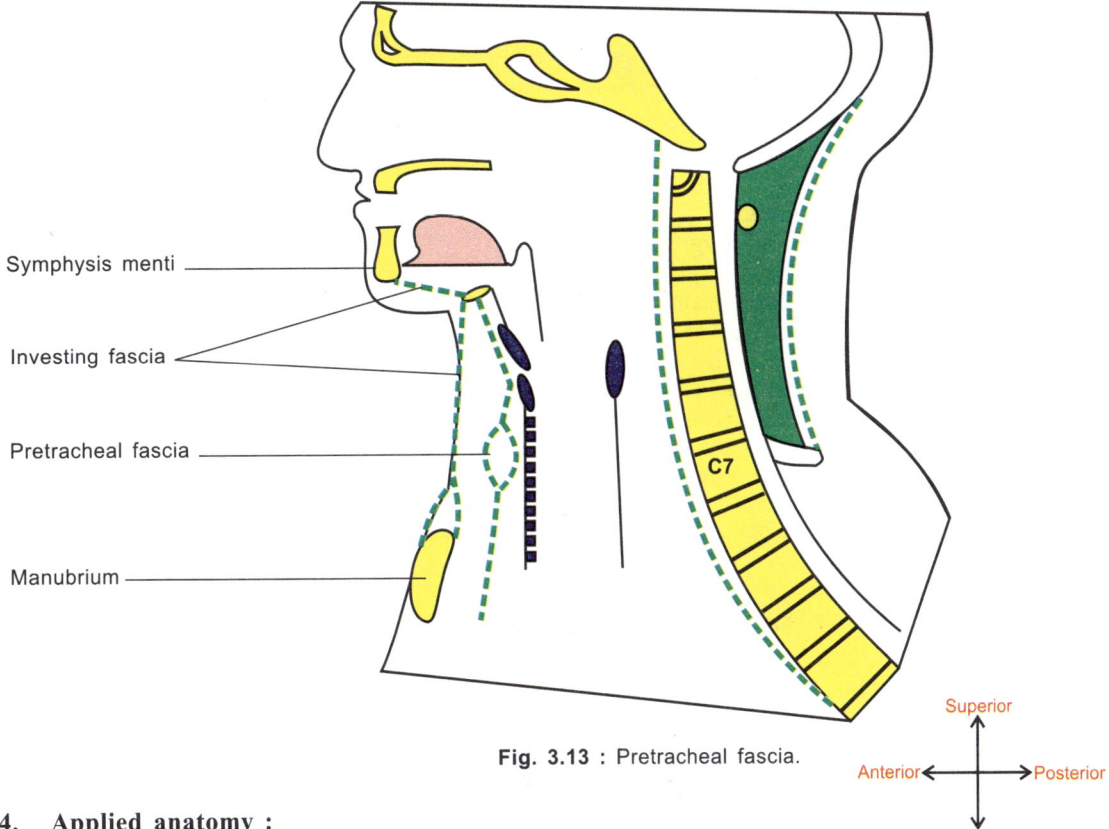

Symphysis menti

Investing fascia

Pretracheal fascia

C7

Manubrium

Superior

Anterior ← → Posterior

Inferior

Fig. 3.13 : Pretracheal fascia.

4. **Applied anatomy :**
    A. Tumors arising from thyroid gland move with degluttination.
    B. The abscess present in front of pretracheal fascia descends in the superior mediastinum.
    C. The abscess present behind the pretracheal fascia descends in the superior mediastinum, to the posterior mediastinum.

SN-5   Ludwigs angina

1. **Introduction :** It is a cellulitis of the floor of the mouth.

2. **Anatomy :** It is limited laterally by two halves of mandible and posteriorly by hyoid bone. This is because of the attachments of investing layer of deep cervical fascia to the base of mandible and hyoid bone.

3. **Site :** A swelling appears below the chin and inside the mouth. It is deep to mylohyoid.

4. **Cause :** It is usually secondary to caries of molar tooth.

5. **Complications :** If infection spreads backwards, it causes oedema of glottis. It may result into asphyxia.

6. **Applied anatomy :** The abscess is drained by a deep incision below the mandible by dividing the mylohyoid muscle.

SN-5   Prevertebral fascia

It is a deep fascia of neck, present in front or anterior to the cervical vertebrae. It forms the floor of the posterior triangle of neck.

1. **Attachments :**
   A. Superiorly : Base of skull.
   B. Inferiorly : Anterior longitudinal ligament of body of third and fourth thoracic vertebrae.
   C. Anteriorly : Retropharyngeal space.
   D. Laterally : Gets lost deep to trapezius.

2. **Features :**
   A. Cervical and brachial plexuses lie behind the prevertebral fascia.
   B. It forms axillary sheath (Cervico axillary canal).
   C. It does not invest subclavian or axillary vein. This lie in loose areolar tissue, free to dilate during increased venous return.

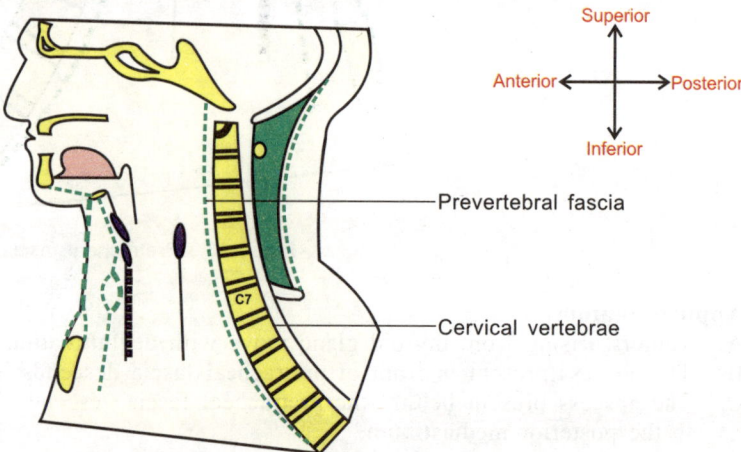

Fig. 3.14 : Prevertebral fascia.

3. **Structures piercing :**
   A. Great auricular nerve.
   B. Lesser occipital nerve.
   C. Transverse cervical and
   D. Supraclavicular nerves.
   } Cutaneous branches of cervical plexus.

4. **Relations :**
   A. Superficial
      a. Accessory nerve.
      b. Lymph nodes of posterior triangle.
   B. Deep :
      a. Muscles forming floor of triangle.
      b. Cervical plexus.
      c. Trunks of brachial plexus.
      d. Third part of subclavian artery.

5. **Functions :** To provide a fix base for gliding movements of pharynx, oesophagus and carotid sheath during movements of neck and during swallowing.

6. **Applied anatomy :**
    A. The abscess formed behind the prevertebral fascia travel down into superior mediastinum upto T_3 -T_4.
    B. The abscess formed infront of prevertebral fascia travel to superior mediastinum and then the posterior mediastinum.

SN-6   Carotid sheath

It is a condensation of deep cervical fascia around carotid vessels and internal jugular vein.

1. **Extent :** It extends from base of skull to the arch of the aorta.

2. **Formation :**
    A. Anterior wall is formed by pretracheal fascia.
    B. Posterior wall is formed by prevertebral fascia.

3. **Thickness :** It is thick around artery and thin around vein to allow free expansion of vein during increased venous return.

4. **Relations :**
    A. Anteriorly, ansa cervicalis is present within the wall or sheath.
    B. Posteriorly, sympathetic trunk is present behind the sheath.

5. **Contents :**
    A. Internal and common carotid arteries.
    B. Internal jugular vein.
    C. Vagus nerve.

6. **Applied anatomy :** It is frequently exposed in block dissection of the neck during surgical removal of deep cervical lymph nodes.

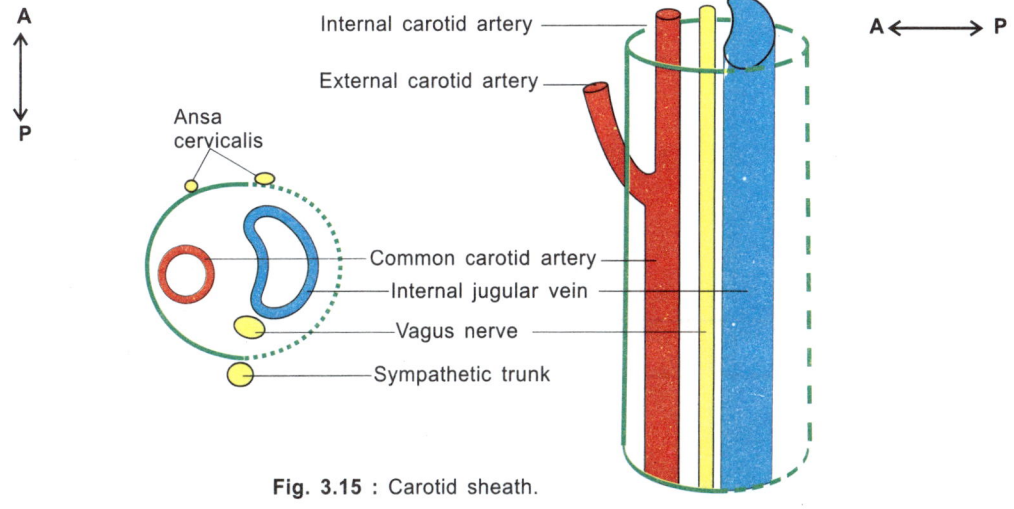

Fig. 3.15 : Carotid sheath.

LAQ-6   **Describe posterior triangle under**
1. Boundaries   2. Roof   3. Floor
4. Contents and   5. Applied anatomy.

1. **Boundaries** :
   A. Anteriorly : Posterior border of sternocleido-mastoid.
   B. Posteriorly : Anterior border of trapezius.
   C. Base : Middle third of clavicle.
   D. Apex : Meeting point of sternocleidomastoid and trapezius at superior nuchal line.

2. **Roof** :
   A. Skin.
   B. Superficial fascia.
   C. Investing layer of deep cervical fascia.
   D. Roof is pierced by -
      a. Nerves
         I. Lesser occipital,
         II. Great auricular,
         III. Transverse cutaneous nerve of neck,
         IV. Supraclavicular nerves.

      b. Veins : External jugular vein and its tributaries.
      c. Lymph vessels.

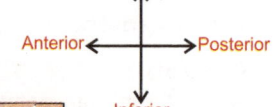

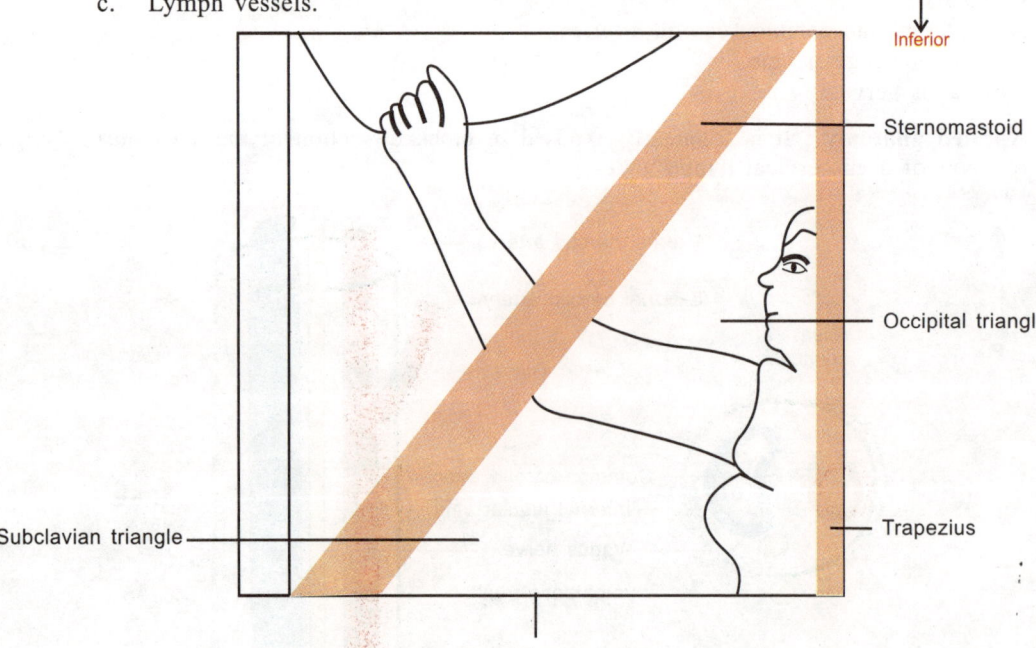

Fig. 3.16 : Boundaries of anterior and posterior triangle.

3. **Floor :** Mainly formed by second layer of muscles of neck (above downwards)
    A. Splenius capitis;
    B. Levator scapulae;
    C. Occasionally by semispinalis capitis at apex;
    D. Scalenus medius;
    E. Scalenus posterior;
    F. Muscular floor is carpeted by prevertebral fascia.

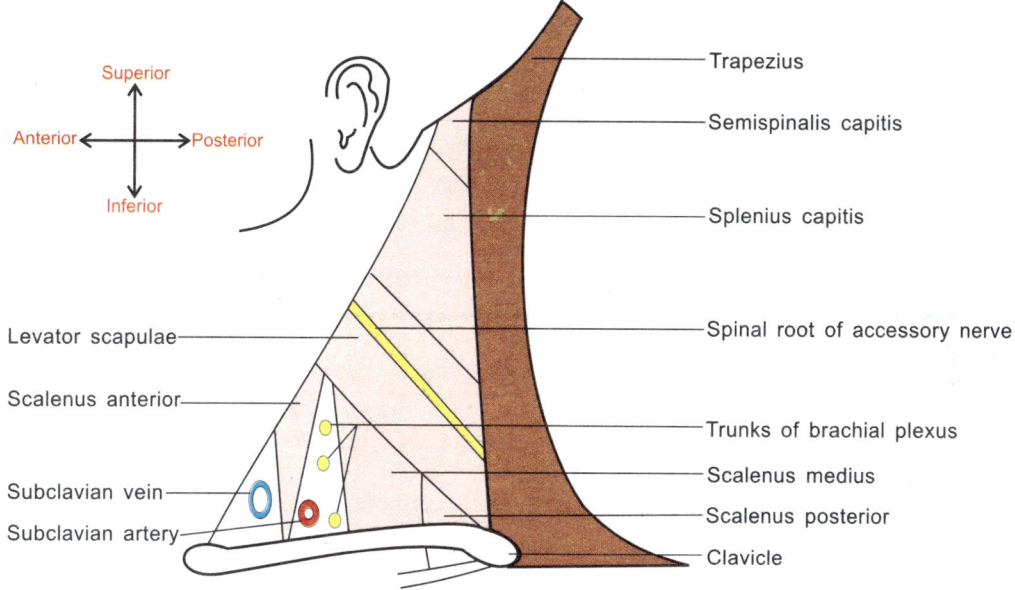

Fig. 3.17 : Floor and contents of the posterior triangle

4. **Contents :** *The spinal accessory nerve and the lymph nodes are the true contents of the posterior triangle and all others are behind or infront of the fascial floor.*
    A. Muscle - Inferior belly of omohyoid
    B. Nerves   **ABC**
        a. **A**ccessory nerve.
        b. Roots, trunks of **b**rachial plexus and their **b**ranches.
            I.   Nerve to rhomboideus.
            II.   Nerve to serratus anterior.
            III. Nerve to subclavius.
            IV.   Suprascapular nerve.
        c. **C**ervical nerves :
            I.   Greater occipital nerve emerges from the apex to pass on the scalp.
            II.   Great auricular nerve.
            III. Lesser occipital nerve.
            IV.   Transverse cervical nerve of neck.
            V.   Supraclavicular nerve.
            Third and fourth cervical nerves supplying trapezius.
    C. Arteries :
        a. Occipital artery emerges from the apex.

   b.   Third part of subclavian artery and branches of subclavian artery.
        I.   Suprascapular   }   Branches of thyrocervical
        II.   Transverse cervical   trunk (1st part of subclavian).
             Transverse cervical artery divides into ascending and descending branch at anterior border of sternocleidomastoid.
   c.   Veins : External jugular vein and its tributaries. Sabclavian vein is lower down and not included in the triangle.
   d.   Lymph nodes -
        I.   Supraclavicular lymph nodes are present along the posterior border of sternomastoid.
        II.   Occipital lymph nodes.

5. **Applied anatomy :**
   A.   Left supraclavicular (Virchow's) lymph nodes are enlarged in malignancy of testis, stomach and other abdominal organs.
   B.   The pressure in the external jugular vein can be recorded in the recumbent position. It is increased in right sided heart failure and in the obstruction of the superior vena cava.
   C.   The retropharyngeal abscess may be expressed in the lower part of posterior triangle.

SAQ-3   Great auricular nerve

1. **Root value :** Ventral ramus of C_2 & C_3 (branches for cervical plexus). C_2 is more important.
    A large trunk passing obliquely upwards over sternocleidomastoid.

2. **Distribution :**
   A.   Skin over angle of mandible.
   B.   Skin over parotid gland.
   C.   Parotid fascia.
   D.   Skin of the lower and lateral surface of ear lobule.
   E.   Skin over mastoid region.

3. **Applied anatomy :** It is palpable and visibly thickened in tuberculoid leprosy.

SN-7   Sternocleidomastoid

Table 3.6 : The table shows the origin and insertion of different parts of sternocleidomastoid.

Particulars	Origin	Insertion
A. Sterno-occipital	Upper part of manubrium sternum.	Lateral two third of superior nuchal line of occipital bone.
B. Sternomastoid		Mastoid process.
C. Cleidomastoid	Upper part of medial surface of clavicle.	Mastoid process.
D. Cleidooccipitalis		Lateral 2/3rd of superior nuchal line of occipital bone.

3. **Relations :**
   A. Superficial - skin containing
      a. Cutaneous nerve -
         I. Great auricular,
         II. Transverse cervical &
         III. Medial supraclavicular.
      b. Vein : External jugular vein
   B. Deep

Table 3.7 : The table shows relations of sternocleidomastoid at different levels.

Structure	At origin	In the middle	At insertion
Muscles	Sternohyoid, Sternothyroid, Omohyoid.	Scalenus medius, Scalenus posterior, Levator scapulae, Splenius capitis, Inferior belly of omohyoid	Splenius capitis, Longus capitis, Posterior belly of digastric. } Deep muscles of neck
Vessels	Anterior jugular vein	Common carotid artery.	Occipital artery.
Nerve	–	Cervical plexus, Brachial plexus, X, XII nerve, Inferior root of ansa cervicalis.	–
Glands	–	Thyroid, lymph node.	–

4. **Nerve supply :**
   A. Motor : Spinal root of accessory nerve (XI - cranial nerve).
   B. Proprioceptive : Second and third ventral rami of cervical spinal nerve.

5. **Action :**
   A. The chief purpose of the muscle is to protract the head (it is a combination of flexion of cervical spine and extension of atlantoaxial joint simultaneously).
   B. *Its contraction tilts the head towards the same side of shoulder and turns the face towards the opposite side.*

6. **Testing of the muscle :**
   A. The face is turned to the opposite side against resistance and the muscle of one side is palpated.
   B. The chin is bent downwards to test the sternocleidomastoid of both sides.

7. **Applied anatomy :**
   A. Congenital torticolis : During difficult labour, undue pulling of the head of the baby causes tearing of the fibers of the sternocleidomastoid. The subsequent fibrosis and contracture is called congenital torticolis.
   B. Torticolis : It is a deformity in which the head is bent to one side (to the side of paralysis) and the chin points towards the opposite side of lesion.

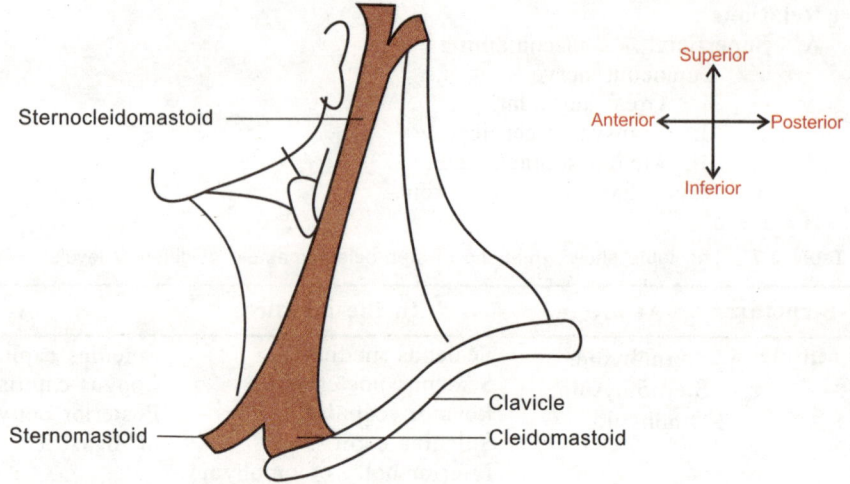

Fig. 3.18 : Origin and insertion of sternocleidomastoid.

LAQ-7	Describe suboccipital triangle under

Describe suboccipital triangle under
1. **Boundaries**   2. **Roof**   3. **Floor**
4. **Contents and**   5. **Applied anatomy.**

1. **Boundaries :**

   A. **Superolaterally :** Superior oblique extends from the back of lateral mass of the atlas to the lateral part of occipital bone between superior and inferior nuchal line.

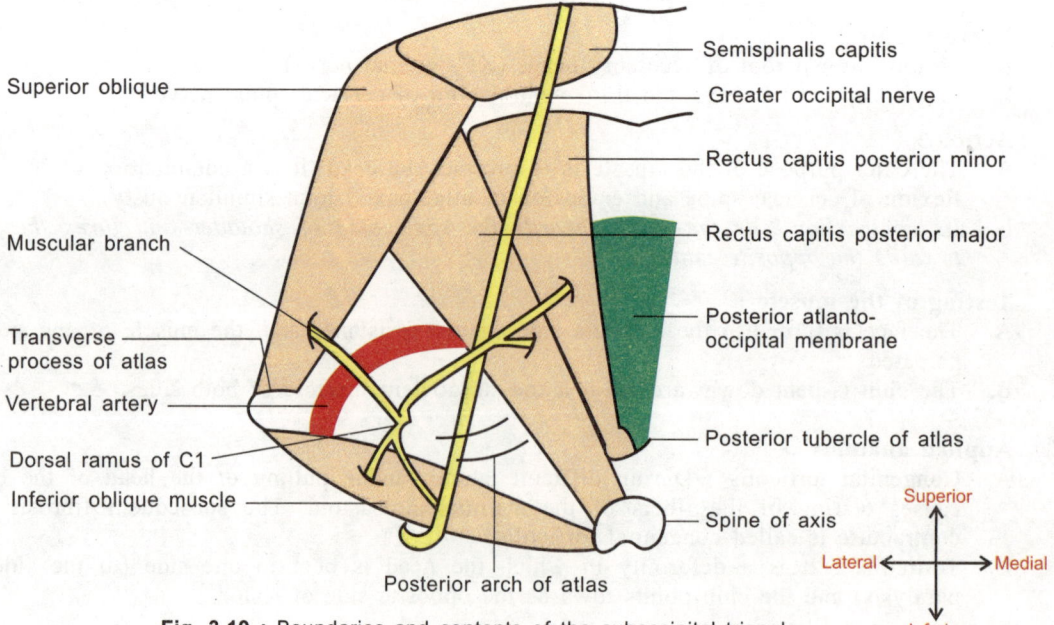

Fig. 3.19 : Boundaries and contents of the suboccipital triangle.

B. Superomedially :
   a. Rectus capitis posterior major is badly named. It is not vertical. It arises from outer surface of the bifid spinous process of the second cervical vertebra and is attached to the lateral part of area below inferior nuchal line. It extends and rotates the head toward the same side.
   b. Rectus capitis posterior minor is the only muscle attached to the posterior arch of atlas. It arises from small fossa near the midline and passes vertically upwards to be inserted into the medial part of the area below the inferior nuchal line. It extends the head.
C. Inferiorly : Oblique capitis inferior is attached between the outer surface of bifid spine of the axis and back of the lateral mass of the atlas.

2. **Floor :**
   A. Posterior arch of the atlas and
   B. Posterior atlanto-occipital membrane.

3. **Roof :** It is formed by semispinalis capitis medially and longissimus capitis laterally. Both muscles are separated by dense fibrous tissue. The structures crossing the roof are
   A. Greater occipital nerve which crosses infero-medially.
   B. Occipital artery which crosses supero-laterally.

4. **Contents :**
   A. Third part of vertebral artery runs across the floor of the triangle.
   B. Dorsal ramus of first cervical nerve (suboccipital nerve) and its muscular branches emerges through the floor of suboccipital triangle.
   C. Suboccipital venous plexus.
   D. Lymphatic plexus.
   E. Fibrofatty tissue.

5. **Applied anatomy:**
   A. Neck rigidity is important sign of meningitis. It is due to spasm of extensor muscles, caused by irritation of nerve roots, present in the sub-arachnoid space.
   B. Cisternal puncture is done through sub-occipital triangle to collect CSF from cisterna-magna. The needle is introduced just above the spine of axis in forward and upward direction.
   C. Posterior cranial fossa can be approached through sub-occipital triangle.

| SN-8 | **Greater occipital nerve** |

1. **Introduction :** Large medial branch of dorsal ramus of C_2.

2. **Root value :** Dorsal ramus of C_2.

3. **Peculiarities :** *Thickest cutaneous nerve of body.*

4. **Distribution :**
   A. Sensory : Skin of scalp over posterior part of ear.
   B. Motor : Semispinalis capitis.

5. **Course and relations :**
   A. Crosses suboccipital triangle.
   B. Pierces semispinalis capitis & trapezius.

C. Runs on back of head & reaches vertex.

6. **Applied anatomy :** In meningitis neck rigidity is caused due to irritation of nerve root.

SAQ-4   External jugular vein

1. **Formation :** External jugular vein is formed by posterior division of retromandibular and posterior auricular vein.

2. **Site :** It begins just below the angle of the mandible or within the parotid gland.

3. **Structures pierced :** It pierces the deep fascia above the clavicle.

4. **Termination :** It drains into subclavian vein behind clavicle.

5. **Peculiarity :** *It is provided with valves.*

6. **Applied anatomy :** It pierces deep fascia above the clavicle to drain into subclavian vein. Its lumen is held open by the deep fascia which is attached to its margin. The air ucked into the lumen of external jugular vein during inspiration produces air mbolism which is a fatal condition.

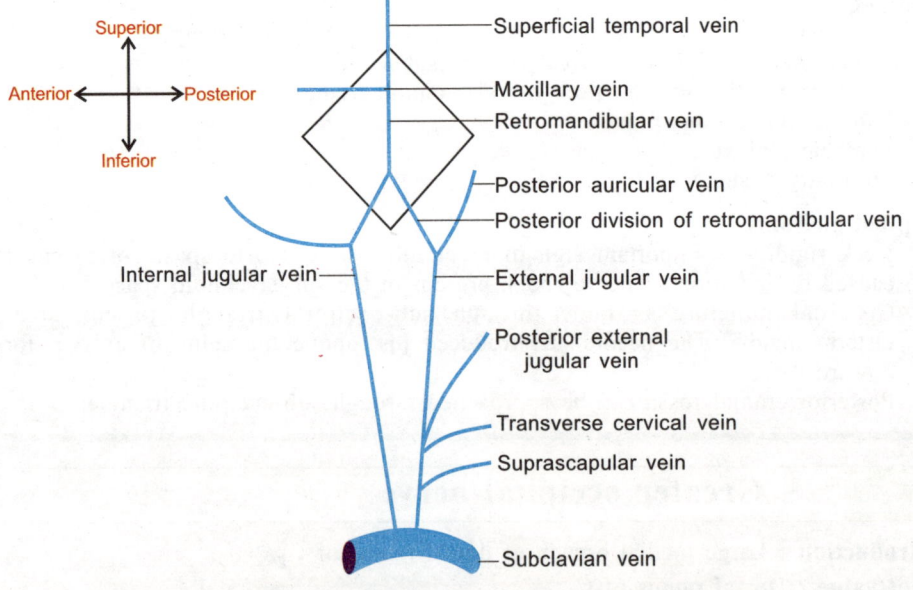

Fig. 3.20 : External jugular vein and its tributaries.

LAQ-8   Describe vertebral artery under
       1.   Origin   2.   Branches and distribution
       3.   Relations and   4.   Applied anatomy.

1. **Origin :** It is a first branch of first part of subclavian artery. It is the largest branch of subclavian artery. It is one of the two principal arteries of the brain. In addition, it also

supplies spinal cord, meninges, surrounding muscles and bones.

2. **Branches and distribution :** It is divided into four parts.
   A. First part is cervical and is horizontal. It extends from the origin to entry into foramen transversarium. It doesn't give important branches.
   B. Second part is vertebral and is vertical. It extends from sixth cervical vertebrae to second cervical vertebrae through foramen transversarium. It gives spinal and muscular branches.
   C. Third part is suboccipital and is horizontal. It is present in the suboccipital triangle. It gives only muscular branches.
   D. Fourth part is cranial and is vertical. It extends from posterior atlanto-occipital membrane to the lower border of pons. It gives
      a. Meningeal branches, supply meninges of posterior cranial fossa.
      b. Branches to brain and spinal cord.

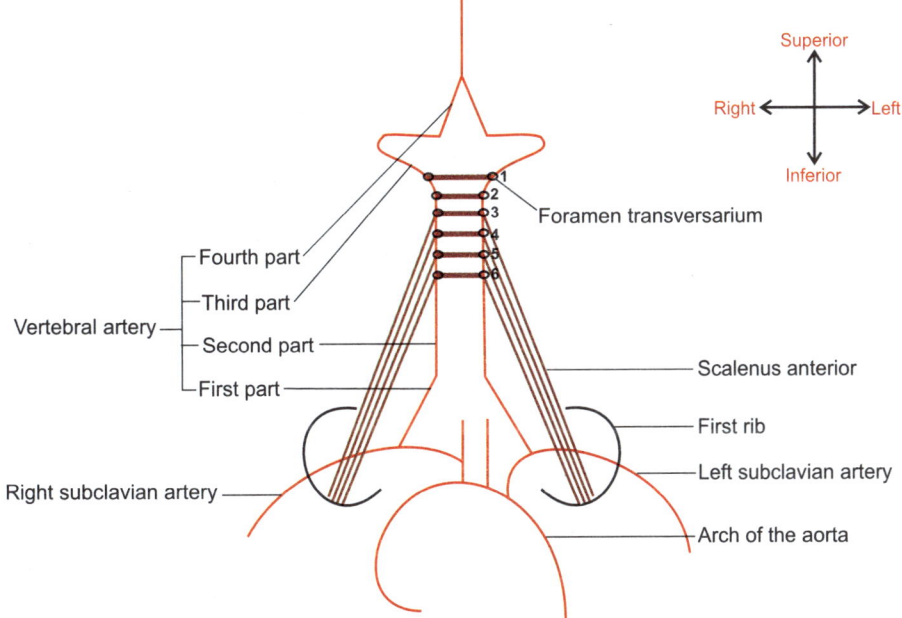

Fig. 3.21 : Vertebral artery and its branches

   I. Posterior spinal artery gives two branches which run on anterior and posterior to dorsal root of spinal nerve.
   II. Anterior spinal artery : It arises from terminal part of vertebral artery and unites as it descends with fellow of the opposite side to form anterior median trunk. It supplies medial part of medulla including pyramid and hypoglossal nuclei.
   III. Posterior inferior cerebral artery : *It is most tortuous artery in the body.* It is largest branch of vertebral artery. It supplies
      i. Lateral part of medulla.
      ii. Fourth ventricle by forming choroid plexus.
      iii. Inferior vermis and inferiolateral surface of cerebellar hemisphere.

3. **Relations :**
   A. The sympathetic plexus of the vertebral artery runs around the artery.
   B. Middle cervical ganglion lies anteromedially.
   C. Inferior cervical ganglion lies posteromedially.

4. **Applied anatomy :**
   A. Medial medullary syndrome : The lesion of the anterior spinal artery is manifested by
      a. Impairment of volitional (desired) movement on the contralateral side due to involvement of cortico spinal tract and
      b. Ipsilateral loss of movements of tongue, wasting of tongue muscles due to involvement of hypoglossal nerve nucleus.
   B. Lateral medullary syndrome (Wallenberg's syndrome) : It is due to the lesion of posterior inferior cerebellar artery. This is manifested by loss of pain and thermal sensibility of the same side of the face and opposite half of the body. Paralysis of the vocal cords, soft palate and pharyngeal muscles of the ipsilateral side.
   C. Subclavian steal syndrome : It takes place in obstruction of the subclavian artery proximal to the origin of vertebral artery. Some amount of blood is stolen from the brain through the vertebral artery of the opposite side to maintain collateral circulation.

| SN-9 | **Lumbar puncture** |

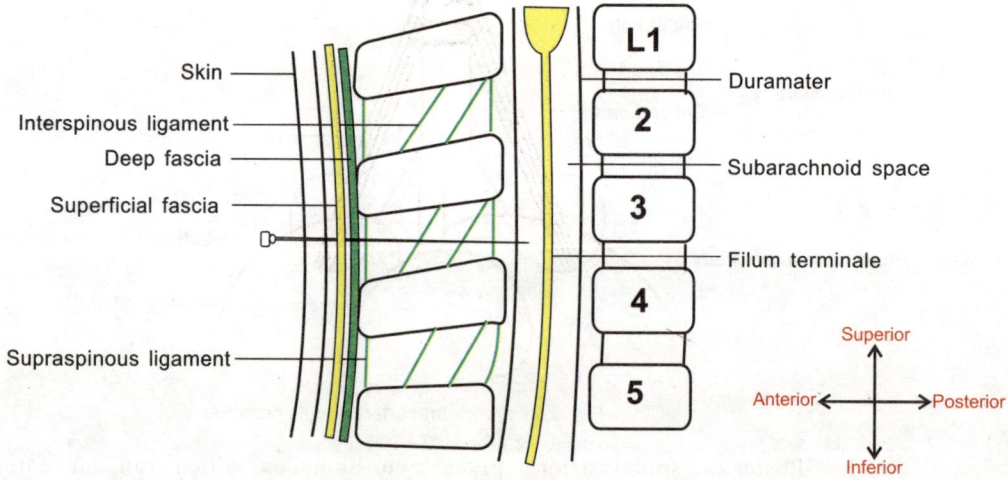

Fig. 3.22 : Lumbar puncture.

1. **Introduction :** It is performed to obtain samples of cerebrospinal fluid for laboratory analysis.

2. **Location :** Spinal cord ends at lower border of first lumbar vertebra. Hence lumbar puncture is done between third and fourth lumbar spine.

3. **Landmark :** A line tangential to the highest points of the iliac crests passes through the lower border of the fourth lumbar vertebra or the interspace between the fourth and fifth lumbar vertebra.

4. **Procedure :** Local anaesthetic drug is injected over the interspace between the fourth & fifth lumbar vertebra and a spinal needle is inserted. Needle passes successively through
   A. Skin.
   B. Superficial fascia.
   C. Supraspinous ligament.
   D. Interspinous ligament (between the paired flaval ligaments).
   E. Epidural space.
   F. Dura and arachnoid to enter the subarachnoid space.

5. **Applied anatomy :**
   A. Biochemical analysis of cerebrospinal fluid to diagnose type of meningitis.
   B. To differentiate extradural & subdural haemorrhage.
   C. For epidural and subdural anaesthesia (spinal anaesthesia).

SAQ-5 — Define venous sinuses and enumerate different venous sinuses

Venous sinuses are defined as 🔑 **SINVS ARE**

Spaces in the cranium lined by endothelium, present.

In between 2 layers of dura mater (endosteal & meningeal) except inferior sagittal and straight sinus which are in between two meningeal layers.

Non compressive in nature, devoid of

Valves and

Smooth muscle.

Absorbs cerebrospinal fluid through arachnoidal granulations

Receives valveless emissary vein, which

Equalises pressure within and outside the skull.

Classification :

Table 3.8 : The table shows paired and unpaired sinuses.

Paired	Unpaired
1. Middle meningeal vein	Anterior intercavernous
2. Sphenoparietal	Posterior intercavernous
3. Cavernous	Basilar venous plexus
4. Superior petrosal	Occipital
5. Petrosquamous	Straight
6. Inferior petrosal	Inferior sagittal
7. Sigmoid	Superior sagittal
8. Transverse	

LAQ-9 — Describe cavernous sinus under
1. Formation   2. Relations   3. Extent
4. Contents   5. Communications & 6. Applied anatomy.

1. **Formation :**
   A. Roof & lateral wall : Meningeal layer of duramater.

B. Floor : Endosteal layer of duramater.
C. Medial wall.
   a. Meningeal layer of duramater &
   b. Endosteal layer of duramater.

2. **Relations :**

Table 3.9 : The table showing relations of the cavernous sinus.

Superiorly	Optic tract. Internal carotid artery. Anterior perforated substance.
Inferiorly	Foramen lacerum.
Medially	Sphenoidal air sinus. Hypophysis cerebri.
Laterally	Uncus of temporal lobe of cerebral hemisphere. Cavum trigeminale with trigeminal ganglion.

3. **Extent :**
Apex of orbit to ⟶ apex of petrous part of temporal bone.

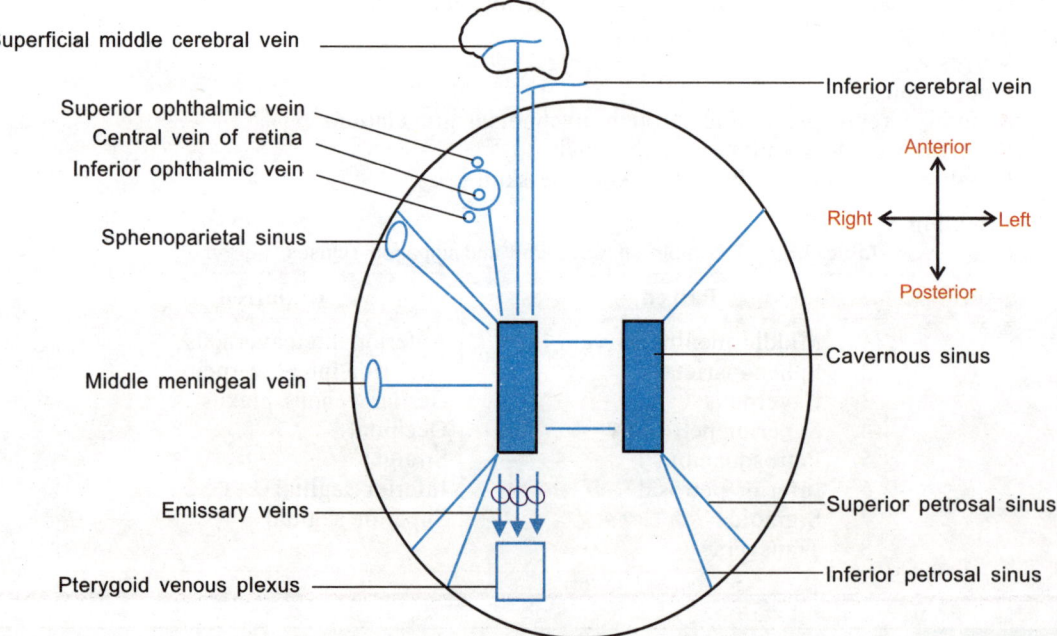

Fig. 3.23 : Tributaries and outgoing channels of cavernous sinus.

4. **Contents :** True content is blood.
Other structures are separated by layer of endothelium.
A. *Structures passing through the sinus.*

a. *Internal carotid artery with sympathetic & venous plexus.*
b. *Abducent nerve (below & lateral to internal carotid artery).*

B. Structures in the lateral wall
   From above downwards

   a. IIIrd - Oculomotor nerve.
   b. IVth - Trochlear nerve.
   c. V_1 - Ophthalmic division of trigeminal.
   d. V_2 - Maxillary division of trigeminal.

C. Incoming channel - From 🔑🔫 **3B**

Table 3.10 : The table shows incoming veins to cavernous sinus.

Brain	a.	Superficial middle cerebral vein.
	b.	Inferior cerebral vein.
Bone	a.	Sphenoparietal sinus.
	b.	Middle meningeal vein.
Eye**b**all	a.	Superior ophthalmic vein.
	b.	Inferior ophthalmic vein.
	c.	Central vein of retina.

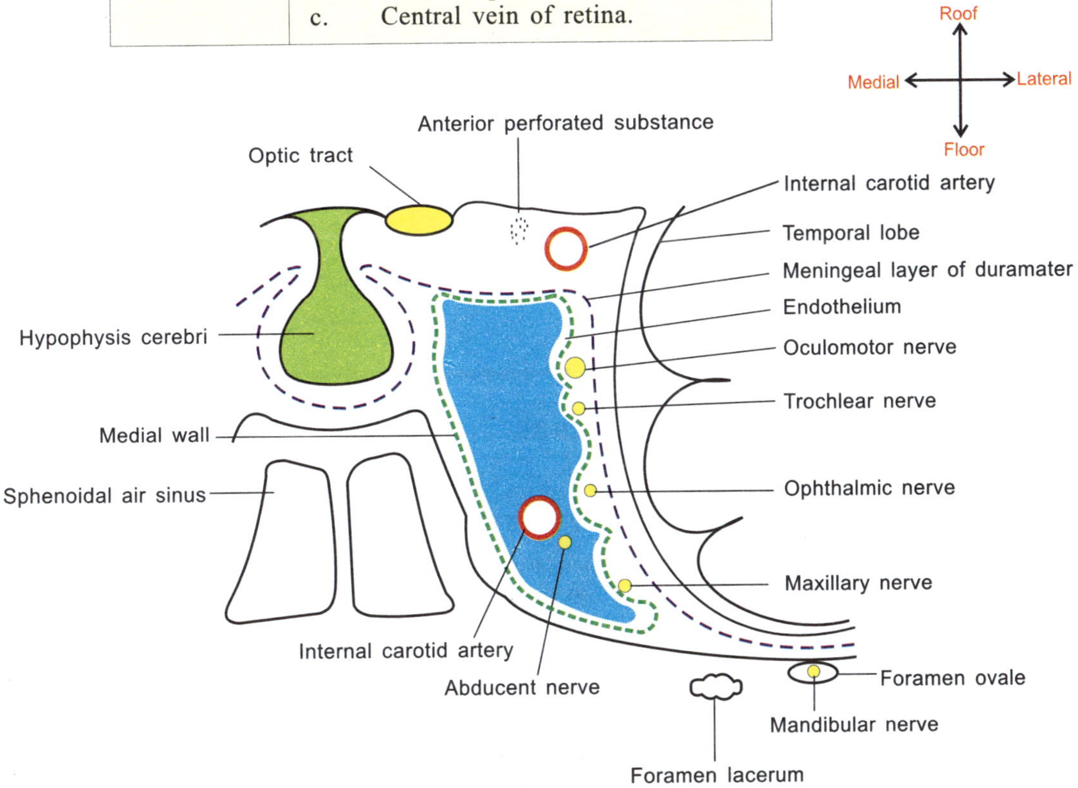

Fig. 3.24 : Boundaries and contents of the cavernous sinus.

5. **Communications :**

    Table 3.11 : The table showing outgoing channels from cavernous sinus.

Region	To	Through
A. Anterior	Facial vein.	Superior ophthalmic vein.
B. Posterior	Transverse. Internal jugular vein.	Superior petrosal sinus. Inferior petrosal sinus.
C. Superior	Superior sagittal sinus.	Superficial middle cerebral vein.
D. Inferior	Pterygoid venous plexus.	Emissary vein passing through. a. Foramen ovale. b. Foramen lacerum. c. Foramen spinosum.
E. Opposite	Cavernous sinus.	a. Anterior intercavernous sinus. b. Posterior intercavernous sinus.

6. **Applied anatomy :**
   A. Thrombosis of cavernous sinus is caused by septic infections in the dangerous area of face. These areas are   🔑   **USA**
      a. **U**pper lip.
      b. **S**eptum of nose and nasal cavities.
      c. **A**djoining area of cheek and paranasal air sinus.
   B. The clinical manifestations of thrombosis in cavernous sinus are
      a. Severe pain in eye.
      b. Ophthalmoplegia.
      c. Oedema of eyelids.
      d. Exophthalmos.
   C. Arterio venous aneurysm. This is caused by rupture of internal carotid artery and results into
      a. Loud systolic thrill.
      b. Unilateral pulsatile exophthalmos.

SN-10   Superior sagittal sinus

Venous sinus situated at convex margin of two layers of falx cerebri.
1. **Extent :** Crista galli to internal occipital protuberance.
2. **Course :** Above the foramen caecum, crista galli ⟶ inner surface of frontal sagittal margins of parietal and squamous part of occipital.
3. **Size :** It becomes progressively larger as it passes backward to internal occipital protuberance.
4. **Fate :** Usually ends in right transverse sinus.
5. **Shape :** Triangular in cross-section.

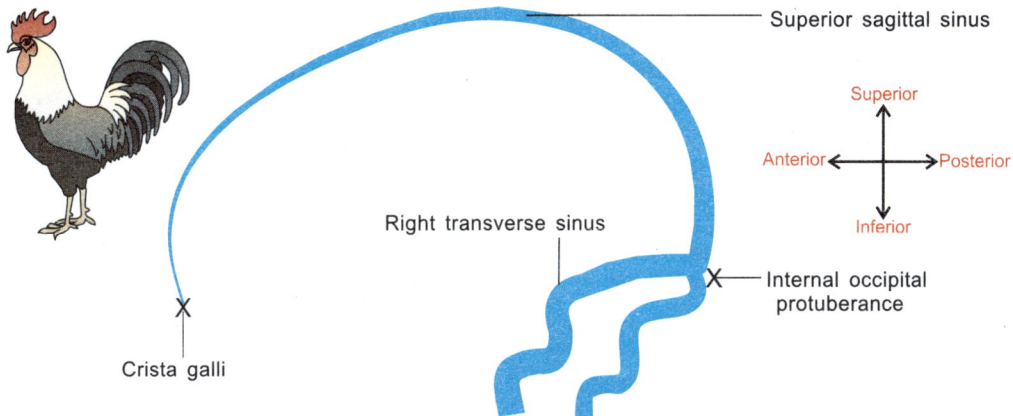

Fig. 3.25 : Extent and termination of superior sagittal sinus.

6. **Features :** Interior of the sinus presents
   A. Opening of superior cerebral veins.
   B. Openings of venous lacunae which are usually three in number.
      (Lacunae are complicated meshwork of veins in which diploic and meningeal veins open).
   C. Projection of arachnoid granulations.
   D. Numerous fibrous strands at inferior angle.

7. **Tributaries :**
   A. Veins from nose.
   B. Superior cerebral vein which are 8 to 12 in number and collects blood from
      a. Superolateral and
      b. Medial surface of cerebral hemisphere.
   C. Diploic and emissary veins through venous lacunae.

8. **Communicates with :**
   A. Veins of scalp through parietal emissary vein.
   B. Veins of nose passing through foramen caecum.
   C. Cavernous sinus through.
      a. Superior anastomotic vein (vein of Trolard).
      b. Superficial middle cerebral vein.

9. **Applied anatomy :**
   Thrombosis :
   Cause: infection of nose, scalp and diploe.
   Result :
   A. Increased intracranial tension.
   B. Paraplegia (due to involvement of paracentral lobule).
   C. Convulsions due to compression of motor area. } Due to obstruction to venous drainage

---

SN-11 | **Sigmoid sinus**

1. **Introduction :** Venous channel in between two folds of dura mater (endosteal and meningeal layer) non compressive in nature lined by endothelium present in cranium and

devoid of
A. Muscular wall.
B. Valve.

2. **Site :** Posterior cranial fossa on parietal, temporal and occipital bone.

3. **Shape :** S shape.

4. **Termination :** It continues as internal jugular vein.

5. **Extent :** Extends from anterior end of transverse sinus - to posterior end of jugular foramen.

6. **Fate :** Continues as internal jugular vein.

7. **Tributaries :** Connects to
    A. Pericranial veins by passing through mastoid & condylar foramen.
    B. Cerebellar vein.
    C. Internal auditory vein.

8. **Applied anatomy :** Infections from posterior cranial fossa can reach to internal jugular vein.

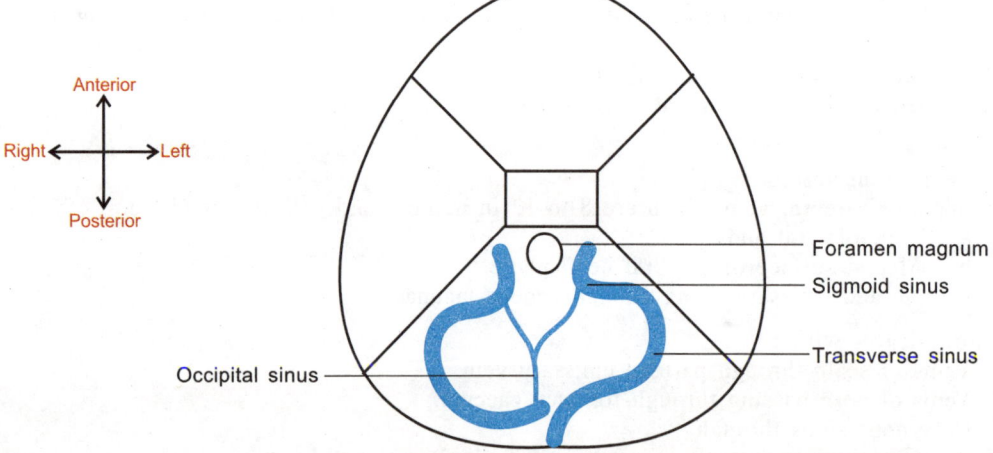

Fig. 3.26 : Sigmoid sinus.

| LAQ-10 | **Describe hypophysis cerebri under**
1. Gross anatomy   2. Blood supply   3. Histology
4. Development &   5. Applied anatomy. |

1. **Gross :**
    A. Situation : Pituitary fossa of the body of sphenoid bone.
    B. Shape : Oval
    C. Size : 8 mm x 12 mm
    D. Weight : 500 mg
    E. Relations
        a. Superior
            I. Diaphragma sellae,

        II.   Optic chiasma,

        III. Tuber cinerium and

        IV. Infundibular recess of third ventricle.

    b.   Inferior : Venous channels.

    c.   Lateral : Cavernous sinus.

2. Blood supply :

   A. Arterial supply :

      a.   Superior hypophyseal artery. $\left.\right\}$ Internal carotid artery

      b.   Inferior hypophyseal artery.

   B. Venous drainage : Short veins emerge on the surface of gland and drains into neighboring dural venous sinuses.

3. Histology :

   A. Anterior lobe : It forms 3/4th of the gland. It consists of

      a.   Chromophilic cells (50%) the cells have affinity to colors.

         I.   Acidophils (alpha cells, about 43% of cells).

         II. Basophils (beta cells, about 7% of cells).

      b.   Chromophobic cells (50%) the cells do not take color.

   B. Intermediate lobe : It is made up of numerous basophil cells and chromophobe cells. They surround colloid material.

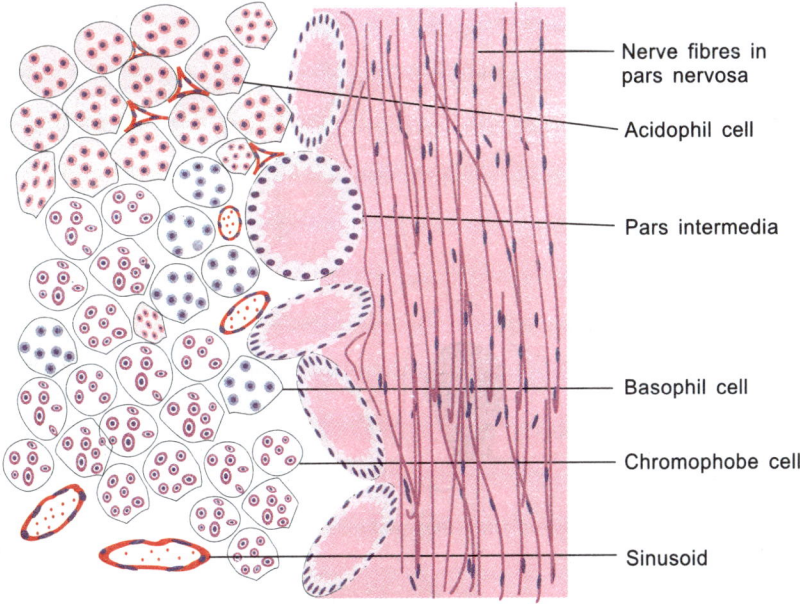

Fig. 3.27 : Histology of pituitary gland.

   C. Posterior lobe : It consists of

      a.   Large number of non myelinated nerve fibers.

      b.   Modified neuroglial cells, called pituicytes.

SN-12   **Development of hypophysis cerebri**

4.   **Development :**
   A.   Chronological age : It develops in the middle of the fourth week of intrauterine life (IUL).
   B.   Germ layer : Ectoderm.
   C.   Site : Roof of the stomodeum.
   D.   Sources :
       a.   Rathke's Pouch : Growing from roof of stomodaeum, (diverticulum of epithelium of primitive pharynx). It gives rises to -
           I.   Adeno hypophysis i.e. pars anterior (pars distalis) and
           II. Pars tuberalis.
       b.   Neuroectoderm : From floor of diencephalon. It give rise to   **IMP**
           I.   Intermediate part.
           II. Median eminence.
           III. Pars posterior.
   E.   **Anomalies :**
       a.   Hypoplasia : Less than normal growth of gland.
       b.   Craniopharyngiomas : Tumour growing from the hypophysial stalk or Rathke's pouch. It is associated with increased intracranial pressure & showing deposition of calcium in the capsule.
       c.   Hyperplasia : More than normal growth.

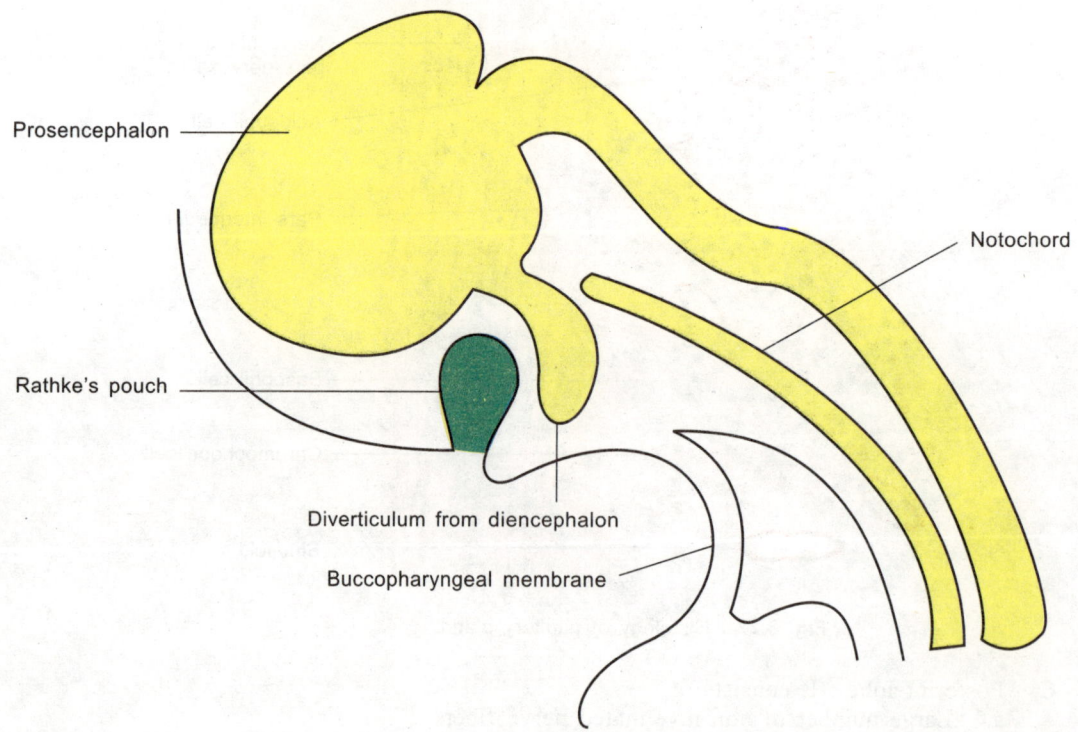

Fig. 3.28 : Development of pituitary gland.

5. **Applied anatomy :**
   A. Pituitary tumour gives rise to two main type of symptoms.
      a. General symptoms : due to pressure over the surrounding structures.
      b. Specific symptoms: Pressure over optic chiasma causes bilateral hemianopia.
         I. Acidophilic adenoma causes acromegaly in adult & gigantism in young individual.
         II. Basophilic adenoma causes cushing syndrome. The damage of the posterior lobe damage causes diabetes insipidus.
   B. Pressure over hypothalamus gives rise to hypothalamic symptoms.

SN-13   Maxillary artery

1. **Introduction :** It is an artery of upper and lower jaws, the muscles of mastication, palate and nose.

2. **Origin :** It is one of the terminal branches of external carotid artery arising within the substance of parotid gland at the neck of mandible.

3. **Course :** It is divided into three parts by lower head of lateral pterygoid muscle.
   A. First part (Mandibular) : It is horizontal and lies below inferior border of lateral pterygoid muscle. It is between neck of mandible & sphenomandibular ligament. Auriculotemporal nerve is related to the first part of artery.
   B. Second part (Pterygoid) : It is oblique and lies superficial or deep to lateral pterygoid muscle.
   C. Third part (Pterygopalatine) : It is horizontal and lies between two heads of lateral pterygoid muscle and deep to pterygomaxillary fissure.

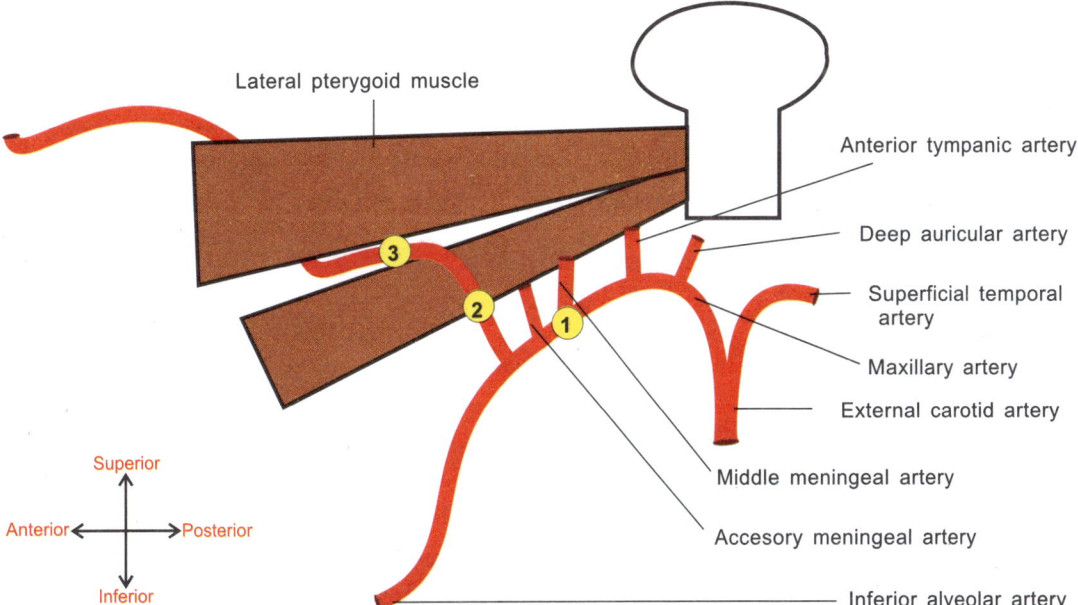

Fig. 3.29 : Branches of maxillary artery.

4. **Branches** : Branches of first & second part accompany the branches of maxillary nerve.

A. First part :   🔑 **DIAMA**

a. Deep auricular artery - supplies skin over outer surface of tympanic membrane.
b. Inferior alveolar artery - passes through mandibular canal.
c. Anterior tympanic artery - supplies inner surface of tympanic membrane.
d. Middle meningeal artery - enters through foramen spinosum and supplies duramater of the middle cranial fossa.
e. Accessory meningeal artery - enters through foramen ovale and supplies duramater of the middle cranial fossa.

B. Second part gives muscular branches to muscles of mastication.

a. Pterygoid.
b. Deep temporal.
c. Massetric.
d. Buccal.

C. Third part : Branches of third part pass through different foramina which enters into pterygopalatine fissure.

a. Posterior superior alveolar.
b. Infra - orbital artery.
c. Greater palatine artery.
d. Pharyngeal branches.
e. Artery of pterygoid canal.
f. Sphenopalatine.

5. **Applied anatomy :**

A. Middle meningeal branch is a largest meningeal branch and clinically is the most important branch of maxillary artery.
B. It may be torn in fracture of the skull producing extra dural haematoma that overlies the motor area of the cerebral cortex.

SN-14   Middle meningeal artery

1. **Origin** : First branch of the first part of maxillary artery in infratemporal fossa.

2. **Relations** : Superficial to sphenomandibular ligament and deep to lateral pterygoid muscle. It is accompanied by

A. Own plexus of sympathetic nerves.
B. Middle meningeal vein, a loyal friend.

3. **Branches :**

A. Ganglionic branches to trigeminal ganglion.
B. Petrosal branch.
C. Superior tympanic branch.
D. Temporal branch.
E. Anastomosing branch.

4. **Course :**

A. It ascends between two roots of auriculotemporal nerve.
B. It enters the middle cranial fossa through foramen spinosum.
C. It runs upwards and forwards on greater wing of sphenoid bone and divides into anterior and posterior division.

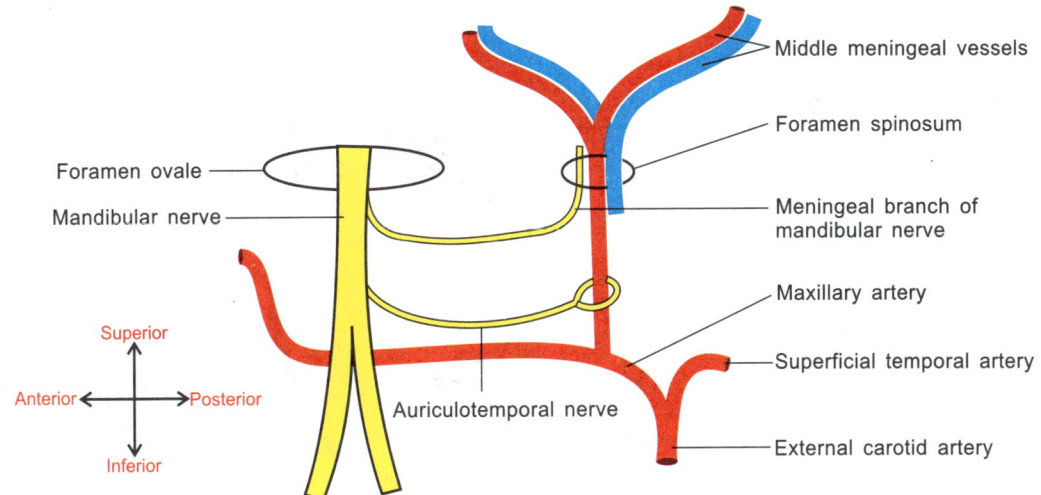

Fig. 3.30 : Middle meningeal artery and its branches.

D. Anterior division is closely related to motor area of brain.

E. Posterior division runs backwards on superior temporal sulcus of brain and ends at posteroinferior angle of parietal bone by dividing into frontal and parietal branches.

5. **Applied anatomy :**

A. Rupture of middle meningeal artery due to injury (foot ball) at pterion causes extra dural haemorrhage.

B. Rupture of anterior division of middle meningeal artery compresses motor area and results into contralateral hemiplegia.

C. Rupture of posterior division of middle meningeal artery results into contralateral deafness.

D. The anterior division is approached by making a hole at pterion (4 cm. above midpoint of zygomatic arch).

SN-15   Superior orbital fissure

Table 3.12 : The table shows the contents of superior orbital fissure.

1. Upper lateral part above the ring	A. Orbital branch of middle meningeal artery (1st part of maxillary artery) B. Meningeal branch of Lacrimal Artery ⚷ MLA C. Lacrimal nerve ⚷ LFT D. Frontal nerve V_1 (Ophthalmic nerve) E. Trochlear nerve (IV) F. Superior opthalmic vein
2. Middle part through the ring	A. Upper division of oculomotor nerve B. Nasociliary nerve C. Lower division of oculomotor nerve D. Abducent nerve
3. Lower medial part below the ring	Inferior ophthalmic vein

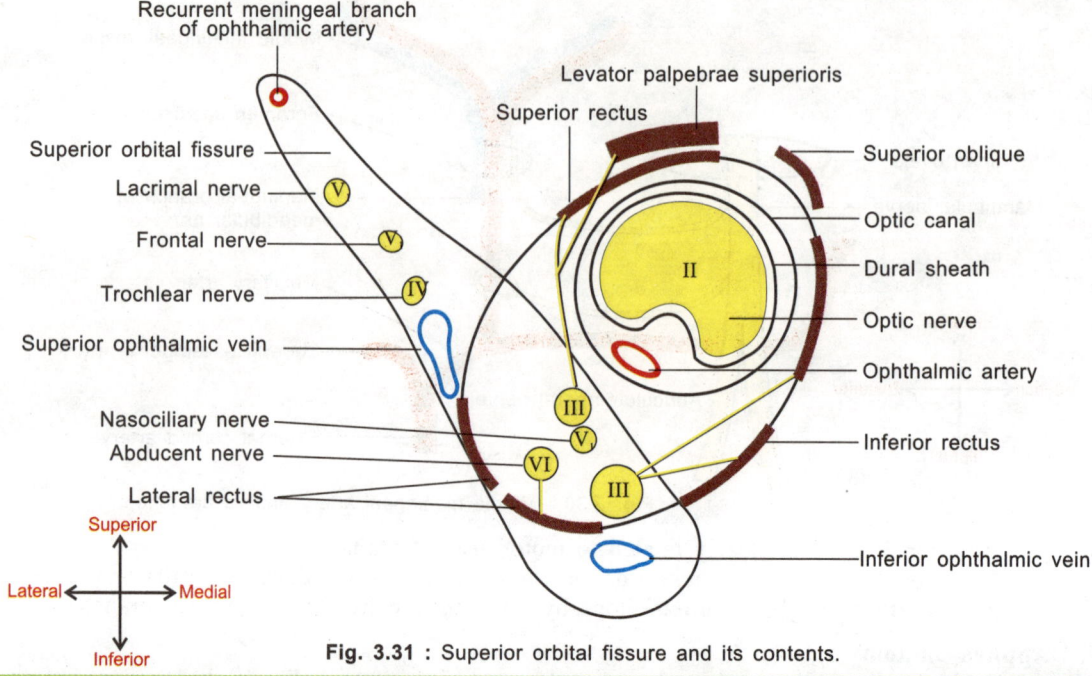

Fig. 3.31 : Superior orbital fissure and its contents.

LAQ-11 Describe extraocular muscles under
1. Attachments 2. Action
3. Nerve supply & 4. Applied anatomy.

1. **Attachments :** Extra ocular muscles are
A. Voluntary muscles
    a. Four recti :
        I. Superior rectus,
        II. Inferior rectus,
        III. Medial rectus and
        IV. Lateral rectus.

Origin of recti : The recti muscles arise from the respective positions of a common tendinous ring. The ring is attached to the orbital surface of the apex of the orbit.
The lateral rectus has an additional small tendinous head, which arises from the orbital surface of greater wing of sphenoid bone.

Insertion of recti : The recti are inserted into the sclera, a little posterior to the sclero corneal junction. The approximately distances of the insertion are

    🔑 **5 6 7 8**

- Medial rectus : 5 mm behind the sclero corneal junction.
- Inferior rectus : 6 mm behind the sclero corneal junction.
- Lateral rectus : 7 mm behind the sclero corneal junction.
- Superior rectus : 8 mm behind the sclero corneal junction.

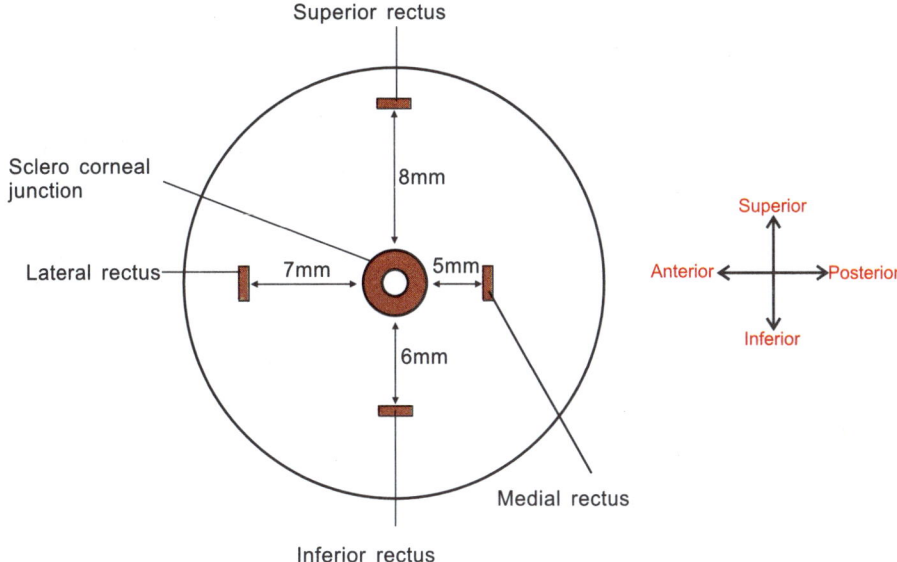

Fig 3.32 : Insertion of recti muscle

b.   Two obliqui :

Table 3.13 : The table shows origin, insertion of the oblique muscles of the eyeball.

Muscle	Origin	Insertion
Superior oblique	Body of sphenoid bone, supero medial to the optic canal.	Posterior superior lateral quadrant of the sclera of the eyeball, behind the equator.
Inferior oblique	Orbital surface of maxilla, lateral to the lacrimal groove.	Posterior inferior lateral quadrant of the sclera of the eyeball, behind the equator.

Levator palpebrae superioris	Orbital surface of lesser wing of the sphenoid bone.	I. Superior lamella :
		    i. Anterior surface of the superior tarsus
		    ii. Skin of the upper eyelid.
		II. Inferior lamella:
		    Upper margin of superior tarsus.

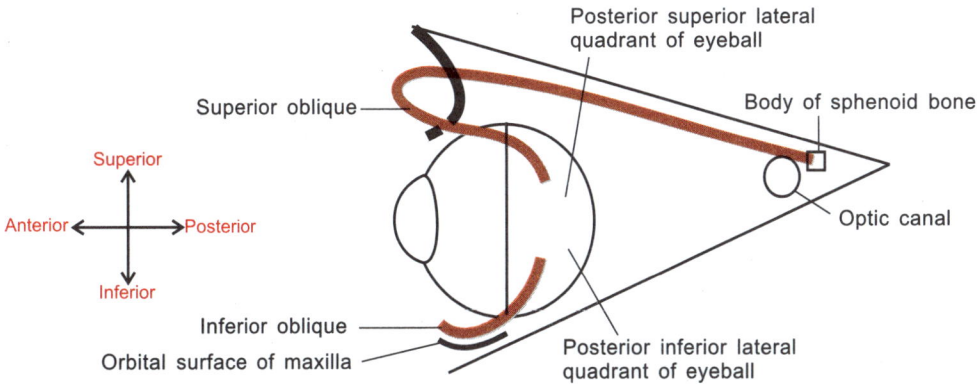

Fig. 3.33 : Origin and insertion of the oblique muscle

B.   Involuntary muscles :
    a.   Superior tarsal muscle is the deep part of levator palpebrae superioris. It is inserted on the upper margin of superior tarsus.
    b.   Inferior tarsal muscle connects the inferior tarsus of the lower eyelid to the fascial sheath of the inferior rectus & inferior oblique. It helps in depression of lower lid.
    c.   Orbitalis muscle bridges the inferior orbital fissure.

2. **Action :**
   A.   Actions of individual muscles :
     a.   Superior rectus : Elevation, adduction, intortion.
     b.   Inferior rectus : Depression, adduction, extortion.
     c.   Inferior oblique : Elevation, abduction, extortion.
     d.   Superior oblique : Depression, abduction, intortion.
     e.   Medial rectus : Adduction.
     f.   Lateral rectus : Abduction.

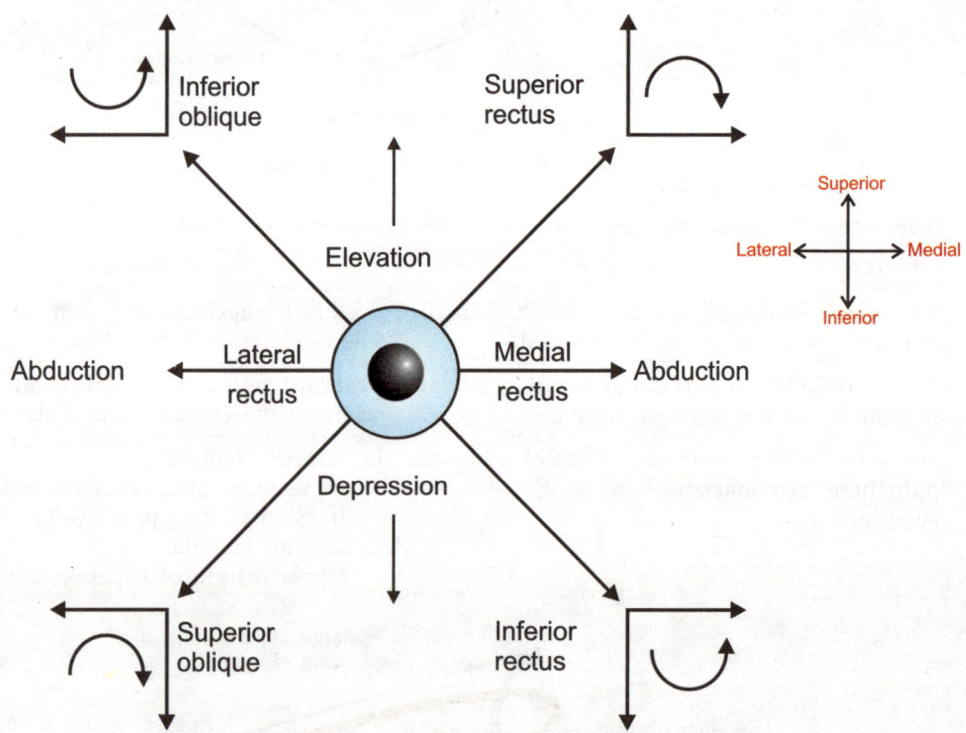

Fig. 3.34 : Actions of recti and oblique muscles.

   B.   Muscles bringing different actions :
     a.   Adduction : Medial rectus, superior rectus and inferior rectus.
     b.   Abduction : Lateral rectus, inferior oblique and superior oblique.
     c.   Elevation : Superior rectus and inferior oblique.
     d.   Depression : Inferior rectus and superior oblique.
     e.   Intortion : Superior rectus and superior oblique.
     f.   Extortion : Inferior rectus and inferior oblique.

3. *Nerve supply* : *All the extra occular muscles of the eyeball are supplied by oculomotor nerve except*

    SO₄ *superior oblique, supplied by trochlear nerve (4th cranial nerve and*

    LR₆ *lateral rectus supplied by abducent nerve (6th cranial nerve)*

(Superior, inferior and medial recti, inferior oblique and levator palpebrae superioris are supplied by oculomotor nerve).

4. **Applied :**

A. The muscles of eyeball are tested in following ways.

Table 3.14 : The table shows initial position of the eyeball for testing movements of the muscles of eyeball.

Muscle	Initial position of eyeball	Movement to be carried
Recti		
Superior	Laterally	Upward
Inferior	Laterally	Downward
Oblique		
Superior	Medially	Downward
Inferior	Medially	Upward

B. Oculomotor nerve lesion produces lateral strabismus and nearly complete ophthalmoplegia of the eyeball as well as ptosis of the eyelid. In addition, the pupil is dilated (mydriasis), and there is loss of accommodation reflex.

C. Trochlear nerve lesion produces diplopia (double vision) when looking downwards. Individuals with diplopia usually experience difficulty and apprehension on descending staircase.

D. Abducent nerve lesion produces medial strabismus (crossed eyes). Weakness or paralysis of a muscle causes squint or strabismus. In this condition the two eyes appear to look in different directions. Diplopia is minimal when looking to the opposite side of the lesion.

E. Nystagmus is characterized by involuntary, rhythmical oscillatory movements of the eyes. This is due to incoordination of the ocular muscles. It may be either vestibular or cerebellar in origin.

LAQ-12   **Describe occulomotor nerve under**

    1. **Functional components**   2. **Nuclei**
    3. **Connections**   4. **Origin**
    5. **Course**   6. **Related ganglion**
    7. **Distribution**   8. **Applied anatomy.**

---

1. **Functional components :**

A. Somatic efferent : Muscles of eyeball.

B. General visceral efferent : It innervates ciliaris and sphincter pupillae muscle.

C. General somatic afferent : Carries proprioceptive sensations from muscles to which it supplies.

2. **Nuclei:**

Table 3.15 : The table shows nuclei and their distribution.

S.No.	Nucleus	Muscles supplying
A.	Raphe	Superior rectus.
B.	Caudal central	Levator palpebrae superioris.
C.	Ventro median	Medial rectus.
D.	Intermediate	Inferior oblique.
E.	Dorso lateral	Inferior rectus.
F.	Edinger Westphal	Sphincter pupillae, & ciliaris.

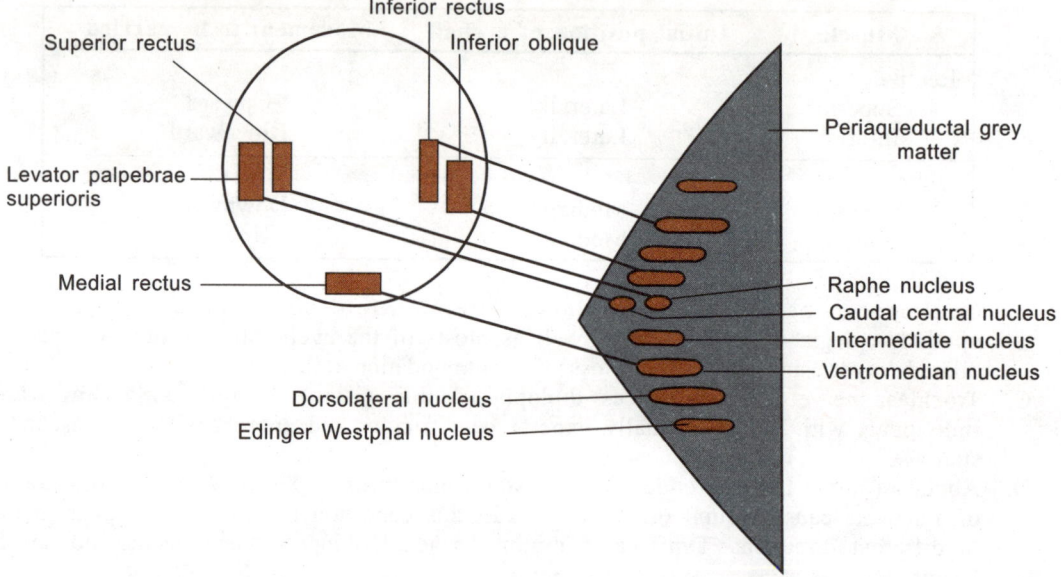

Fig. 3.35 : Nuclei of oculomotor nerve.

3. **Connections of nucleus :**

A. Afferent : Central connections
   Cerebral cortex (area 4,6,8) ⟶ Corona radiata ⟶
   Genu of internal capsule ⟶ Oculomotor nuclei.

B. Efferent : Peripheral connections
   a. Muscles of eyeball.
   b. Collateral connections 🗝 PCMC
      I. **P**retectal nucleus.
      II. **C**orticonuclear tracts of both sides.
      III. **M**edial longitudinal bundle.
      IV. **C**orticobulbar or tectobulbar tract.

4. **Origin :** Oculomotor nucleus, which lies in the grey matter of upper part of midbrain.

5. **Course :**

A. Intra-neuronal : Oculomotor nucleus ⟶ tegmentum ⟶ red nucleus ⟶ medial part of substantia nigra and emerges out of brainstem on medial side of crus cerebri through oculomotor sulcus.

B. Extra-neuronal : It pierces the pia mater and lies in subarchnoid space.
In subarachnoid space it lies between
  a. Posterior cerebral artery.
  b. Superior cerebellar artery and passes on to
     I. Lateral side of posterior communicating artery and pierces arachnoid mater
        and lies in free and attached margin of tentorium cerebelli.
     II. Lateral to posterior clinoid process & pierces the dura mater.
     III. Traverses the roof & descends in the lateral wall of cavernous sinus, receives
          few filaments from internal carotid artery and communicates with ophthalmic
          division of trigeminal nerve.
     IV. Cavernous sinus : Relations from above downwards are third and fourth nerve,
          ophthalmic and maxillary division of trigeminal nerve.
     V. Nerve divides into upper & lower division at anterior end of cavernous sinus.

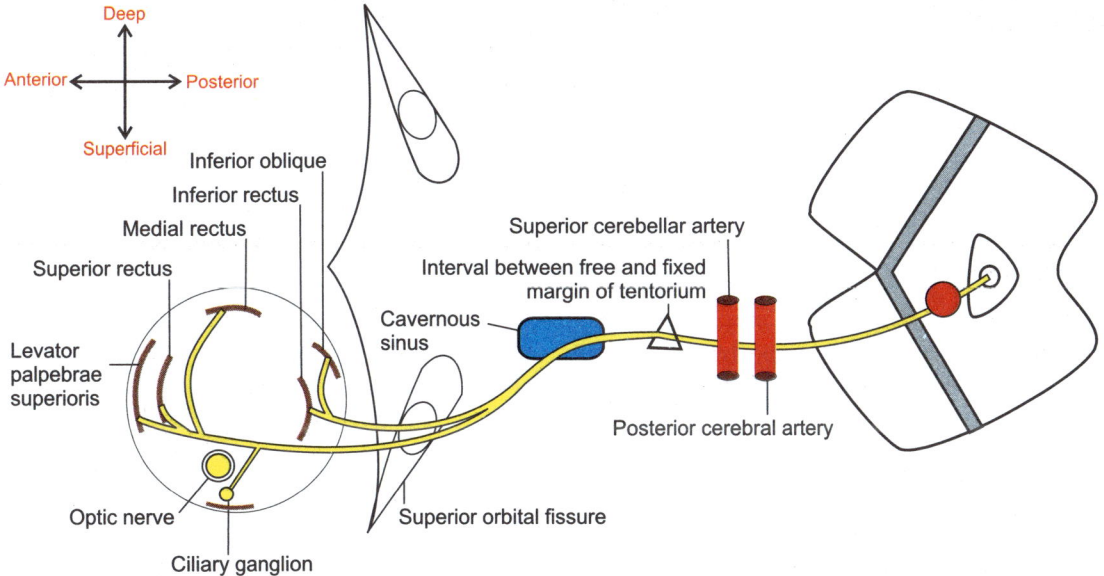

Fig. 3.36 : Course of oculomotor nerve.

6. **Related ganglion :** Ciliary ganglion, a peripheral parasympathetic ganglion.

7. **Distribution :**
   A. Motor
      a. Upper division
         I. Levator palpebrae superioris
         II. Superior rectus
      b. Lower division
         I. Inferior rectus
         II. Inferior oblique
         III. Medial rectus
   B. Parasympathetic to ciliary ganglion supplies sphincter pupillae and ciliaris muscle,
      through the branch of inferior oblique.

8. **Applied Anatomy :**
   A. Infra nuclear paralysis of oculomotor nerve results into 🗝 APPLiED
      a. Loss of accommodation.
      b. Ptosis.
      c. Protrusion of eyeball.
      d. Lateral squint.
      e. Embolus in cavernous sinus may produce third nerve paralysis.
      f. Diplopia.
      g. Dilatation of pupil.
   B. In paralysis of oculomotor nerve, patient cannot look upwards, downwards or medially.
   C. Third nerve is usually affected due to syphilitic periarteritis of posterior cerebral and superior cerebellar arteries as the nerve passes between the arteries.
   D. Weber's syndrome.

SAQ-6   Weber's syndrome

Introduction : A condition which includes
1. Upper motor neuron lesion of cortico spinal tract in crus cerebri of the midbrain.
2. Lower motor neuron lesion of third nerve, supplying the muscles of eyeball.
   It results into
   A. Contralateral hemiplegia and
   B. Ipsilateral paralysis of muscles of eyeball supplied by oculomotor nerve.

SN-16   Ciliary ganglion

1. **Introduction :** Collection of cell bodies of parasympathetic nerve supplying sphincter pupillae muscle situated at the apex of the orbit.

2. **Size :** Pin head.

3. **Content :** Cell bodies of multipolar neuron.

4. **Situation :** Apex of the orbit.

5. **Relation :**
   A. Medially : Optic nerve.
   B. Laterally : Lateral rectus muscle.

6. **Connections :** three roots
   A. Motor (parasympathetic)
      a. Preganglion fibres : Edinger-Westphal nucleus - lower division of third nerve - ciliary ganglion - Fibres are relayed.
      b. Postganglionic fibres : are carried by short ciliary nerve & supply
         I. Sphincter pupillae and
         II. Ciliaris muscle.
   B. Sensory : Nasociliary fibres pass through ciliary ganglion without relay.
   C. Sympathetic fibers pass through the ciliary ganglion without relay.
      a. Preganglionic : Spinal nerve to superior cervical sympathetic ganglion.
      b. Postganglionic : Plexus around internal carotid artery ⟶ short ciliary nerve ⟶ blood ⟶ vessels of eyeball & supply the muscle dilator pupillae.

7. **Branches :** 8 to 10 short ciliary nerves.

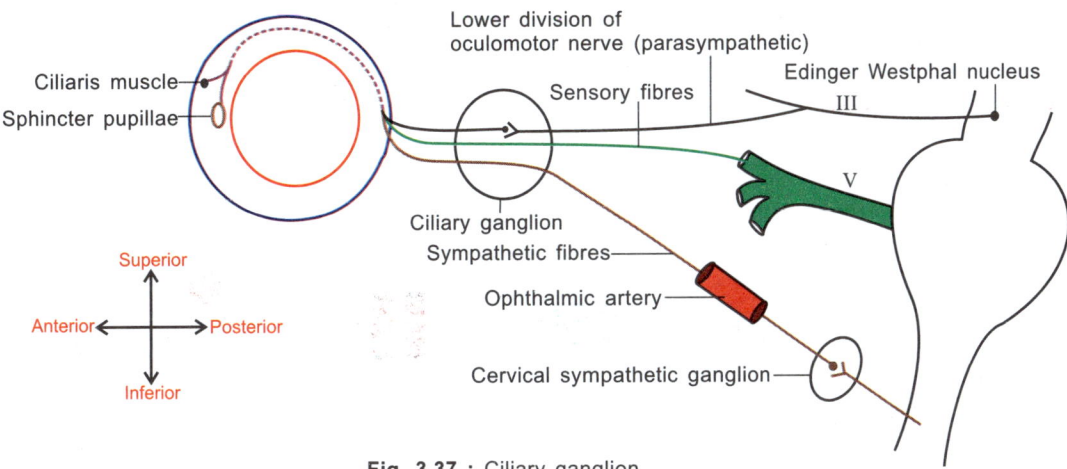

Fig. 3.37 : Ciliary ganglion.

8. **Peculiarity :** Postganglionic parasympathetic fibres are myelinated.

9. **Applied anatomy :**
    A. Complete division of oculomotor nerve is manifested as
        a. Ptosis : Drooping of eyelid.
        b. External strabismus : Due to unopposed action of lateral rectus.
        c. Dilated and fixed pupil.
        d. Loss of accommodation.
        e. Apparent protrusion of eyeball due to flaccid paralysis of most of ocular muscles.
        f. Diplopia where false image is higher than true image.
    B. Neurosyphilis : Periarteritis of posterior cerebral and superior cerebellar arteries will result into lesion of oculomotor nerve.
    C. Weber's syndrome : Contralateral hemiplegia (upper motor neuron lesion) and ipsilateral paralysis of muscles supplied by oculomotor nerve.

LAQ-13 **Describe trochlear nerve under**
1. **Functional components** 2. **Nucleus**
3. **Course and distribution and** 4. **Applied anatomy.**

1. **Functional components :**
    A. Somatic efferent, for movement of the eyeball.
    B. General somatic afferent, for proprioceptive impulses from the superior oblique muscle. These impulses are relayed to the mesencephalic nucleus of the trigeminal nerve.

2. **Nucleus :** The trochlear nucleus is situated in the ventromedial part of the central grey matter of the midbrain at the level of inferior colliculus.

3. **Course and distribution :**
    A. The trochlear nerve emerges from the superior medullary velum near the frenulum veli just below the inferior colliculus. *It is the only cranial nerve which emerges on the dorsal aspect of the brainstem.*

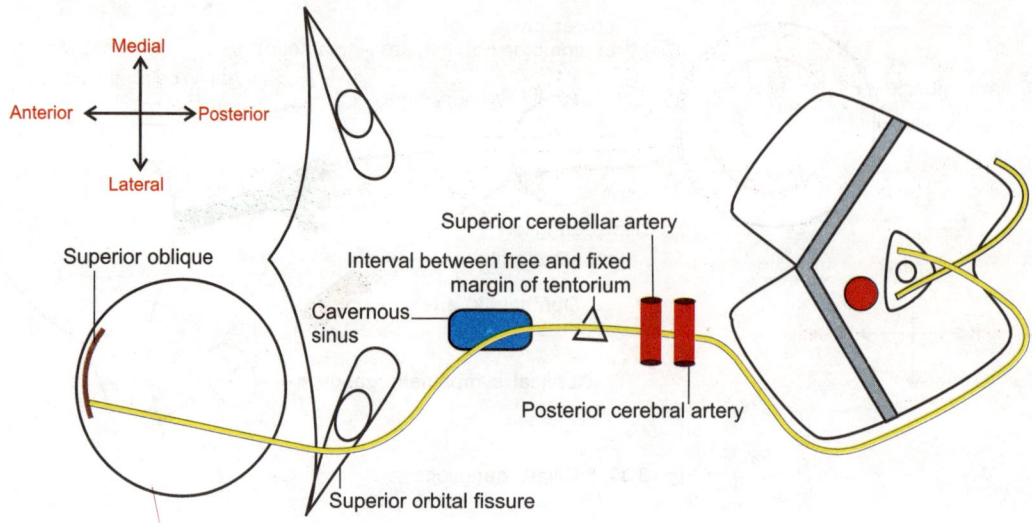

Fig. 3.38 : Course of trochlear nerve.

B. It winds round the superior cerebellar peduncle and the cerebral peduncle just above the pons. It passes between the posterior cerebral and superior cerebellar arteries to appear ventrally lateral to the cerebral peduncle.

C. It enters the cavernous sinus by piercing the posterior corner of its roof. Next it runs forwards in the lateral wall of the cavernous sinus between the oculomotor and ophthalmic nerves. In the anterior part of the sinus it crosses over the third nerve.

D. It enters the orbit through the lateral part of the superior orbital fissure.

E. In the orbit, it passes medially above the origin of levator palpebrae superioris and ends by supplying the superior oblique muscle through its orbital surface.

4. **Applied anatomy :** When the trochlear nerve is damaged, diplopia occurs on looking downwards, vision is single, so long as the eyes look above the horizontal plane.

LAQ-14	**Describe abducent nerve under**
	1. **Functional components** 2. **Nucleus**
	3. **Course and distribution and** 4. **Applied anatomy.**

This is the sixth cranial nerve. It supplies the lateral rectus muscle of the eyeball.

1. **Functional components :**
    A. Somatic efferent, for lateral movement of the eyeball.
    B. General somatic afferent, for proprioceptive impulses from the lateral rectus muscle. These impulses reach the mesencephalic nucleus of the trigeminal nerve.

2. **Nucleus :** The abducent nucleus is situated in the lower part of the pons, in the floor of the fourth ventricle, deep to the facial colliculus.

3. **Course and distribution :**
    A. The nerve is attached to the lower border of the pons, opposite the upper end of the pyramid (of the medulla).

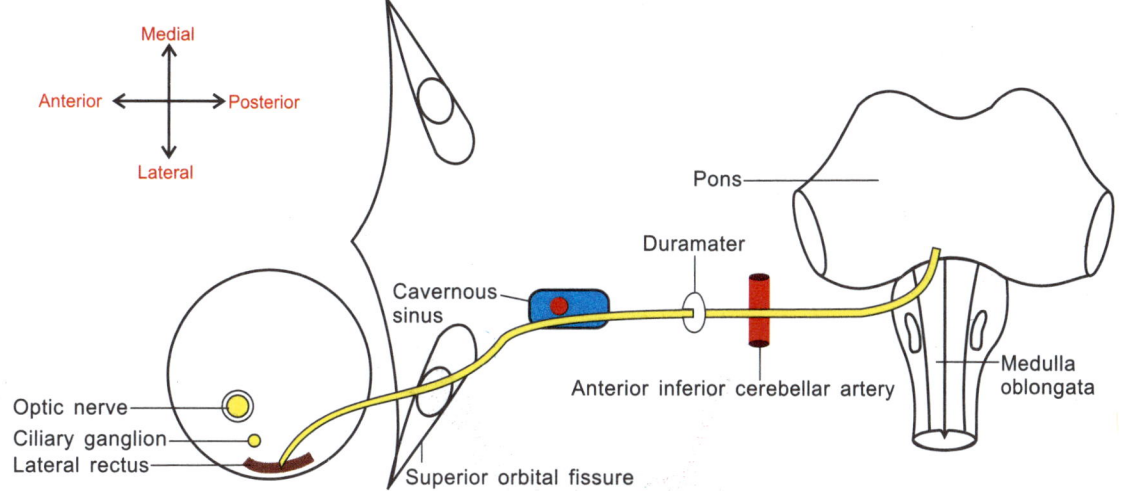

Fig. 3.39 : Course of abducent nerve.

B. It runs upwards, forwards and laterally through the cisterna pontis (and usually dorsal to the anterior inferior cerebellar artery) to reach the cavernous sinus.

C. It enters the cavernous sinus by piercing its posterior wall at a point lateral to the dorsum sellae and superior to the apex of the petrous temporal bone. As the nerve crosses the superior border of the petrous temporal bone it passes beneath the petrosphenoidal ligament, and bends sharply forwards. In the cavernous sinus at first it lies lateral to the internal carotid artery and then inferolateral to it.

D. It enters the orbit through the middle part of the superior orbital fissure. Here it lies inferolateral to the oculomotor and nasociliary nerves.

E. In the orbit it ends by supplying the lateral rectus muscle. It enters the ocular surface of the muscle.

4. **Applied anatomy :** Paralysis of the abducent nerve results in:
A. Medial (internal or convergent) squint and
B. Diplopia.

LAQ-15 **Describe digastric triangle under**
1. **Boundaries**   2. **Roof**   3. **Floor**
4. **Contents and**   5. **Applied anatomy.**

1. **Boundaries :**
Anteroinferiorly : Anterior belly of digastric.
Posteroinferiorly : Posterior belly of digastric and stylohyoid.
Superiorly (base) :
A. Base of mandible.
B. Line joining the angle of the mandible to the mastoid process.

2. **Roof :**
A. Skin

B.   Superficial fascia contains 🔑 **3C**
a.   **C**utaneous vein (tributaries of external jugular vein).
b.   **C**utaneous branches of great auricular vein.
c.   **C**ervical branch of facial nerve.
C.   Deep fascia encloses submandibular salivary gland.

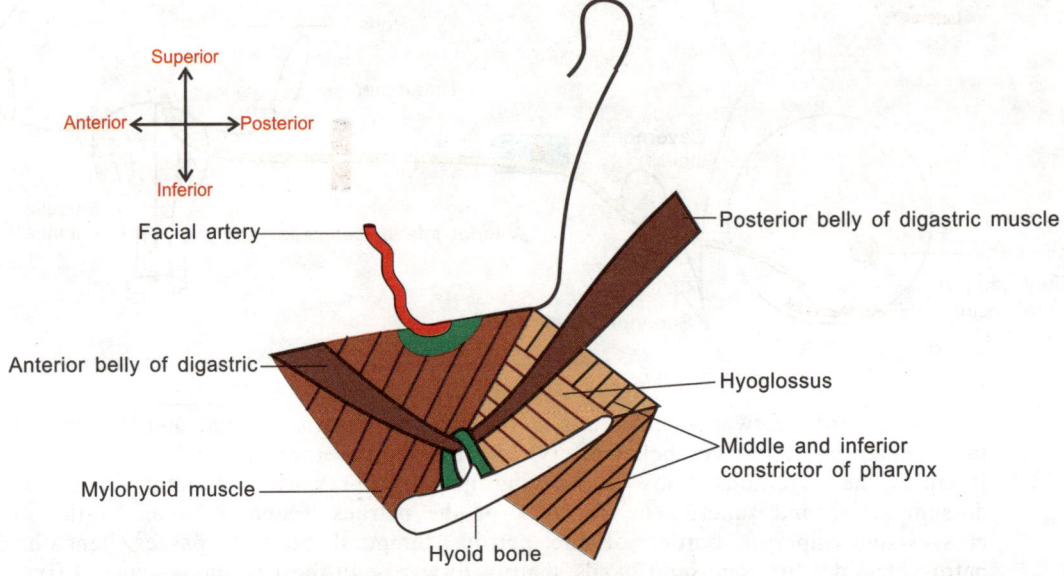

Fig. 3.40 : Boundaries of digastric triangle.

3.   **Floor:** From anterior to posterior
A.   Mylohyoid.
B.   Hyoglossus.
C.   Middle constrictor of pharynx.

4.   **Contents :** They are studied into
A.   Anterior part of the triangle.
a.   Structures superficial to mylohyoid.
I.   Submandibular salivary gland (superficial).
II.   Submandibular lymph nodes.
III. Submental artery.
IV. Mylohyoid vessels & nerve.
V.   Facial vein.
b.   Structures deep to mylohyoid : Submandibular salivary gland (deep).
B.   Posterior part of triangle.

Table 3.16 : The table shows structures present in the posterior part of the digastric triangle.

Superficial	Deep (Styloid)		Deepest
Parotid gland	a.	Styloid process	Internal carotid artery
External carotid artery	b.	Styloglossus	Internal jugular vein
	c.	Stylopharyngeus	X Vagus nerve.
	d.	IX (glossopharyngeal)	
	e.	X (pharyngeal branch)	

5. **Applied anatomy :** An infection in the submandibular region is limited to a triangular area. Bounded posteriorly by the hyoid bone; and anterolaterally on each side by the two halves of mandibular base. This is so because the investing layer of deep cervical fascia is attached to theses bones. The triangular swelling is called Ludwig's angina. Collection of the pus may push the tongue upwards.

LAQ-16 **Describe carotid triangle under**
1. Boundaries   2. Roof   3. Floor
4. Contents and   5. Applied anatomy.

1. **Boundaries :**
   A. Superiorly : Posterior belly of the digastric muscle and the stylohyoid.
   B. Anteroinferiorly : Superior belly of the omohyoid.
   C. Posteriorly : Anterior border of upper half of the sternomastoid muscle.

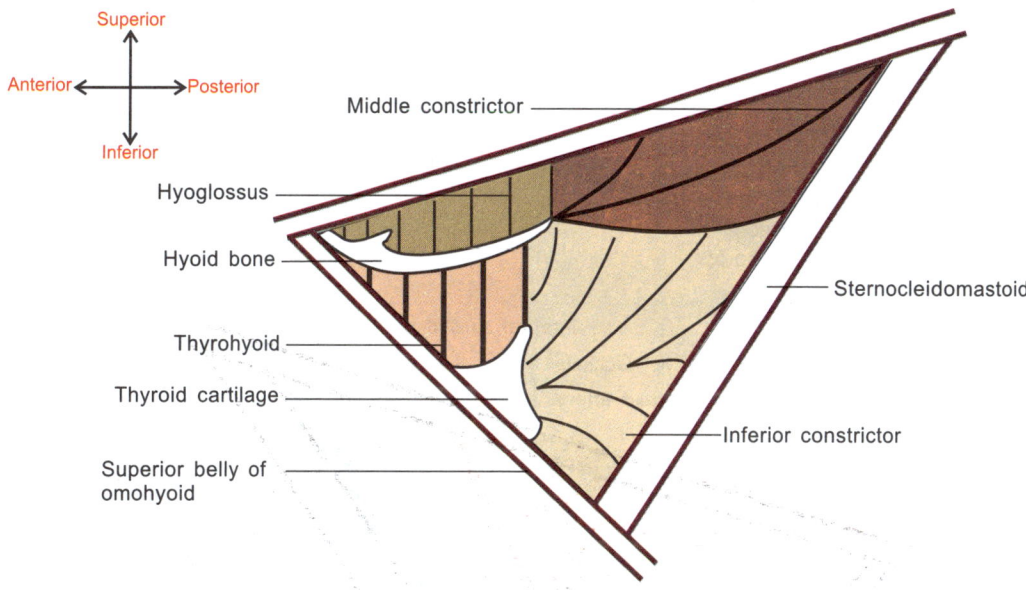

Fig. 3.41 : Boundaries and floor of carotid triangle.

2. **Roof :**
   A. Skin.
   B. Superficial fascia. It contains
      a. Platysma muscle,
      b. Cervical branch of the facial nerve and
      c. Transverse cutaneous nerve of the neck.
   C. Investing layer of deep cervical fascia.

3. **Floor :** It is formed by  **HIT**
   A. **H**yoglossus.
   B. **I**nferior and middle constrictors of pharynx.
   C. **T**hyrohyoid muscle.

4. **Contents :**
    A. Carotid sheath and its contents :
        a. Common carotid artery.
        b. Internal carotid artery.
        c. Internal jugular vein.
        d. Vagus nerve. It is present posteromedially.
    B. Relations of carotid sheath :
        a. Anterior wall : Ansa cervicalis.
        b. Posterior wall : Sympathetic trunk.
    C. External carotid artery and its first five branches :
        a. Ascending pharyngeal artery,
        b. Superior thyroid artery,
        c. Lingual artery,
        d. Facial artery,
        e. Occipital artery.
    D. Carotid body and carotid sinus.
    E. Tributaries of internal jugular vein :
        a. Pharyngeal vein,
        b. Lingual vein,
        c. Common facial vein.
    F. Nerves :
        a. Vagus nerve with its superior laryngeal branch,
        b. Spinal accessory nerve,
        c. Hypoglossal nerve.
    G. Deep cervical lymph nodes :

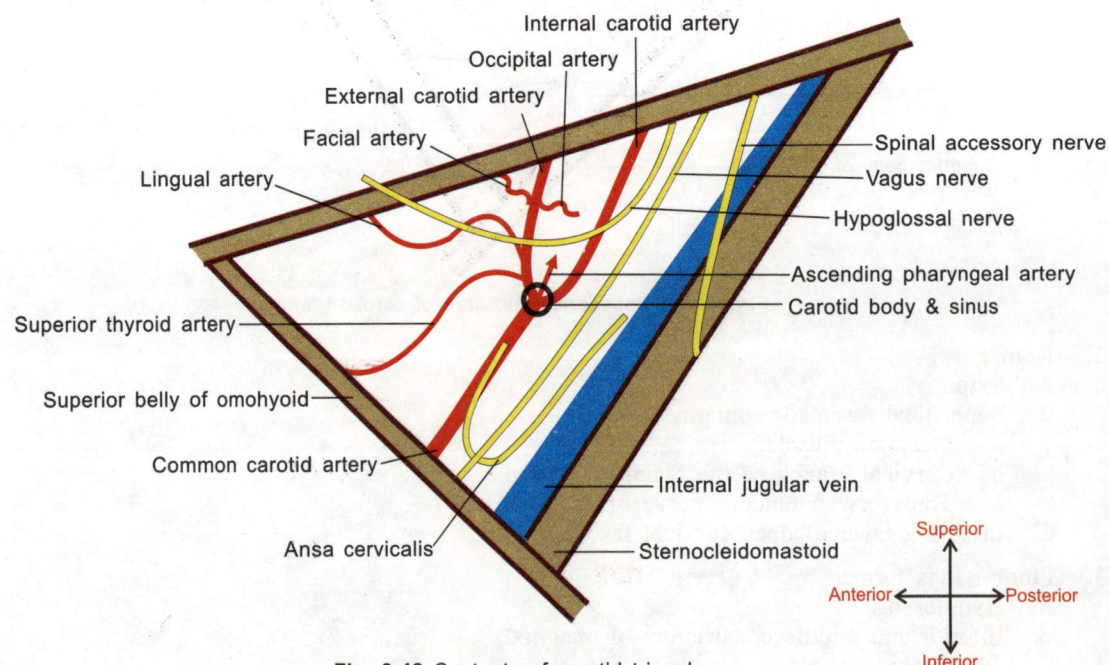

Fig. 3.42 Contents of carotid triangle.

5. **Applied anatomy :**
   A. A strong carotid pulse is palpable in the carotid triangle inferior to the level of Adam's apple by gently pressing the common carotid artery against the underlying vertebra.
   B. In the elderly, atheromatous plaques may be dislodged by such palpations. Hence pulsation should be felt on the right side since a stroke induced in the right cerebral hemisphere is less devastating.

SN-18 External carotid artery

1. **Origin :** It is one of the terminal branch of the common carotid artery.

2. **Extent :** From the upper border of thyroid cartilage to the neck of mandible.

3. **Branches :** All the branches of external carotid artery lie above the level of angle of jaw, and hence, supply the face rather than neck. The exception is superior thyroid artery, which falls down on the job. It is afraid of heights and reaches down to grab the thyroid.
   A. Medial : Ascending pharyngeal.
   B. Dorsal : Occipital and posterior auricular.
   C. Ventral : Superior thyroid, lingual and facial.
   D. Terminal : Superficial temporal and maxillary.

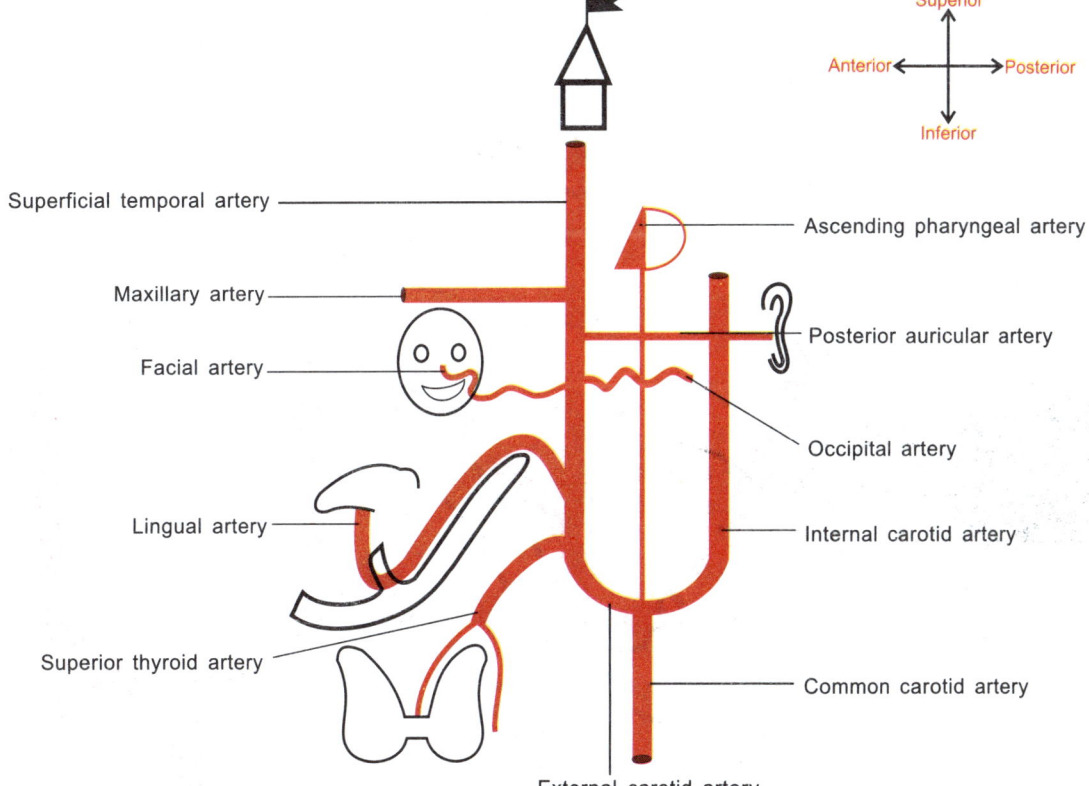

Fig. 3.43 : Branches of external carotid artery.

4. **Course :** It lies anterior and medial to internal carotid artery at its origin. It passes deep to the posterior belly of digastric and stylohyoid muscle and enters parotid gland and divides into terminal branches.

5. **Relations :**
   A. Superficial:
      a. In the carotid triangle, it is overlapped by sternomastoid and crossed by hypoglossal and lingual nerve and facial vein.
      b. In the digastric triangle it is related to posterior belly of digastric and stylohyoid muscle.
      c. In parotid gland : It is overlapped by retromandibular vein.
   B. Deep :
      a. Constrictor muscles of pharynx.
      b. Superior laryngeal nerve & its two branches internal and external laryngeal nerve.
      c. Internal carotid artery.

SN-18 **Lingual artery**

1. **Origin :** It is the second ventral branch of external carotid artery, arises opposite the tip of greater cornu of hyoid bone.

2. **Course and relations :** It is divided into three parts by hyoglossus muscle.
   A. First part (lateral to hyoglossus), extends from external carotid artery to the tip of greater cornu of hyoid bone. It forms upward loop to avoid rupture during the movements of hyoid bone.

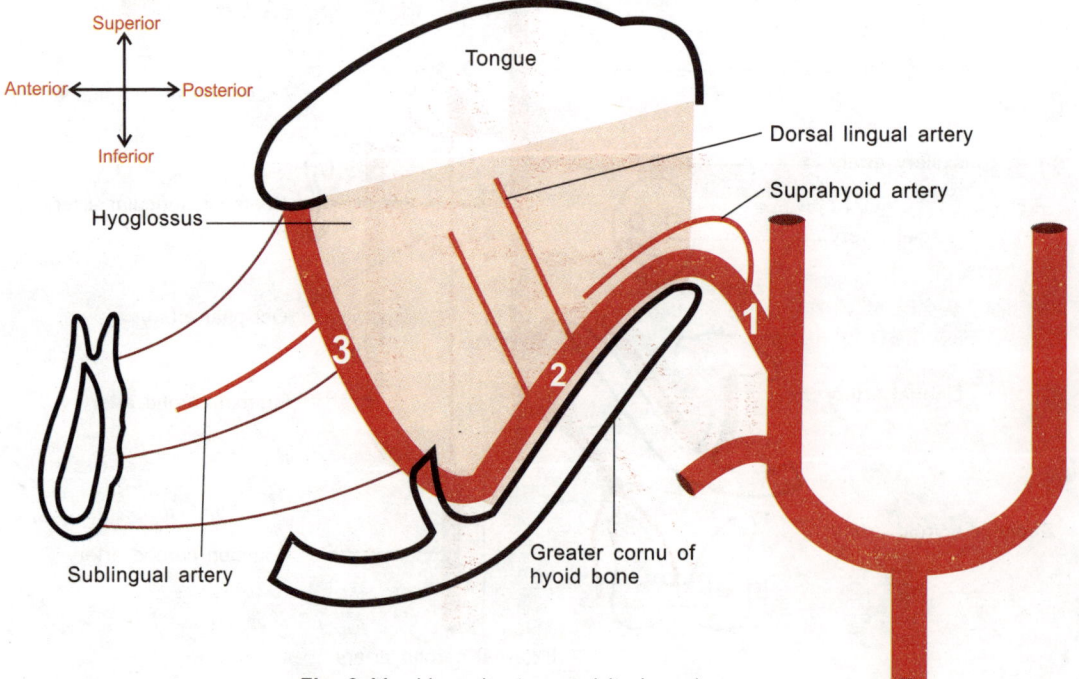

Fig. 3.44 : Lingual artery and its branches.

    B.   Second part lies deep to the hyoglossus muscle and on the upper border of greater cornu of hyoid bone. It lies superficial to middle constrictor.

    C.   Third part runs along anterior border of hyoglossus muscle. It is also called deep lingual artery.

3.   Branches :
    A.   First part : Suprahyoid artery.
    B.   Second part : Dorsal lingual artery.
    C.   Third part : Sub-lingual artery.

4.   Applied anatomy: In surgical removal of tongue, the first part of the artery is ligated before it gives any branch to tongue or tonsil.

SN-19   **Facial artery**

The chief artery of the face.

1.   Peculiarity : The artery is tortuous for the movement of pharynx and muscles of face.

2.   Origin : It is third ventral branch of external carotid artery arising above level of the tip of greater cornu of hyoid bone.

3.   Course : It is divided into cervical and facial.

    A.   It runs **s**uperficial to **s**uperior constrictor of the pharynx and **d**eep to posterior belly of **d**igastric (🔑 **d for d**) and to the ramus of mandible, at the anterior border of the masseter muscle.

        It grooves the submandibular gland.

    B.   It enters the face by winding round the base of the mandible and pierces deep cervical fascia at the junction of ramus and body of mandible. It runs upward half an inch lateral to angle of mouth and ascends by the side of nose and anastomoses with ophthalmic.

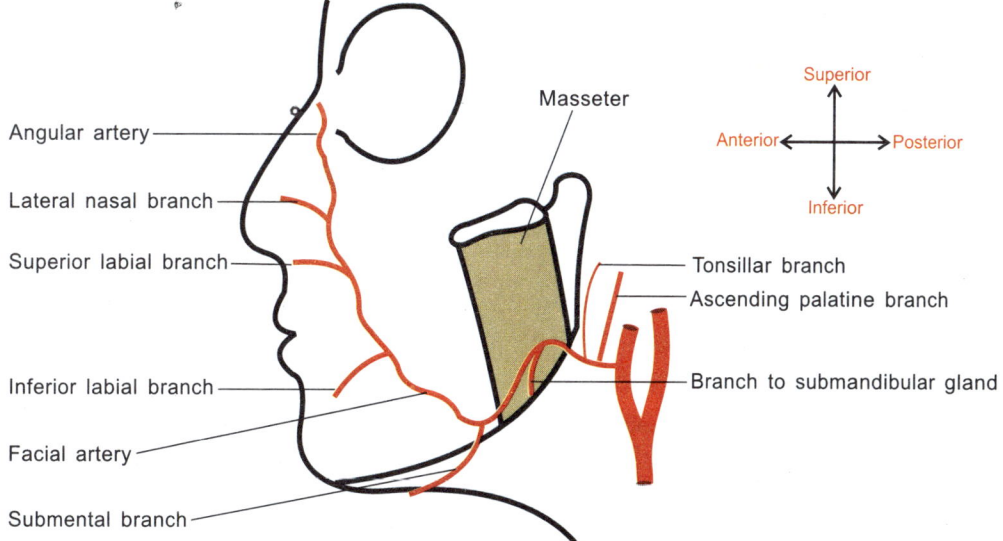

Fig. 3.45 : Facial artery and branches.

4. **Branches :**
   A. Cervical part :
      a. Ascending palatine,
      b. Tonsillar,
      c. Sub-mental and
      d. Glandular.
   B. Facial part :
      a. Inferior labial,
      b. Superior labial,
      c. Lateral nasal.

5. **Applied anatomy :** The wounds of face bleed profusely but heal quickly because of rich blood supply and profuse anastomosis.

SN-20   Ansa cervicalis (Ansa hypoglossi)

Ansa loop, *cervical* nerve

1. **Introduction :** A loop formed by ventral rami of cervical nerves.

2. **Formation :** It is formed by first, second and third ventral rami of cervical nerves.

3. **Roots :**
   A. Superior root is formed by first cervical nerve.
   B. Inferior root is formed by second and third cervical nerve.

4. **Relation :** It lies on the anterior wall of carotid sheath.

5. **Distribution :**
   A. Superior root : Superior belly of omohyoid.
   B. Ansa cervicalis :
      a. Sternohyoid,
      b. Sternothyroid and
      c. Inferior belly of omohyoid.

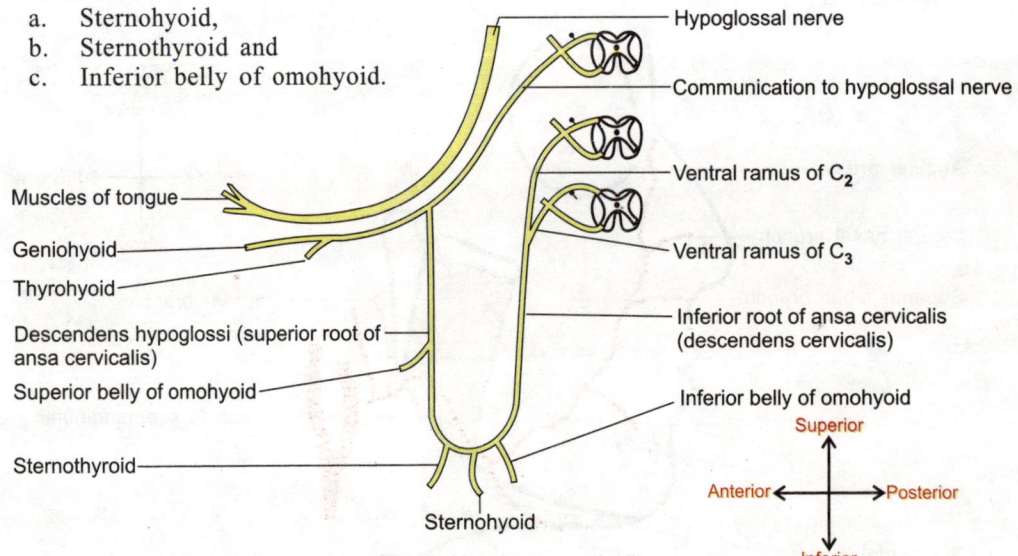

Fig. 3.46 : Ansa cervicalis.

LAQ-17 Describe parotid gland under
1. **Morphology** 2. **Relations** 3. **Blood supply**
4. **Lymphatics** 5. **Nerve supply** 6. **Development**
7. **Histology and** 8. **Applied anatomy.**

1. **Morphology :** It is largest salivary gland.
   A. Weight : 25 gm.
   B. Shape is like an inverted pyramid.
   C. Covering : Consists of inner true capsule, formed by condensation of fibrous tissue formed by peripheral part of gland.
   D. Outer false capsule : Formed by investing layer of deep cervical fascia.
   Presenting parts
   a. Apex.
   b. Base.
   c. Borders: Anterior, medial & posterior.
   d. Surface: Superficial, anteromedial and posteromedial.

2. **Relations :** **Table 3.17 :** The table shows relations of parotid gland.

	Structure related	Structure emerging (Superficial to deep)
A. Apex	Posterior belly of digastric	a. Cervical branch of facial nerve b. Anterior and posterior division of retromandibular vein
B. Base	a. External acoustic meatus b. Posterior part of TM joint	a. Temporal branch of facial nerve b. Superficial temporal vein c. Superficial temporal artery d. Auriculotemporal nerve
C. Surface a. Superficial	I. Skin II. Superficial fascia III. Posterior fibres of platysma IV. Superficial group of lymph node	Great auricular nerve supplying I. Skin over the angle of mandible II. Parotid fascia
b. Anteromedial	I. **M**asseter ☛ **4M** II. Posterior ramus of **m**andible III. **M**edial pterygoid IV. **M**axillary artery	

c. Posteromedial	☛ **3 processes**
	I. Mastoid **p**rocess
	  i. Sternocleidomastoid
	  ii. Splenius capitis
	  iii. Longissimus capitis
	II. Styloid **p**rocess
	  i. Stylohyoid
	  ii. Stylopharyngeus
	  iii. Styloglossus
	III. Transverse **p**rocess of atlas:
	  Rectus capitis lateralis
		I. Auriculotemporal nerve
		II. Facial nerve
		III. External carotid artery
		IV. Posterior division of retro-mandibular vein.

	Structure related	Structure emerging (Superficial to deep)

D. Borders
  a. Anterior
	-	I.
		  i. Branches of facial nerve
		    - Zygomatic branch
		    - Upper buccal branch
		    - Lower buccal branch
		    - Mandibular branch
		  ii. Transverse facial vessels
		II. Accessory parotid gland and its duct
		III. Parotid duct

b. Posterior	I. Sternocleidomastoid II. Posterior auricular branch of facial nerve. III. Posterior auricular vessels.	-
c. Medial	Pharynx	-

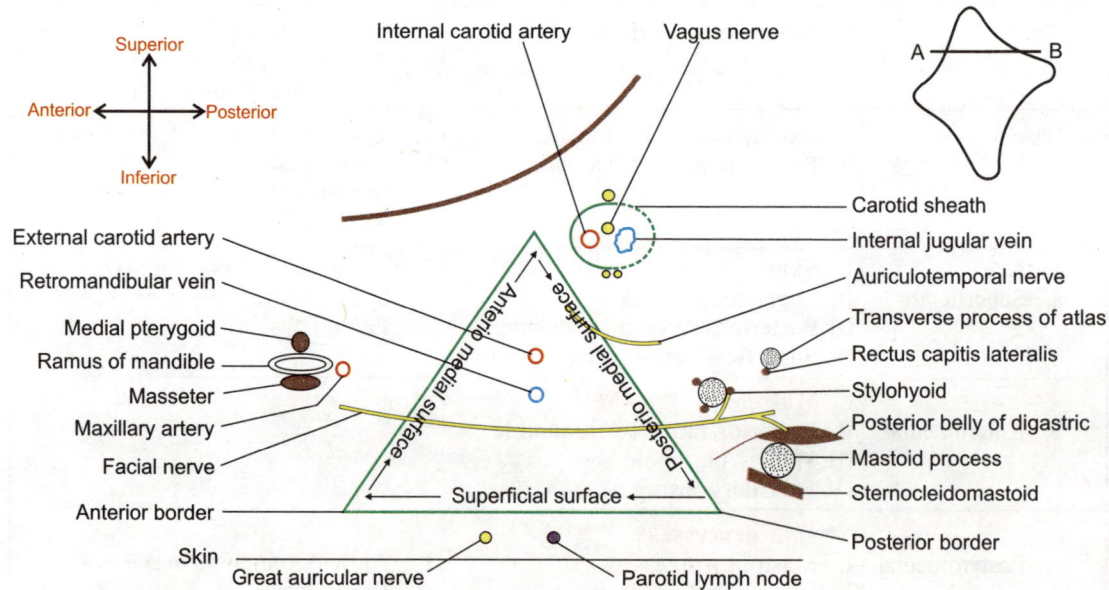

Fig. 3.47 : Parotid gland and its ralations.

3. **Blood supply:**
    A. Arterial: Branches of external carotid artery (E C A).
    B. Venous: Tributaries of external jugular vein (E J V).

4. **Lymphatic**
    A. Afferent lymphatics drain into parotid group of lymph nodes.
    B. Efferent lymphatic drains to jugulo-digastric group of deep cervical lymph node.

5. **Nerve supply :**
    A. Gland
        a. Sensory : Auriculotemporal nerve branch of mandibular nerve.
        b. Motor :
            I. Secretomotor : (parasympathetic).
                i. Preganglionic fibres arises from inferior salivatory nucleus. It travels via glossopharyngeal nerve - tympanic branch of glossopharyngeal nerve - tympanic plexus - lesser petrosal nerve - otic ganglion - fibres relay.
                ii. Postganglionic : Auriculotemporal nerve.
            II. Vasomotor (sympathetic)
                i. Preganglionic fibres arises from spinal cord : Superior cervical sympathetic ganglion.
                ii. Postganglionic : Plexus around external carotid artery to parotid gland.
    B. Parotid fascia : Great auricular nerve.

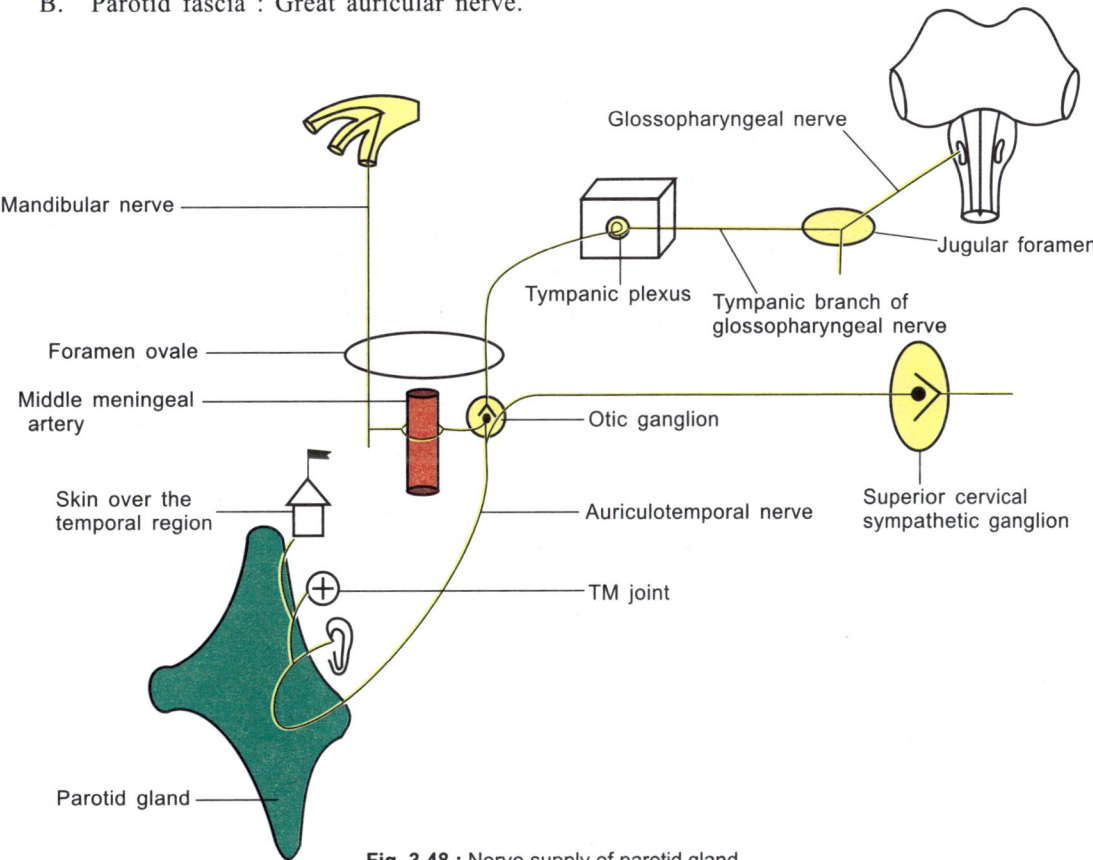

Fig. 3.48 : Nerve supply of parotid gland.

6. **Development :**

    A. Chronological age : sixth and seventh week of intrauterine life.

    B. Germ layer : It develops from ectoderm.

    C. Site : Primodial oral cavity.

D.   Source : It develops as a furrow between the mandibular and the maxillary arches at the site of future angle of the mouth. The groove is converted into the tube. The blind end of the tube branches rapidly in the substance of the cheek. As the fusion of the mandibular and maxillary arch takes place, its anterior end get shifted backwards. The end which remains like a tube forms the parotid duct and the posterior end rapidly undergoes branching and forms the glandular substance.

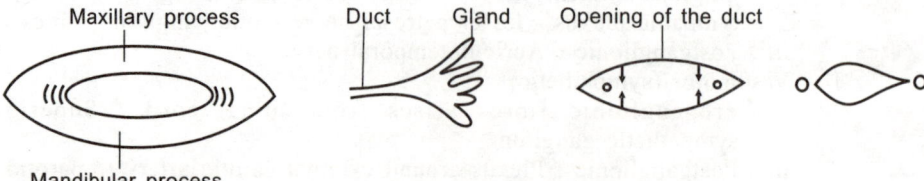

Fig. 3.49 : Development of parotid gland.

7.   **Histology :**
    A.   Compound tubulo - alveolar gland.
    B.   Acini are lined by serous cells.
    C.   Myoepithelium cells are present.

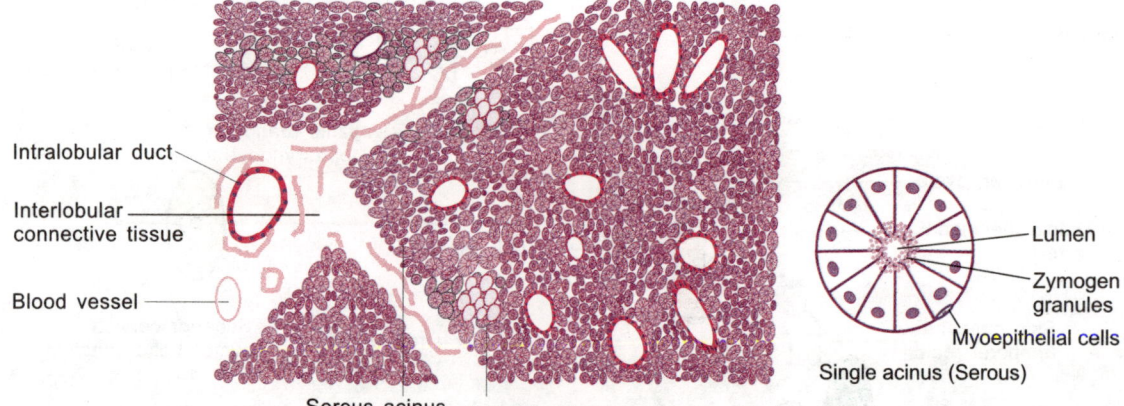

Fig. 3.50 : Histology of parotid gland.

8.   **Applied anatomy :**
    A.   Parotiditis : Inflammation of parotid gland is very painful due to unyielding nature of parotid fascia. Mumps is viral infection of parotid gland, which is usually bilateral and self - limiting. There are no complications in children because gonads are not developed in children. If it occurs in adult, the complications are oophoritis in female, orchitis in male and pancreatitis in both sexes.
    B.   Parotid abscess is drained by taking transverse incision over parotid gland to avoid injury to the branches of facial nerve (Hilton's Method).
    C.   Mixed parotid tumor : It is slow growing, benign painless tumour and does not involve facial nerve.
    D.   Frey's syndrome : Sometimes penetrating wound of parotid gland damages auriculo-temporal nerve and great auricular nerve. During regeneration, auriculotemporal nerve joins with great auricular nerve. Therefore stimulation of parotid gland brings stimulation of great auricular nerve. This results into sweating on the parotid gland.

SN-21	**Parotid duct (Stenson's duct)**

1. **Introduction :** It is thick walled tube, which carries secretion of gland to vestibule of mouth.

2. **Formation :** By union of two vertical ducts (formed by ductules).

3. **Size :** Of crow quill.

4. **Length :** 5 cm., **width :** 3 mm.

5. **Course :**
   A. Begins - From middle of anterior border of parotid gland and
      a. Runs on masseter muscle
      b. First bend : It directs medially at the anterior border of masseter and pierces buccal pad of fat, buccopharyngeal fascia and buccinator muscle.
      c. Second bend : It is between buccinator and mucous membrane of oral cavity.
      d. Third bend : It pierces mucous membrane and enters vestibule of mouth.
   B. Ends by opening on the
      a. *Summit of raised papilla.*
      b. *Opposite the crown of upper second molar tooth.*
      c. *Within vestibule of mouth.*

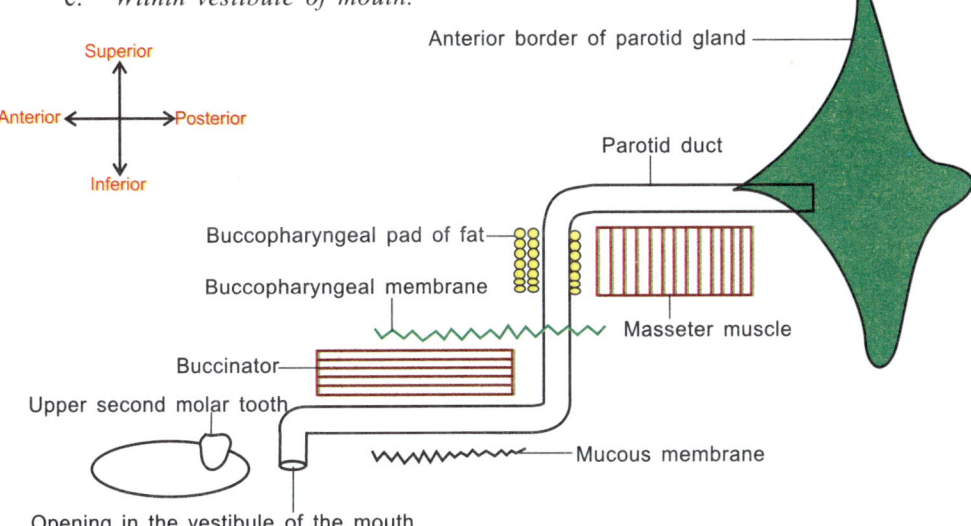

Fig. 3.51 : Course of parotid duct.

6. **Structure :**
   A. Outer fibroelastic coat and smooth muscle.
   B. Inner mucous membrane which is lined by stratified cuboidal epithelium.

7. **Blood Supply :** A branch of external carotid artery.

8. **Venous Drainage :** Veins drain into external jugular vein.

9. **Lymphatics :** Superficial and deep cervical group of lymph node.

10. **Nerve supply :** Auriculotemporal nerve.

11. **Development :**
    A. Germ layer : Ectoderm.
    B. Source : Stomodeum.
    C. Site : Furrow between the mandibular and maxillary arches at the site of future angle of mouth.

12. **Applied anatomy :**
    A. Oblique passage of duct between mucous membrane and the buccinator serves as a valve like mechanism and prevents inflation of the duct during violent blowing.
    B. Parotid duct is palpated and rolled on the firm anterior edge of masseter muscle.

| **LAQ-18** | **Describe facial nerve under** |

> 1. **Functional components** 2. **Connections**
> 3. **Course and relations** 4. **Branches &**
> 5. **Applied anatomy.**

1. **Functional components :**

Table 3.19 : The table shows functional components, nucleus and functions of facial nerve.

Functional components	Nucleus and its location	Functions
A. Special visceral efferent SaVE - BRANCHES ☛ bran = branches ches = arches	Motor nucleus situated at lower part of pons.	Branchial arch (muscles of facial expression) a. Muscles of facial expression, scalp and ear. b. Stapedius. c. Posterior belly of digastric. d. Stylohyoid. e. Buccinator f. Platysma
B. General visceral efferent GiVE - Glands Glands = salivary and lacrimal glands	a. Superior salivary nucleus, located at lower part of pons b. Lacrimatory nucleus, overlapped by superior Salivary nucleus.	a. Secremotor fibers to submandibular and sublingual salivary glands b. Secretomotor fibers to the lacrimal gland.
C. Special visceral afferent SVAd - Taste	Nucleus solitarius present at the junction of pons and medulla oblongata.	Taste sensation from anterior 2/3rd of tongue.
D. General somatic afferent	Sensory nucleus situated at the rostral end of the nucleus solitarius in the medulla oblongata. The cell bodies of these fibers are located in the geniculate ganglion of the facial nerve.	a. General sensation from the skin of concha of external ear. b. Proprioceptive sensations from muscles supplied by the nerve.

2. **Connections :**
   A. Central connection : Cerebral cortex from areas 4, 6, 8.
   B. Corticonuclear fibres : Corona radiata - Genu of the internal capsule.

3. **Course and relations :**
   A. Intra-neuronal :
      a. Motor root arises from motor nuclei of facial nerve situated in deep part of pons. It winds around abducent nucleus and forms facial colliculus, which is due to neurobiotaxis. The nerve fibers have a tendency to migrate in the direction from which they receive their stimuli.
      b. Sensory root (Nervus intermedius) formed by
         I. Superior salivatory nucleus & lacrimatory nucleus.
         II. Nucleus solitarius both roots emerges at the junction of pons and olive.
   B. Extra-neuronal : divided into 3 parts
      a. First part : It passes through the internal acoustic meatus and reaches anterosuperior angle of the medial wall of the middle ear cavity and bends to form second part.
         It forms a bulging at the bend called geniculate ganglion.
      b. Second part : It runs horizontally backwards along medial wall of tympanic cavity.
         I. It lies above promontory and fenestra vetibuli and runs to the.
         II. Posterior part of medial wall.
      c. Third part : Runs vertically downwards through stylomastoid foramen.
   C. Extra cranial : Turns anteriorly and pierces the posteromedial surface and emerges from anteromedial surface of parotid gland.
   D. Terminates in the parotid gland : by dividing into terminates branches.

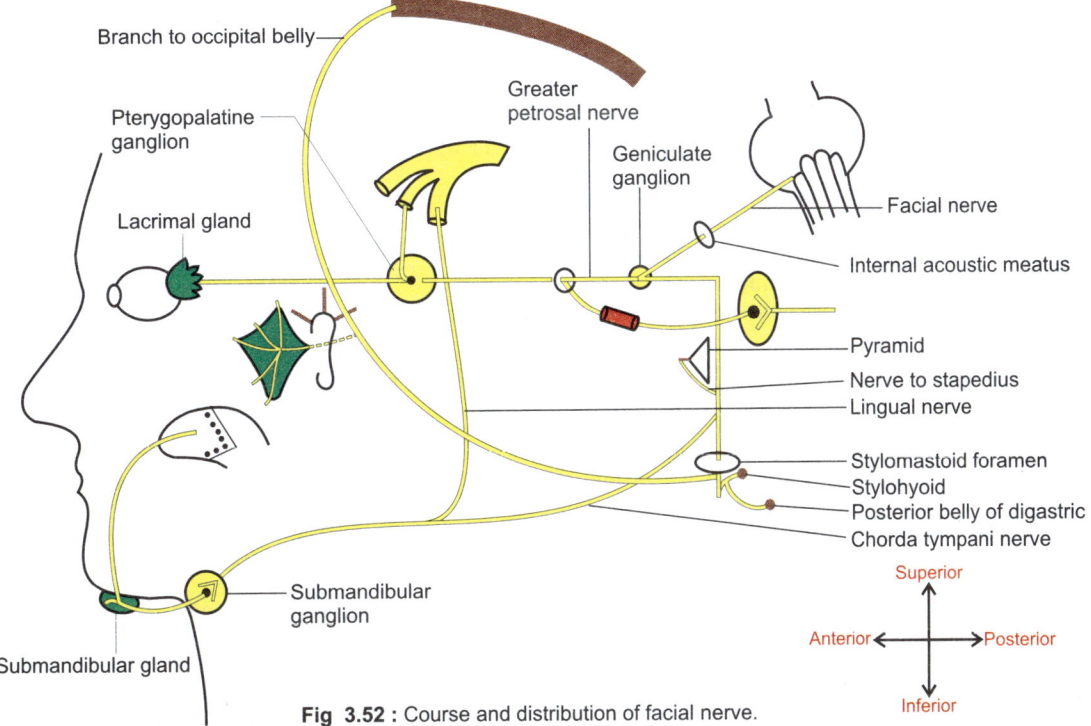

Fig 3.52 : Course and distribution of facial nerve.

4. **Branches :**
   A. Intracranial
      a. First part : No branches.
      b. At the junction of first and second part, greater petrosal nerve arises which carry secretomotor fibres to the lacrimal gland, deep petrosal nerve to pterygoid canal pterygopalatine ganglion → relay → zygomaticotemporal nerve → lacrimal gland.
      c. Second part :
         I. Sympathetic branches to middle meningeal artery.
         II. Branch to lesser petrosal nerve, by which it reaches the otic ganglion.
      d. Third part :
         I. Stapedial branch to stapedius through small canal.
         II. Chorda tympani joins lingual nerve and carries taste fibres from tongue. It also carries secretomotor fibres to submandibular gland.
         III. Communicating to vagus.
   B. Extracranial
      a. Posterior auricular branch. It gives communicating branch to great auricular and lesser occipital. It divides into
         I. Auricular branch, which supplies auricularis posterior.
         II. Occipital branch, which supplies occipital belly of occipitofrontalis.
      b. Digastric branch supplies posterior belly of digastric.
      c. Stylohyoid branch supplies stylohyoid muscle.
   C. Terminal branches
      a. Temporal
         I. Frontal belly of occipitofrontalis.
         II. Muscles of ear
         III. Corrugator supercilii
      b. Zygomatic : Orbicularis oculi.
      c. Buccal
         I. Upper : (lower zygomatic).
            i. Zygomatic major.
            ii. Zygomatic minor.
            iii. Levator labii superioris.
            iv. Levator labii superioris alaquae nasi.
            v. Levator Anguli oris.
         II. Lower :
            i. Buccinator.
            ii. Orbicularis oris.
      d. Mandibular branch supplies risorius muscles.
      e. Cervical branch supplies platysma.

5. **Applied anatomy :** **Table 3.20 :** The table shows effects of lesion of upper motor and lower motor.

Particulars	Lower motor neuron lesion (Infranuclear palsy)	Upper motor neuron lesion (Supranuclear palsy)
Site	Below the facial nerve nucleus.	Above the facial nerve nucleus.
Cause of lesion	A. Damage in the parotid gland. B. Bell's palsy. C. Lesion in the middle ear. D. Tumours in the internal acoustic meatus.	Lesion in the genu of internal capsule is due to cerebral haemorrhage.
Muscles paralysed.	Ipsilateral muscles of the whole face are paralysed.	Contralateral muscles of lower half of face are paralysed.

SN-22   Lower motor neuron lesion

1. **Lesion of facial nerve distal to stylomastoid foramen :** The lesion of facial nerve is due to vertical incision of the parotid gland.

2. **Lesion of facial nerve at the stylomastoid foramen :** It results in Bell's palsy. The 'Bell's palsy' is the lower motor neuron type of facial palsy (paralysis of muscles of facial expression). It occurs due to inflammation of facial nerve in the facial canal at the stylomastoid foramen.

   The exact cause is not known, but it is thought to be due to viral infection, causing inflammation and oedema of facial nerve with its consequent compression in the facial canal. Pain of variable intensity behind the ear precedes facial weakness which develops over a 48 hour period.

   Characteristic features (on the side of paralysis)
   A. Facial asymmetry : due to unopposed action of muscles of opposite side.
   B. Loss of wrinkles on forehead : due to paralysis of fronto-occipitalis.
   C. Inability to close the eye (wide palpebral fissure) : due to paralysis of orbicularis oculi.
   D. Inability to move the angle of the mouth upwards and laterally during laughing : due to paralysis of zygomaticus major.
   E. Loss of nasolabial furrow : due to paralysis of levator labii superioris alaquenasi.
   F. Accumulation of food in the vestibule of the mouth : due to paralysis of the buccinator.
   G. Dribbling of saliva : due to paralysis of orbicularis oris.
   H. Inability to inflate the cheek properly : due to paralysis of buccinator muscle.

3. The lesion in the vertical course of the facial nerve within the mastoid bone results in the loss of taste sensation on the anterior two-third of the tongue on the side of the lesion. There is loss of secretion from submandibular salivary gland; however, lacrimation and the stapedius reflex would be normal.

4. A lesion in the middle ear segment of the nerve (tympanic) does not affect lacrimation but results into ipsilateral hyperacusis, loss of secretion of submandibular gland on the side and loss of taste sensation on the same side of the lesion.

5. A lesion at or proximal to the geniculate ganglion (translabyrinthine) produces diminished lacrimation on the same side as well as disturbance in function of the other branches. After regeneration, the parasympathetic secretomotor fibers intended for salivary glands grow, and join the secretomotor fibers intended to supply the lacrimal gland; the anticipation of food then produces lacrimation, instead of salivation (syndrome of crocodile tears). The specific feature of this syndrome is paroxysmal lacrimation during eating.

SN-23   Upper motor neuron lesion

Lesion above the facial nerve nucleus in the pons or above involves corticonuclear fibers. The main cause is lesion in the internal capsule.

The supranuclear lesions produce upper motor neuron type of paralysis. The muscles only of the lower half of the face are paralysed. The muscles of the upper half of the face are normal beacuse they are bilaterally innervated.

Effects of upper motor neuron lesion : *The patient is able to wrinkle the skin of his forehead, but he is not able to perform the actions of the muscles of lower half of the face (as they have unilateral innervation from the cerebral hemisphere hence paralyzed).*

LAQ-19 Describe infratemporal fossa under
1. Boundaries & 2. Contents.

1. **Boundaries :**
   A. Roof : It is formed by
      a. Infratemporal surface of greater wing of sphenoid bone it has following foramen from anterior to posterior.
         I. Foramen ovale which transmits 🗝—🐀 MALE.
            i. **M**andibular nerve (V_3).
            ii. **A**ccessory meningeal artery (a branch of maxillary artery).
            iii. **L**esser petrosal nerve (a branch of tympanic plexus).
            iv. **E**missary vein connects cavernous sinus to pterygoid venous plexus.
         II. Foramen spinosum transmits 🗝—🐀 3 M.
            i. **M**iddle meningeal artery.
            ii. **M**iddle meningeal vein.
            iii. **M**eningeal branch of mandibular nerve.
      b. Squamous part of temporal bone.
   B. Anterior wall is formed by
      a. Posterior surface of maxilla.
      b. Inferior orbital fissure.
   C. Medial wall is formed by
      a. Lateral surface of lateral pterygoid plate.
      b. Tensor palati.
      c. Superior constrictor.
      d. Pterygo maxillary fissure.

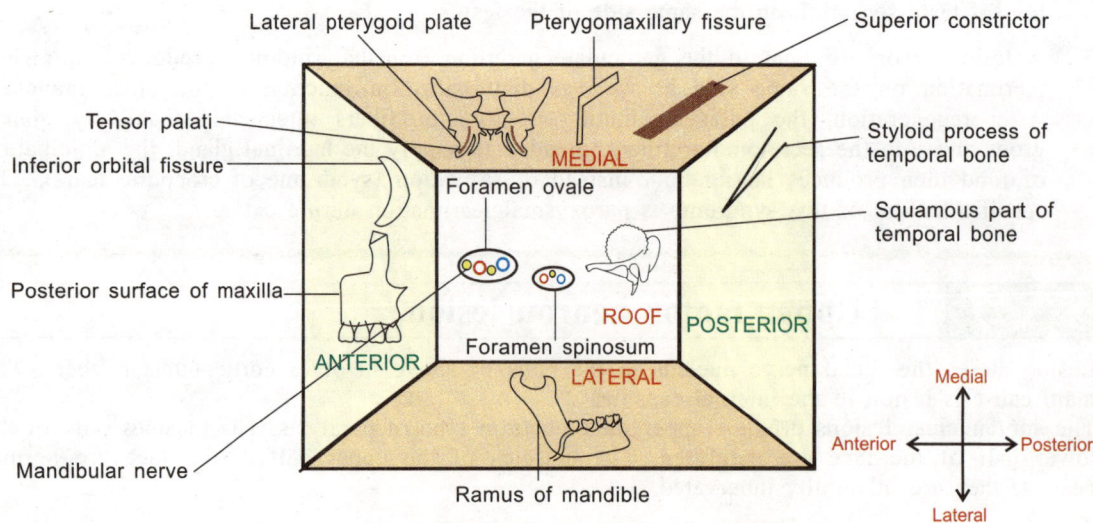

Fig. 3.53 : Boundries of infra temporal fossa

   D. Posterior wall is formed by
       a. Styloid process of temporal bone.
       b. Carotid sheath.
   E. Lateral wall is formed by
       a. Ramus of mandible.
       b. Coronoid process.

2. **Contents :**
   A. Muscles :
       a. Temporalis.
       b. Medial pterygoid.
       c. Lateral pterygoid.
   B. Artery :
       Maxillary artery and its branches
       a. Branches of first part   DIAMA
           I.   **D**eep auricular,
           II.   **I**nferior alveolar,
           III. **A**nterior tympanic,
           IV.   **M**iddle meningeal and
           V.   **A**ccessory meningeal.
       b. Branches to muscles of mastication.
           I.   Massetric branch,
           II.   Temporal branch.
           III. Pterygoid branch and
           IV.   Buccal branch.
   C. Pterygoid venous plexus.
   D. Nerves :
       a. Branches of mandibular division of trigeminal nerve.
           I.   Branches from main trunk.
                 i.   Branch to medial pterygoid.
                 ii. Meningeal branch.
           II.   Branches from anterior trunk (mainly motor)
                 i.   Massetric branch.
                 ii. Branch to lateral pterygoid.
                 iii. Deep temporal branch.
                 iv. Buccal branch.
           III. Branches from posterior trunk.
                 i.   Lingual branch.
                 ii. Auriculotemporal.
                 iii. Inferior alveolar.
       b. Chorda tympani nerve
       c. Posterior superior alveolar branch of maxillary nerve.
   E. Ganglion : Otic ganglion.

LAQ-20   Describe temporomandibular joint under
1. Classification   2. Ligaments
3. Movements & muscles bringing movements   4. Relations
5. Nerve supply &   6. Applied anatomy.

1. **Classification :**
   A. **Structurally :** Simple, complex, condylar, multiaxial, saddle shaped, atypical synovial joint.
   - a. **Simple :** Two bones namely mandible and temporal bone take part in the formation of TM joint.
     - I. Mandibular fossa on the inferior surface of the squamous part of temporal bone.
     - II. Head of mandible.
   - b. **Complex :** Joint cavity is separated by articular disc into upper menisco temporal lower menisco mandibular
   - c. **Condylar :** Left and right condyles of the head of mandible forms a bicondylar articulation.
   - d. **Multiaxial :** Protraction, retraction, elevation, depression and side to side movement.
   - e. **Saddle shaped :** Surfaces are convex and concave.
   - f. **Atypical synovial :** The articular surfaces of the head of mandible and mandibular fossa of temporal bone are not covered by hyaline cartilage, but are covered by fibro cartilage. Here collagen fibres predominate and cartilage cells are few.
   B. **Functionally :** Diarthrosis.

2. **Ligaments :** The ligaments can be divided into

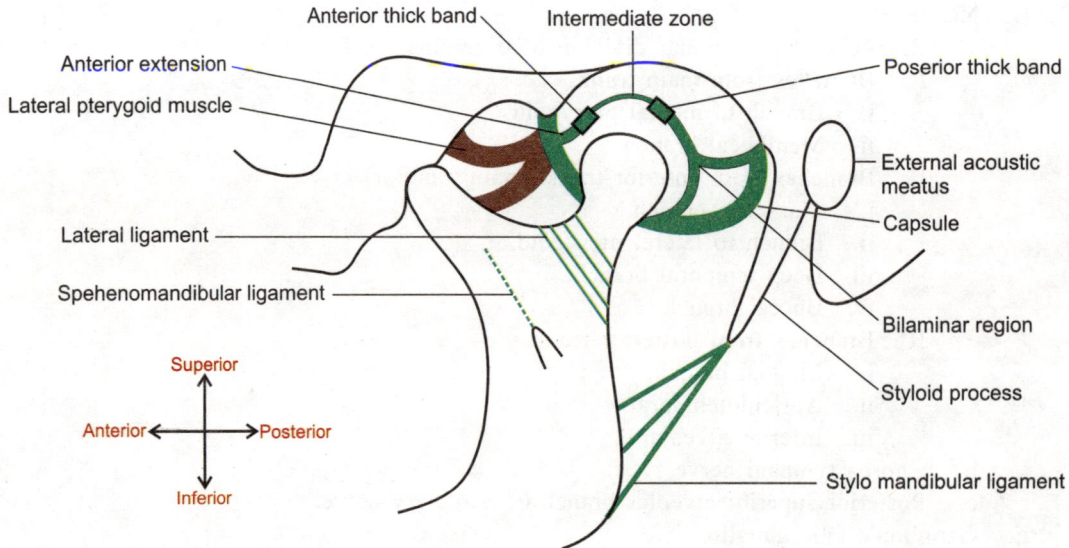

Fig. 3.54 : Articular disc and ligaments of temporomandibular joint.

A. Main ligaments
    a. Fibrous capsule
        I. Attachments
            i. Above :
                - Anteriorly : Anterior to articular tubercle.
                - Posteriorly : Posterior to the squamotympanic fissure.
                - Medially and laterally : To the margins of the mandibular fossa.
            ii. Below : Around neck of mandible
        II. Nature of the capsule
            i. Loose and lax above the disc,   **L** and **L**
            ii. Tense and thick below the disc.   **T** and T
        III. Peculiarities
            i. It is spacious, lax and strong.
            ii. It gives attachment to lateral pterygoid muscle.
    b. Articular disc : It is oval in shape and fibro-cartilage in nature.
        I. Morphologically it represents lateral pterygoid muscle.
        II. It is attached
            i. Anteriorly near the head of mandible.
            ii. Peripherally to the inside of the fibrous capsule.
        III. Parts :
            i. Anterior extension.
            ii. Anterior thick band.
            iii. Intermediate thin part.
            iv. Posterior thick band.
            v. Posterior bilaminar extension.
        IV. Variation in thickness : It is thick peripherally and thin in the center.
        V. Peculiarity : Gives attachment to lateral pterygoid muscle.
        VI. Functionally it divides the joint cavity into upper and lower compartment.
            i. The movement in the upper compartment is gliding.
            ii. The movement in the lower is rotatory and gliding.
    c. Lateral TM ligament
        I. It is a stout band of fibrous tissue.
        II. It covers lateral aspect of capsule and strengthens it.
        III. It extends from tubercle of root of zygoma to neck of the mandible.
        IV. It tightens in retraction and protraction and relaxes in the rest position.
    d. Synovial membrane
        I. It lines the fibrous capsule above and below the disc but does not cover the disc.
        II. It lines non articular surface of articulating bones.
        III. In new born, even the articular surfaces are covered by synovial membrane.
B. Accessory ligament :
    a. Sphenomandibular ligament :
        I. Introduction : It is an accessory ligament of temporomandibular joint, which lies on a deep plane away from fibrous capsule.
        II. Attachment: Arises from spine of sphenoid bone to the lingula of mandible.
    b. Stylomandibular ligament :
        I. It is a specialized band of deep cervical fascia.
        II. It stretches from the apex and adjacent anterior aspect of styloid process to the angle of mandible and posterior border.
        III. It is considered only accessory to the joint and of uncertain function.

3. **Movements and muscles bringing movements :**
   There are three sets of mandibular movements at the TM joint. These are
   A. Depression and elevation.
      a. *Depression is produced mainly by the lateral pterygoid.* The digastric, geniohyoid and mylohyoid muscles help when the mouth is opened wide or age against resistance.
      b. Elevation is produced by the masseter, the temporalis, and the medial pterygoid muscles of both sides.
   B. Side to side movement (gliding movement).
      Lateral or side to side movements are produced by the medial and lateral pterygoids of each side acting alternately.
   C. Protraction and retraction.
      a. Protrusion is done by the lateral (principally its inferior head) and medial pterygoids.
      b. Retraction is produced by the posterior fibers of the temporalis. It may be resisted by the middle and deep fibers of the masseter, the digastric and geniohyoid muscles.

4. **Relations :**
   A. Lateral :
      a. Skin and fascia,
      b. Parotid gland and
      c. Temporal branches of facial nerve.
   B. Medial :
      a. Tympanic plate of temporal bone,
      b. Spine of sphenoid; and sphenomandibular ligament,
      c. Auriculotemporal and chorda tympani nerve and
      d. Middle meningeal artery.

5. **Nerve supply :**
   A. Auriculo temporal nerve, a branch of posterior division of mandibular nerve.
   B. Masseteric nerve, a branch of the mandibular nerve.

6. **Applied anatomy :**
   A. *Forward dislocation is commonest form of displacement.*
      With the mouth open, the condyles are in the articular eminence and sudden violence, even muscular spasm (a convulsive yawn), may displace one or both temporomandibular joint.
   B. *Anterior dislocation readily occurs in the edentulous i.e. person without teeth.* It is easily reduced, the joint is less stable because the increased elevation of the edentulous mandible permanently elongates lateral ligament.
   C. The reduction of the TM joint is easily achieved by pressing down on the molar teeth with thumbs placed in the mouth, and at the same time pushing the chin upward and backward. The downward pressure on the molar teeth overcomes the tension of the temporalis and massetar muscles which are in spasm; and the upward and backward pressure on the chin helps the head of mandible to put into original position.
   D. *The great strength of the lateral temporomandibular ligament prevents the head of the mandible from passing backward and fracturing the tympanic plate when a severe blow falls on the chin.*
   E. The articular disc of the temporomandibular joint may become partially detached from

the capsule, and this results in its movement becoming noisy and producing an audible click during movements at the joint.

SN-24   Sphenomandibular ligament

1. **Introduction :** It is an accessory ligament of temporomandibular joint, which lies on a deep plane away from fibrous capsule.

2. **Attachment :** From spine of sphenoid bone to the lingula of mandible.

3. **Relations :**
    A. Laterally :   **MAIL**
        a. **M**axillary artery.
        b. **A**uriculotemporal nerve.
        c. **I**nferior alveolar nerve.
        d. **L**ateral pterygoid muscle.
    B. Medially :
        a. Medial pterygoid muscle.
        b. Chorda tympani nerve.
        c. Wall of the pharynx.

4. **Development :** Mesoderm of first pharyngeal arch, remnant of dorsal part of Meckel's cartilage.

5. **Applied anatomy :** Fracture of neck of mandible or dislocation of temporomandibular joint ruptures sphenomandibular ligament. This leads to loss of taste sensations due to injury to chorda tympani nerve.

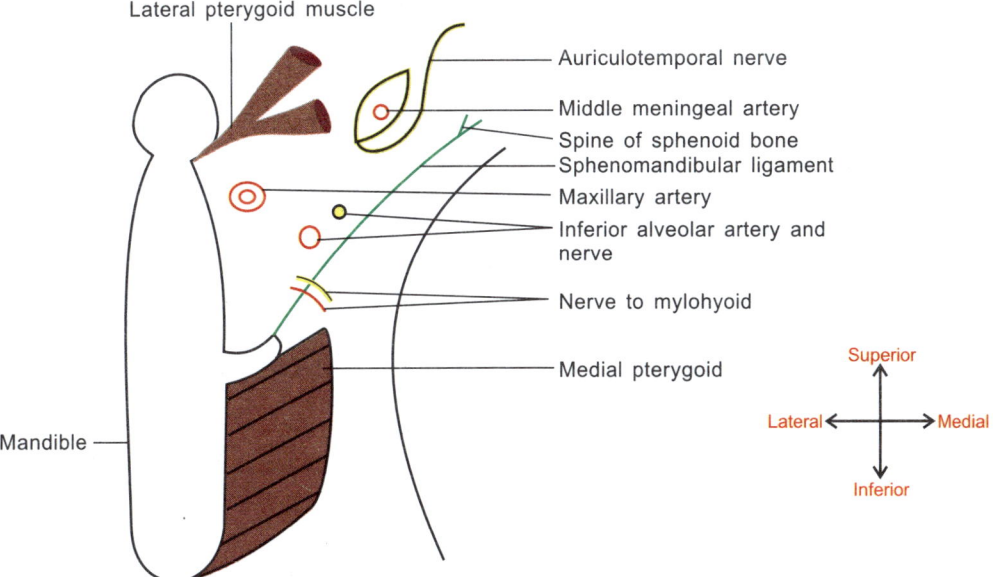

Fig. 3.55 : Relations of sphenomandibular ligament.

LAQ-21   **Describe muscles of mastication under**
  1.   **Origin**   2.   **Insertion**
  3.   **Action   &**   4.   **Nerve supply.**

Table 3.21 : The table shows origin, insertion and action of muscles of mastication.

Muscle	1. Origin	2. Insertion	3. Action

A. Masseter: It has three parts.	a. Superficial part
	  I. Anterior two-third of lower border of zygomatic arch.
	  II. Zygomatic process of maxilla.
	b. Intermediate part: Middle third of zygomatic arch.
	c. Deep part: Medial surface of zygomatic arch.
		All the fibers fuse and insert into the lateral surface of ramus of mandible.	Elevates the mandible to close the mouth and clenches the teeth.

B. Temporalis:	Whole of the temporal fossa between inferior temporal line and infratemporal crest of the greater wing of sphenoid bone.	Main insertion is on the anterior and posterior border of coronoid process.	a. Upper and anterior fibers elevate the mandible. b. Posterior fibers retract the mandible..
C. Lateral pterygoid: It has two heads.	a. Superior head arises from infratemporal surface and crest of the greater wing of sphenoid bone. b. Inferior head arises from lateral surface of lateral pterygoid plate.	a. Pterygoid fovea on the anterior surface of the neck of the mandible. b. Articular disc of TM joint. c. Capsule of TM joint.	a. It is indispensable for the active opening of the mouth. b. Both pterygoid acting together, protrude the mandible. c. Both the pterygoids contract alternately to produce side to side movements of the mandible.

D. Medial pterygoid: It has two heads.	a. Superficial head:
	  I. Tuberosity of maxilla.
	  II. Pyramidal process of palatine bone.
	b. Deep head:
	  I. Medial surface of lateral pterygoid plate
	  II. Pterygoid fossa.
		a. Rough area on the medial surface of angle of mandible.
		b. Adjoining part of the ramus of mandible.
		c. Area below and behind the mandibular foramen.
			a. Moves the mandible upward, forward and medially and closes the moth.
			b. *It is a great chewing muscle.*
			c. Both the pterygoids contract alternately to produce side to side movements of the mandible.

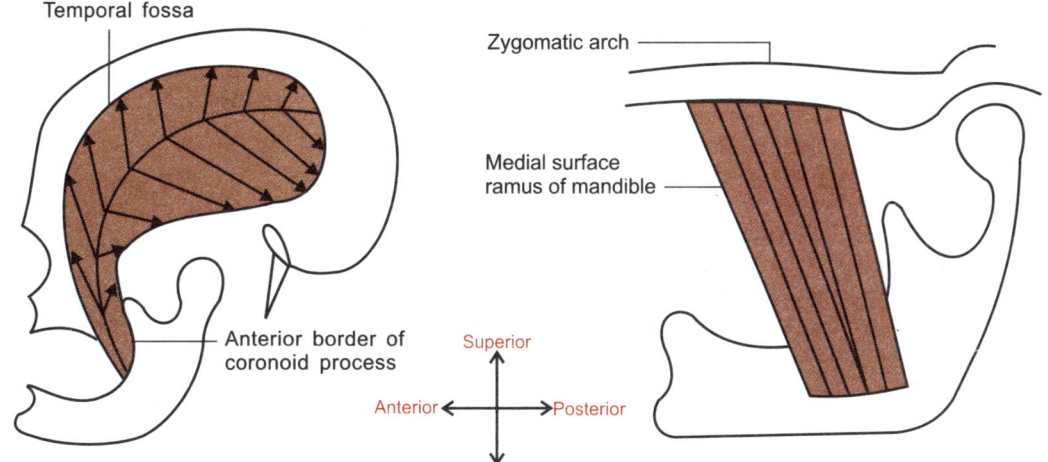

Fig. 3.56 : Attachment of temporalis muscle.

Fig. 3.57 : Attachment of masseter muscle.

4.   **Nerve supply :** *All the muscles of mastication are supplied by branches from anterior trunk of mandibular nerve except medial pterygoid which is supplied by branch from main trunk of mandibular nerve.*

LAQ-22   **Describe mandibular nerve under**
                1.   Origin   2.   Course and relations
                3.   Branches &   4.   Applied anatomy

1.   **Origin :** This nerve arises from trigeminal, the fifth cranial nerve.

2.   **Course and relations :** It begins in the middle cranial fossa by large sensory root and a small motor root. Both the roots join just before entering into foramen ovale. It emerges through foramen ovale as a mixed nerve. The main trunk lies in the infratemporal fossa. After a short course, the main trunk divides into anterior and posterior division.

3.   **Branches :**
      A.   From the main trunk :
           a.   Meningeal branch supplies duramater of the middle cranial fossa.
           b.   Nerve to the medial pterygoid supplies
                I.   Medial pterygoid muscle,
                II.   Tensor palati muscle and
                III.   Tensor tympani muscle.
      B.   From the anterior trunk : It is mainly motor except buccal branch, which is sensory.
           a.   Masseteric nerve supplies masseter muscle and TM joint.
           b.   Deep temporal supplies temporalis muscle.
           c.   Nerve to the lateral pterygoid supplies lateral pterygoid muscle.
           d.   Buccal nerve supplies the skin and mucous membrane related to buccinator.
      C.   From the posterior trunk : It is mainly sensory except nerve to mylohyoid, which is motor.

  a. Auriculotemporal nerve divides into
     I. Auricular part supplies the
       i.   Skin of the tragus.
       ii. Upper part of pina.
       iii. External acoustic meatus.
       iv. Tympanic membrane.
     II. Temporal part supplies skin of the temporal region.
     III. Articular branch to TM joint.
     IV. Parotid branch to the parotid gland.
  b. Lingual.
  c. Inferior alveolar which gives
     I. Nerve to mylohyoid
     II. Mental nerve.

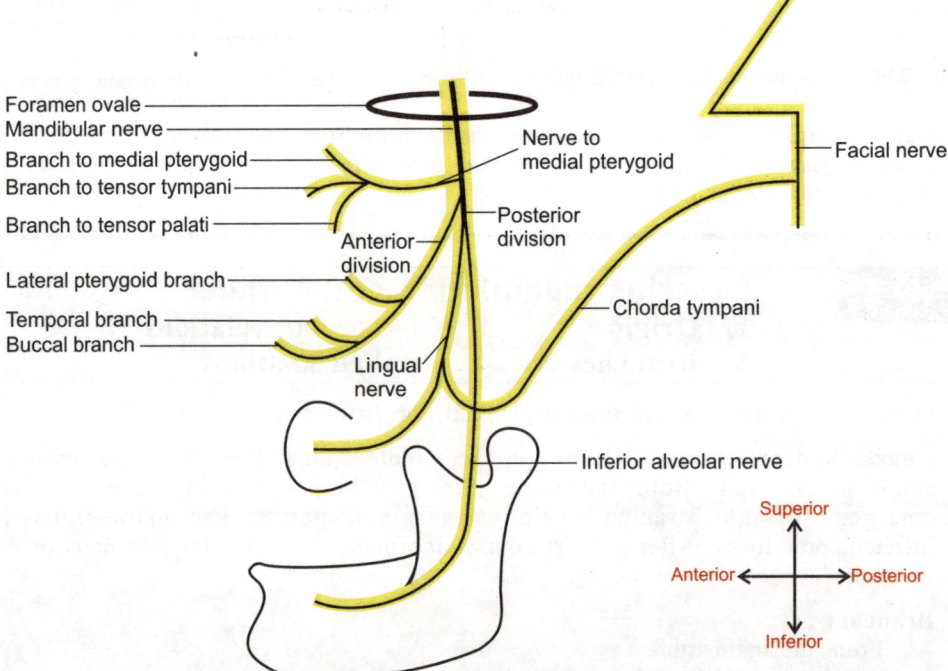

Fig. 3.58 : Mandibular nerve and its branches.

4. **Applied anatomy :**
  A. A lesion at the foramen ovale involves mandibular nerve and results in paraesthesia along the mandible, the lower (mandibular) teeth, and the side of face. There is also paralysis of muscles of mastication and loss of jaw-jerk reflex as this nerve supplies both afferent and efferent limbs for the jaw jerk reflex.
  B. Mandibular neuralgia : The pain along the distribution of mandibular division of trigeminal nerve is called mandibular neuralgia. It is often difficult to treat. This is treated by division of the sensory root of trigeminal nerve.
  C. The motor part of mandibular is tested by asking the patient to clench the teeth.

SN-25   Otic ganglion

It is collection of cellbodies of parasympathetic nerve supplying parotid gland situated in the peripheral part of cranium.

    A.   Topographically it is related to the mandibular nerve.

    B.   Functionally it is related to glossopharyngeal nerve.

1.   **Size :** 2 - 3 mm in size.

2.   **Situation :** Infratemporal fossa.

3.   **Relations :**

    A.   Superiorly : Foramen ovale.

    B.   Anteriorly : Medial pterygoid muscle.

    C.   Posteriorly : Middle meningeal artery.

    D.   Medially : Tensor palati.

    E.   Laterally : Mandibular nerve.

4.   **Connections :**

    A.   Parasympathetic or motor root

        a.   Preganglionic : Inferior salivary nucleus - glossopharyngeal nerve - tympanic branch of glossopharyngeal nerve - forms tympanic plexus along with caroticotympanic branch of internal carotid artery - a lesser petrosal branch is given - passes through foramen ovale - otic ganglion - relay.

        b.   Postganglionic - auriculotemporal nerve - parotid gland.

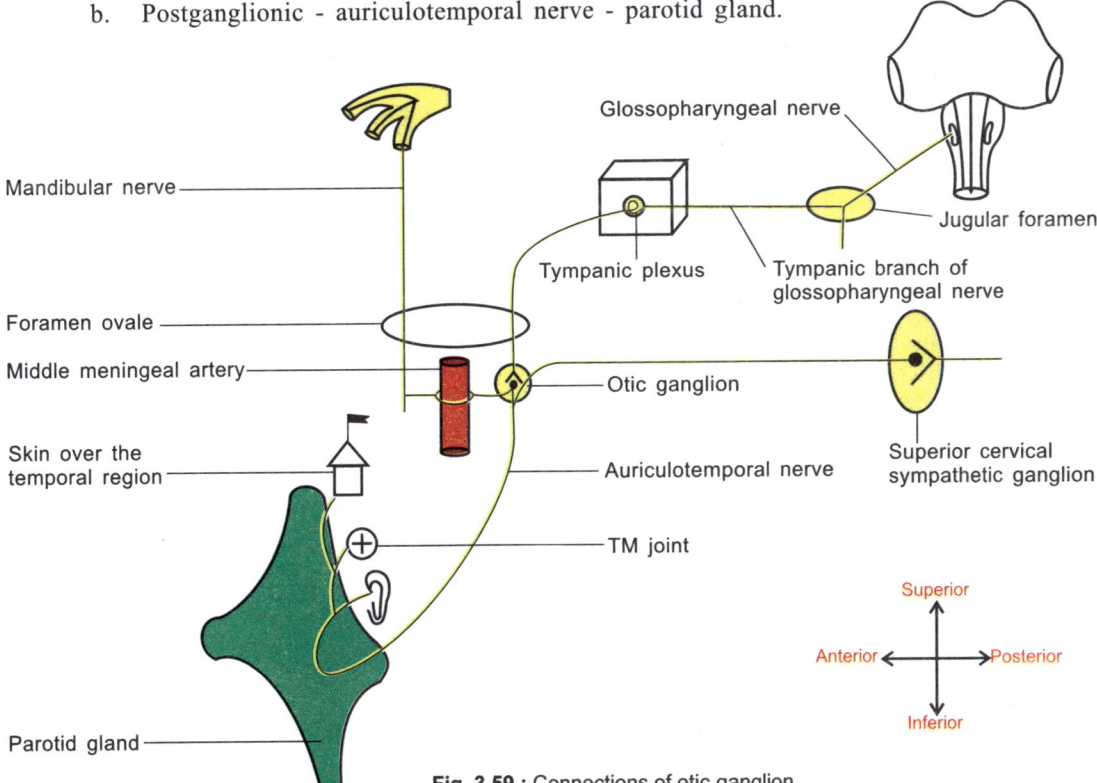

Fig. 3.59 : Connections of otic ganglion.

B. Sensory : Auriculotemporal nerve passes through otic ganglion without interrupting.
C. Sympathetic :
    a. Preganglionic : spinal nerve - superior cervical sympathetic ganglion.
    b. Postganglionic : plexus around external carotid artery.

5. Branches :
A. Auriculotemporal nerve to parotid gland.
B. Nerve to medial pterygoid pass through the otic ganglion and supply the
    a. Tensor palati and
    b. Tensor tympani.
C. The otic ganglion is connected to the chorda typmpani nerve and the nerve of pterygoid canal. This communicating channel possibly forms an alternate route of the taste pathway from the anterior two-third of trunk to the geniculate ganglion of the facial nerve.

6. Applied anatomy : Injury to the auriculotemporal nerve manifests in the loss of saliva.

LAQ-23 **Describe submandibular gland under**
    1. Morphology   **2. Relations**
    3. Blood supply   **4. Lymphatic drainage**
    5. Nerve supply and   **6. Applied anatomy.**

1. Morphology :
This is a large salivary gland situated in the anterior part of digastric triangle. It extends upto stylomandibular ligament.
A. Division : The gland is divided by mylohyoid muscle into
    a. Large superficial part and
    b. Small deep part.
B. Ends : It presents two ends :
    a. Anterior and
    b. Posterior.
C. Presents three surfaces :
    a. Inferior,
    b. Lateral &
    c. Medial.

2. Relations :
A. Superficial part :
    a. Relation to inferior surface :
        I. Skin,
        II. Superficial fascia,
        III. Platysma,
        IV. Deep fascia,
        V. Common facial vein,
        VI. Cervical branch of facial nerve,
        VII. Submandibular lymph node.
    b. Relation to lateral surface :
        I. Submandibular fossa of mandible,

II. Medial pterygoid muscle and
III. Facial artery.

c. Medial surface is extensive and divided into 3 parts :
   I. Anterior
      i. Mylohyoid muscles,
      ii. Mylohyoid vessels,
      iii. Mylohyoid nerve and
      iv. Submental branch of facial artery.
   II. Intermediate
      i. Hyoglossus,
      ii. Lingual nerve,
      iii. Submandibular ganglion,
      iv. Hypoglossal nerve and
      v. Intermediate tendon of digastric.
   III. Posterior
      i. Styloglossus,
      ii. Stylopharyngus,
      iii. Digastric,
      iv. Middle constrictor of pharynx and
      v. Hypoglossal nerve, lingual artery.

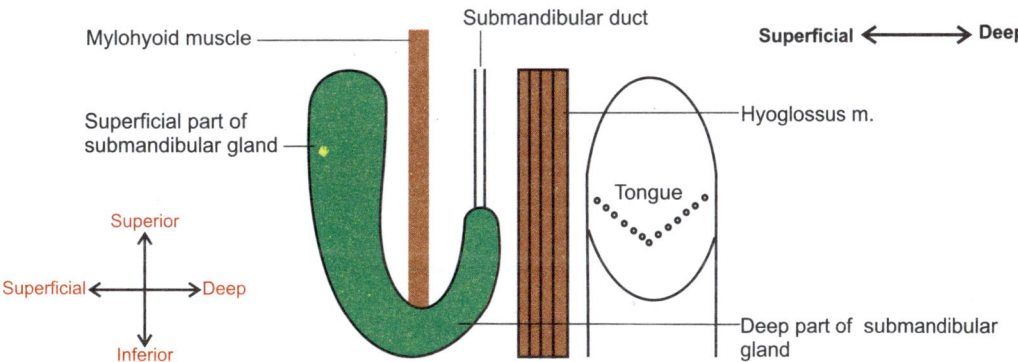

Fig. 3.60 : Superficial and deep part of submandibular gland.

B. Deep Part :
  a. Laterally : Mylohyoid.
  b. Medially : Hyoglossus and styloglossus

3. Blood supply :
A. Arterial supply : Facial artery.
B. Venous drainage : Common facial or lingual vein.

4. Lymphatic drainage : Submandibular lymph nodes.

5. Nerve supply :
A. Secretomotor fibres : Arises from superior salivatory nucleus.
  a. Preganglionic fibers pass through facial nerve, geniculate ganglion, chorda tympani and the lingual nerve to reach submandibular ganglion.
  b. Post ganglion fibers arise from ganglion and enter submandibular gland.
B. Sensory fibres reach the ganglion through lingual nerve.

C. Sympathetic fibres arise from superior cervical sympathetic ganglion.
These fibres do not relay in the submandibular ganglion

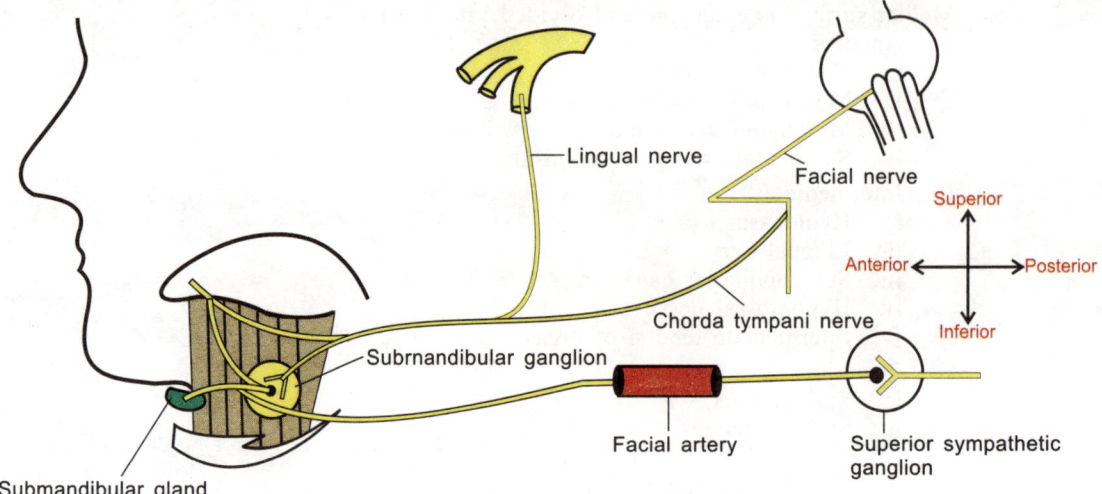

Fig. 3.61 : Nerve supply of submandibular gland.

6. **Applied Anatomy :**
A. The submandibular gland is excised by an incision one inch below the angle of jaw. Since the mandibular branch of facial nerve is closely related.
B. The secretion of the submandibular gland is more viscus, hence the incidence of calculi is more common in the submandibular gland.
C. A stone in the submandibular duct (Wharton's duct) can be palpated bimanually in the floor of the mouth and can even be seen if sufficiently large.

SN-26   Submandibular ganglion

1. **Introduction :** It is a collection of cell bodies present in the course of parasympathetic nerve supplying the submandibular and sublingual gland.
A. It is topographically connected to lingual nerve.
B. It is functionally connected to facial nerve.

2. **Gross :**
A. Shape : Fusiform.
B. Situation : On hyoglossus muscle.
C. Relations :
a. Superior : Lingual nerve.
b. Inferiorly : Deep part of submandibular gland.
D. Connections :
a. Parasympathetic.
I. Preganglionic fibres : Superior salivatory nucleus - facial nerve - chorda tympani joins with lingual nerve - submandibular ganglion - relay.
II. Postganglionic fibres : Unnamed branches - to submandibular or sublingual gland.

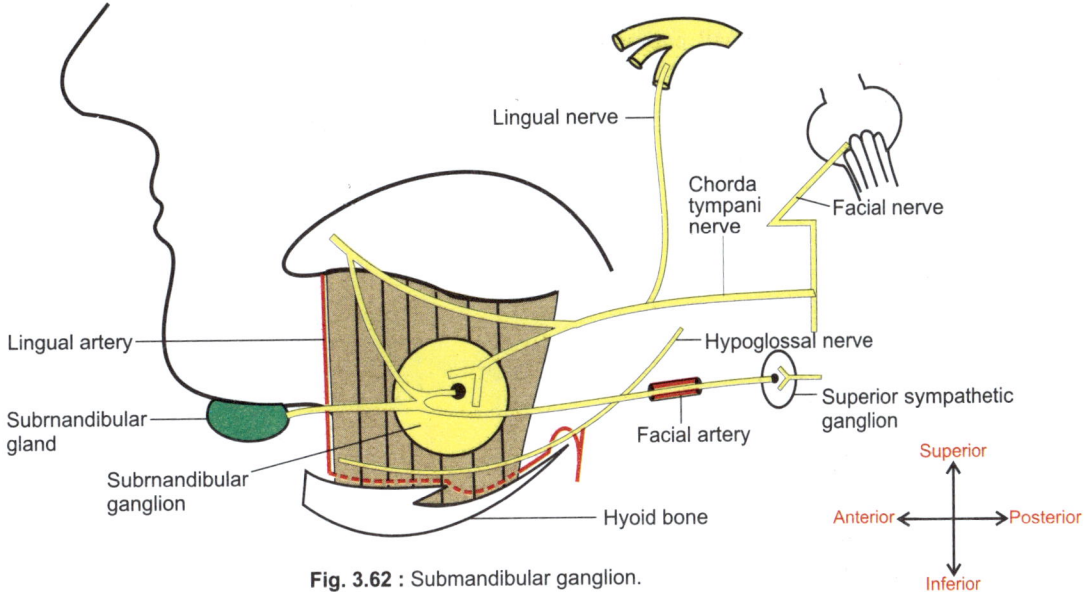

Fig. 3.62 : Submandibular ganglion.

   b.   Sympathetic fibres :
       I.   Preganglionic fibers arise from : Spinal nerves - superior cervical sympathetic ganglion - fibers relay in the ganglion.
      II.   Postganglionic fibers form the plexus around external carotid artery - (lingual artery) the fibers do no relay.
   c.   Sensory : Lingual nerve, branch of submandibular nerve.
  E.   Branches : Five to six branches enter the submandibular gland, sublingual and anterior lingual gland.

LAQ-24 **Describe thyroid gland under**
1. Gross   **2. Histology**
3. Development and   **4. Applied anatomy.**

(*Thyreos* shield, *cides* form)
1. **Gross :**
  A. Situation :
    a. It is situated in front of $C_{5, 6, 7}$ and T_1 vertebrae.
    b. Each lobe extends from oblique line of thyroid cartilage to the sixth tracheal ring.
    c. The isthmus extends from the second to the third tracheal ring.
  B. Dimensions and weight :
    a. Each lobe measures **2" x 1" x 1"**.
    b. The isthmus measures ½" x ½"
    c. Weight : About 25 gms.
  C. Capsules :
    a. True capsule : It is condensation of peripheral connective tissue of gland.
    b. False capsule : It is condensation of pretracheal layer of deep cervical fascia.

D. Surfaces :
   a. Glands   LMP compare the surfaces of a long bone.
       I.   Lateral
       II. Medial
       III. Posterior
   b. Isthmus
       I.   Anterior
       II. Posterior
E. Borders :
   a. Glands
       I.   Anterior
       II. Posterior
   b. Isthmus
       I.   Upper
       II. Inferior
F. Relations of thyroid Gland :
   a. Relations to surface
       I.   Lateral   4S
          I.   Sternothyroid,
          Ii.   Sternohyoid,
          iii. Superior belly of omohyoid and
          iv   Sternomastoid.

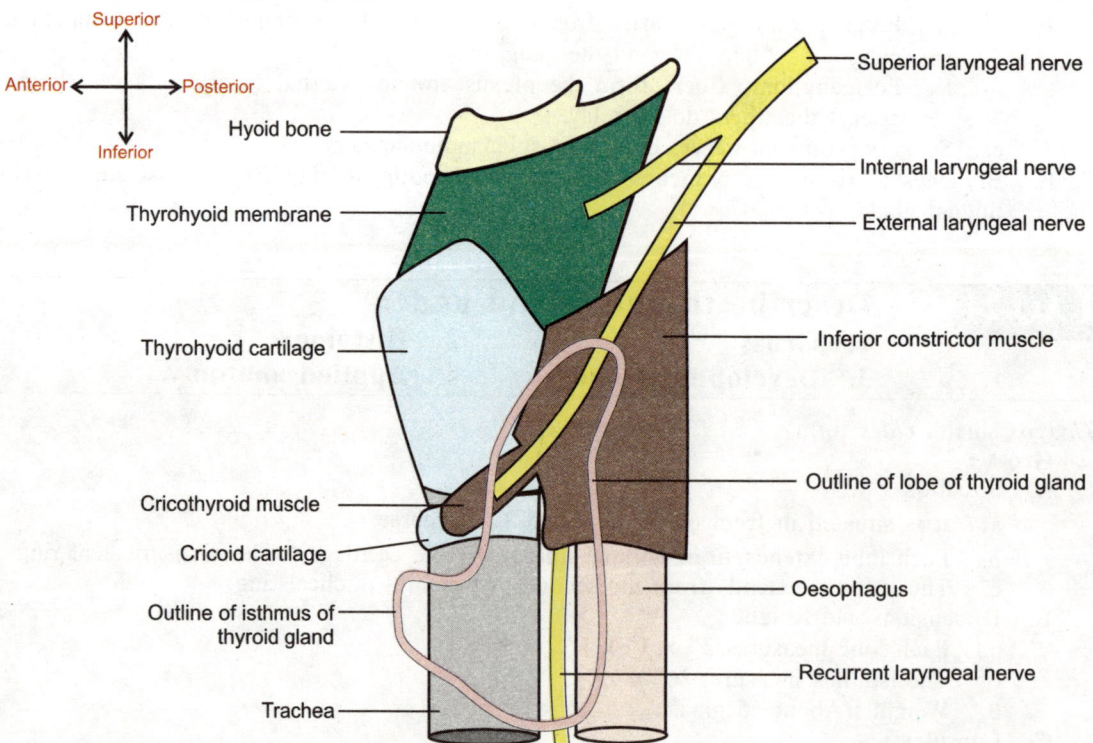

Fig. 3.63 : Structures related to medial and lateral surface of thyroid gland.

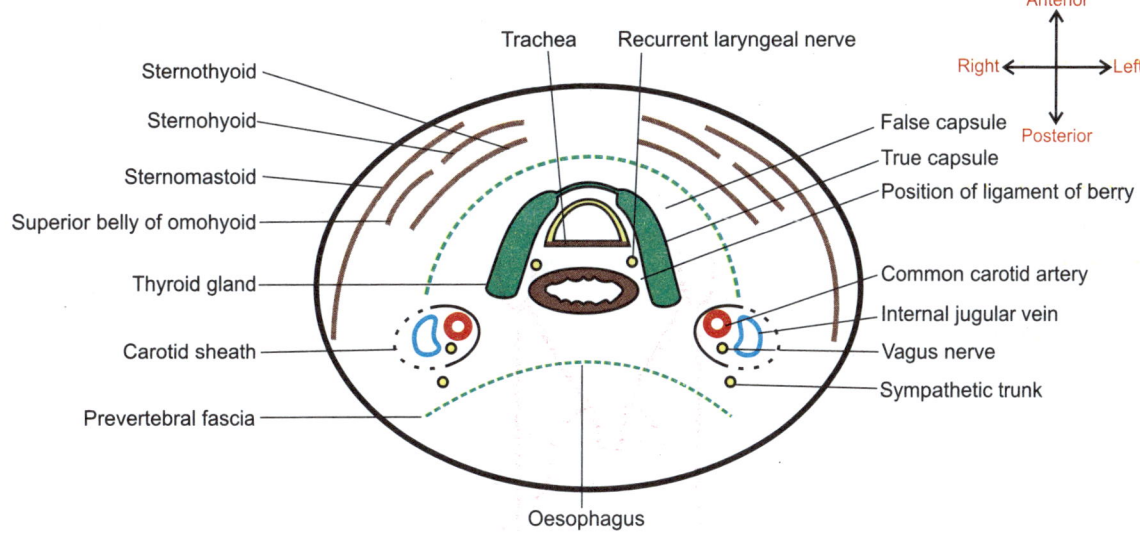

Fig. 3.64 : Relations at the level of the isthumus of the thyroid gland.

II. Medial
  i. **M**uscles :
   - Inferior constrictor and
   - Cricothyroid.
  ii. **T**ubes :
   - Trachea and
   - Oesophagus.
  iii. **N**erves :
   - External and
   - Recurrent laryngeal.
III. Posterolateral : Carotid sheath.
 b. Relations to border
  I. Anterior : Superior thyroid artery (anterior branch).
  II. Posterior : Parathyroid gland is important structure. 🔑🗝 **ITA**
   i. **I**nferior thyroid artery.
   ii. **T**horacic duct (only on left side).
   iii. **A**nastomosis between superior & inferior thyroid artery.
G. Blood Supply :
 a. Arterial : 🔑🗝 **ITA**
  I. *Inferior thyroid artery : It supplies blood to the major part of the thyroid gland i.e. (Two-third of lateral lobes and half of the isthmus).* It is a branch of thyrocervical trunk (a branch of subclavian artery) penetrates deep surface of gland and anastomoses with descending branch of superior thyroid artery on posterior border of thyroid gland. *It is closely related to recurrent laryngeal nerve near the gland.* It supplies
   i. Lower two-third of lobe of the gland and
   ii. Lower half of isthmus.
  II. Superior thyroid artery (a branch of external carotid) descends upto apex of

thyroid gland and divides into anterior and posterior branch, which descends along anterior and posterior border. The anterior branch anastomoses with artery of opposite side on superior border of isthmus. Posterior branch anastomoses with inferior thyroid artery on posterior border. *It is closely related with external laryngeal nerve.* It supplies

i.   Upper one-third of the gland and
ii. Upper half of isthmus.

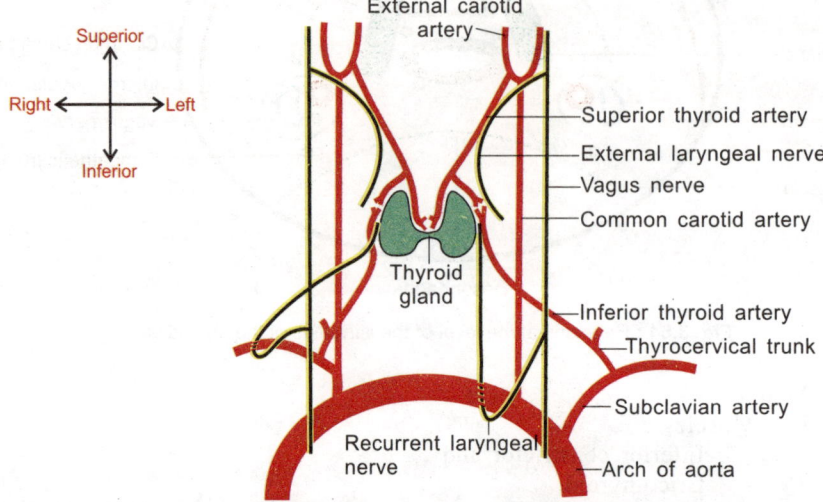

Fig. 3.65 : Arterial supply of thyroid gland.

III. Thyroid ima : It either arises from brachiocephalic trunk or arch of aorta. It supplies isthmus of thyroid gland.

IV. Numerous accessory thyroid arteries, branches of oesophageal and tracheal arteries. These branches supply the gland from the medial or deep surface.

b.   Venous Drainage : The veins of the thyroid gland form plexus which is situated deep to the capsule and drain as follows

I.   Superior thyroid vein : It drains into internal jugular vein.
II. Middle thyroid vein : It drains into internal jugular vein.
III. Inferior thyroid vein : It drains into left branchiocephalic vein.

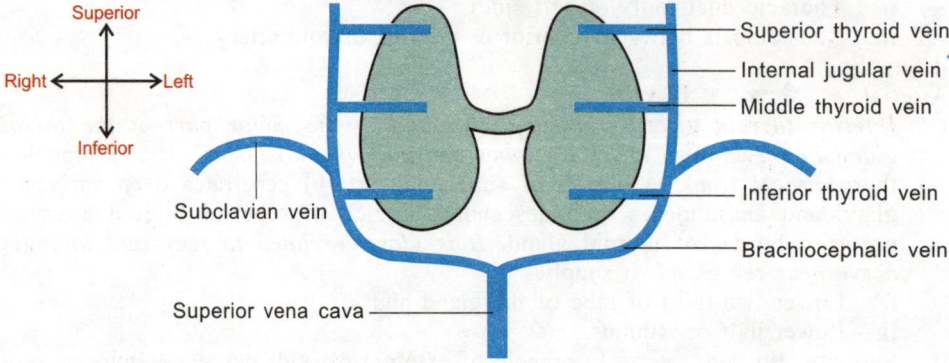

Fig. 3.66 : Venous drainage of thyroid gland.

H.   Lymphatic Drainage : They are arranged into
     a.   Upper group : Prelaryngeal and jugulo digastric.
     b.   Lower group : Pretracheal group along recurrent laryngeal nerve.
I.   Nerve supply : They are derived
     a.   Mainly from middle cervical sympathetic ganglion.
     b.   Partly by superior and inferior sympathetic ganglion.
     c.   Function : Vasoconstriction.

2.   Histology :

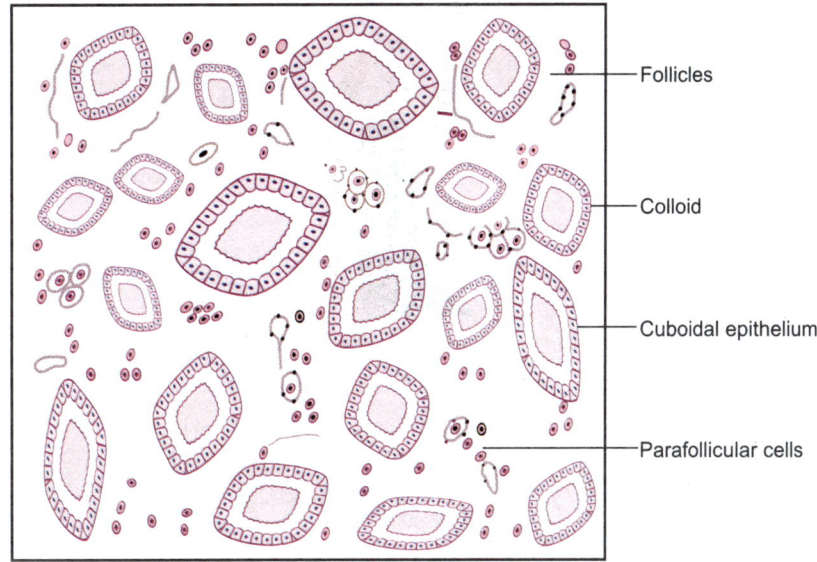

Fig. 3.67 : Histology of thyroid gland.

A.   Lumen of follicles, shows colloid material.
B.   Follicles are lined by cuboidal epithelium.
C.   There are clear or light cells called parafollicular cells which produce calcitonin.
D.   They are polyhedral with oval, eccentric nuclei.
E.   They are present between follicular cells and lie on basement membrane.

3.   Development :
A.   Chronological age : It develops in the fourth week of intrauterine life.
B.   Germ layer : It develops from endoderm diverticulum, the thyro glossal duct.
C.   Site : Floor of the pharynx behind the tuberculum impar of the developing tongue.
D.   Sources : It develops as a median thyroid diverticulum extending from foramen caecum
     to thyroid cartilage. The distal part becomes bifid within which the duct divides into a
     series of double cellular plates. The duct disappears, its cephalic end persists as a
     foramen caecum and its caudal end occasionally forms the pyramidal lobe.
E.   Anomalies :   🔑   **ITA**
     a.   **I**ncomplete descent of thyroid gland.
     b.   **T**hyroglossal duct.
     c.   **T**hyroglossal cyst.
     d.   **A**genesis of thyroid gland.

4. **Applied anatomy :**

A. 🔑 **ITA** *During thyroidectomy __inferior__ thyroid artery should be __tied away__ from the gland to avoid injury to recurrent laryngeal nerve and superior thyroid artery should be tied near the gland to avoid the injury to the external laryngeal nerve.*

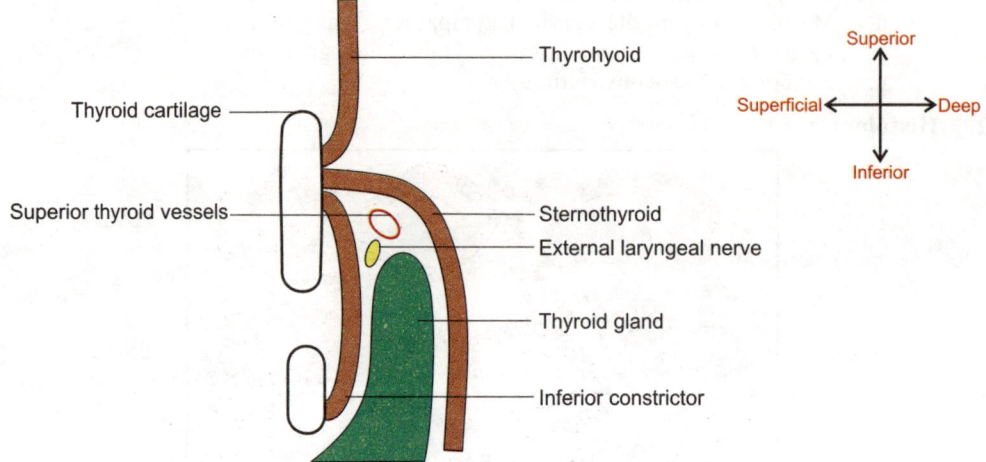

Fig. 3.68 : Attachments of sternothyroid muscle showing prevention of upward enlargement of thyroid gland.

B. Thyroid gland is enclosed in the pretracheal fascia, which is attached to the trachea and larynx. The posterior wall of the larynx is the anterior wall of pharynx. During deglutination, the pharynx moves, so that larynx also moves. Hence, swellings arising from thyroid gland also move. *This is an important diagnostic feature to differentiate swelling arising from thyroid gland and swelling arising from other structures in the midline.*

C. The upward enlargement of thyroid gland is prevented by sternothyroid muscle as it is attached to oblique line of thyroid cartilage. *Hence all the swellings of thyroid gland enlarge downwards.*

D. A dense capsule is present deep to true capsule. Hence during thyroidectomy, true capsule is also removed along with the thyroid gland, to avoid bleeding.

E. Partial thyroidectomy is preferred over total thyroidectomy, to avoid postoperative myxoedema. Usually posterior parts of both lobes of thyroid glands are left to avoid hypoparathyroidism.

F. Benign tumors are characterized by displacement and compression of neighboring structures.

G. Malignant tumors of thyroid gland are characterized by invasion and erosion of neighboring structures namely recurrent laryngeal nerve.

SN-27   Thyroglossal duct

1. **Introduction :** A duct extending from the foramen caecum of tongue to thyroid primordium. It is present in embryonic life. It is formed by endoderm of third and fourth pharyngeal arches.

2. **Fate :** Distal part usually differentiates to form pyramidal lobe and thyroid gland and the remainder part obliterates.

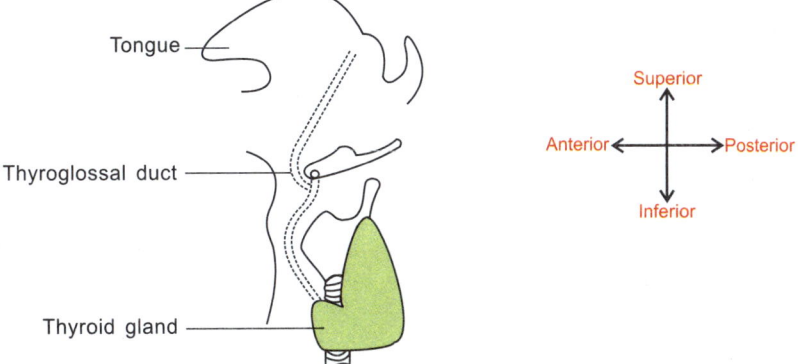

Fig. 3.69 : Thyroglossal duct.

3. **Chronological age :** At seventh week of intra uterine life.

4. **Applied anatomy :** Persistence of fragment of thyroglossal duct results into thyroglossal cysts or fistula.

Refer the Fig of thyroglossal cyst.

SN-28   Thyroglossal cyst

1. **Aetiology :** It results from persistence of a portion of a thyroglossal duct.

2. **Incidence :** It is the commonest congenital anomaly.

3. **Site :** Below the level of hyoid bone.

4. **Age :** It is evident in the late teens presumably because the lining becomes secretory.

5. **Clinical manifestation :**
    A. It presents as a swelling along the course of duct.
    B. There is reoccurrence of thyroglossal cyst if the whole of the thyroglossal duct is not removed.

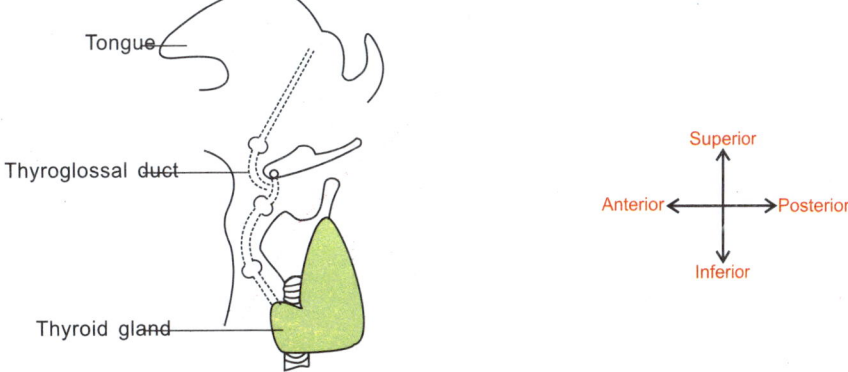

Fig 3.69A : Thyroglossal cyst.

SN-29 Parathyroid gland

These are two pairs (superior and inferior) of small endocrine glands.

1. **Site :** On posterior border lateral of lateral lobe of thyroid gland. They are present within the capsule of thyroid gland.

2. **Gross :**
    A. Weight : 50 mg. each.
    B. Dimensions : 6 x 4 x 2 mm.
    C. Position :
        a. Superior parathyroid gland is more constant in position and lies at the middle of posterior border of lateral lobe of thyroid gland. It lies inside the true capsule and dorsal to recurrent laryngeal nerve.
        b. The inferior parathyroid gland is ventral to the recurrent laryngeal nerve. The position of inferior parathyroid gland is variable. It may be :
            I.   Outside the false capsule of thyroid gland and above the inferior thyroid artery.
            II. Within the false capsule of thyroid gland and below the inferior thyroid artery near the lower pole of thyroid lobe.
            III. Within the substance of the thyroid gland near its posterior border.

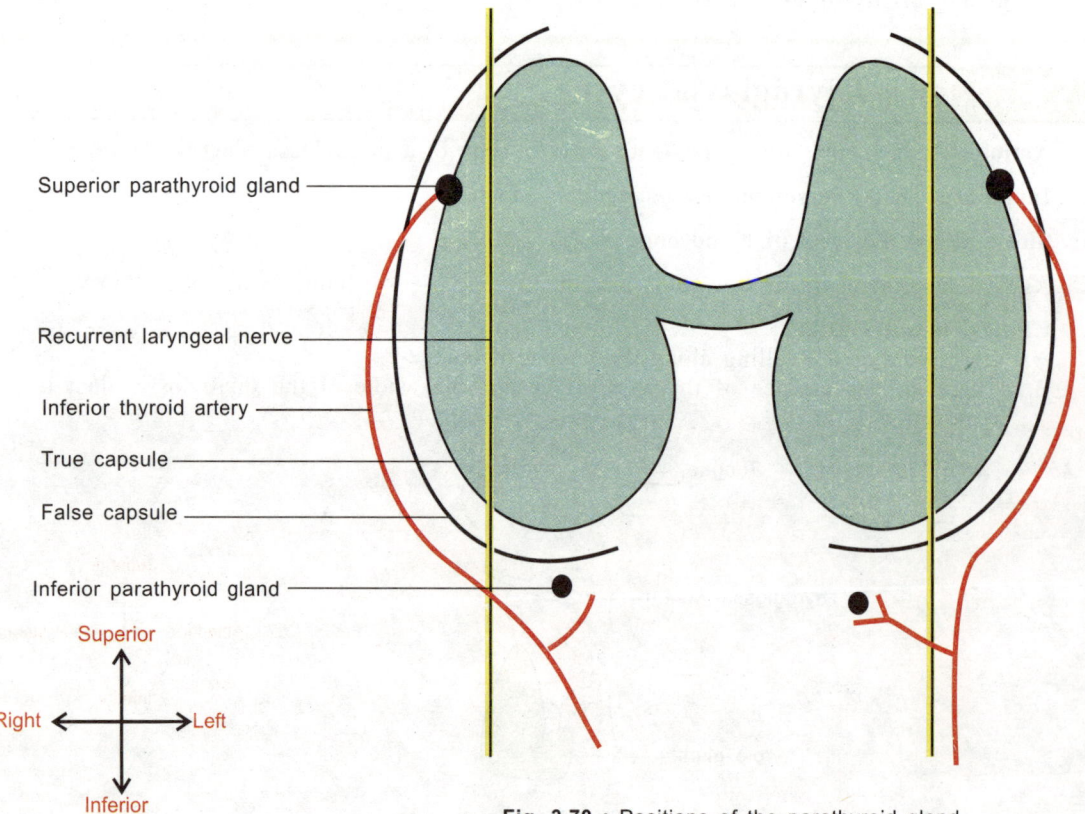

Fig. 3.70 : Positions of the parathyroid gland.

D. Blood supply : It has rich blood supply.
   a. Arterial supply :
      I. Inferior thyroid artery.
      II. Anastomosis between superior and inferior thyroid artery.
   b. Venous drainage by :
      I. Superior thyroid vein drains into internal jugular vein.
      II. Middle thyroid vein drains into internal jugular vein.
      III. Inferior thyroid vein drains into left brachiocephalic vein.
E. Applied anatomy :
   a. Tumors of the parathyroid gland, present outside the false capsule, grow downward and descend in the posterior mediastinum of thorax.
   b. Tumors of parathyroid gland present within the false capsule, grow downwards and descend into superior mediastinum of thorax.

SN-30   Subclavian artery

1. **Introduction :** It is the main artery of upper limb and supplies considerable part of neck and brain.

2. **Origin :** On the right side it arises from brachiocephalic trunk. On the left side it arises from arch of aorta.

3. **Extent :** It extends from sternoclavicular joint to outer border of first rib.

4. **Course and relations :** The artery is divided into three parts by scalenus anterior muscle.

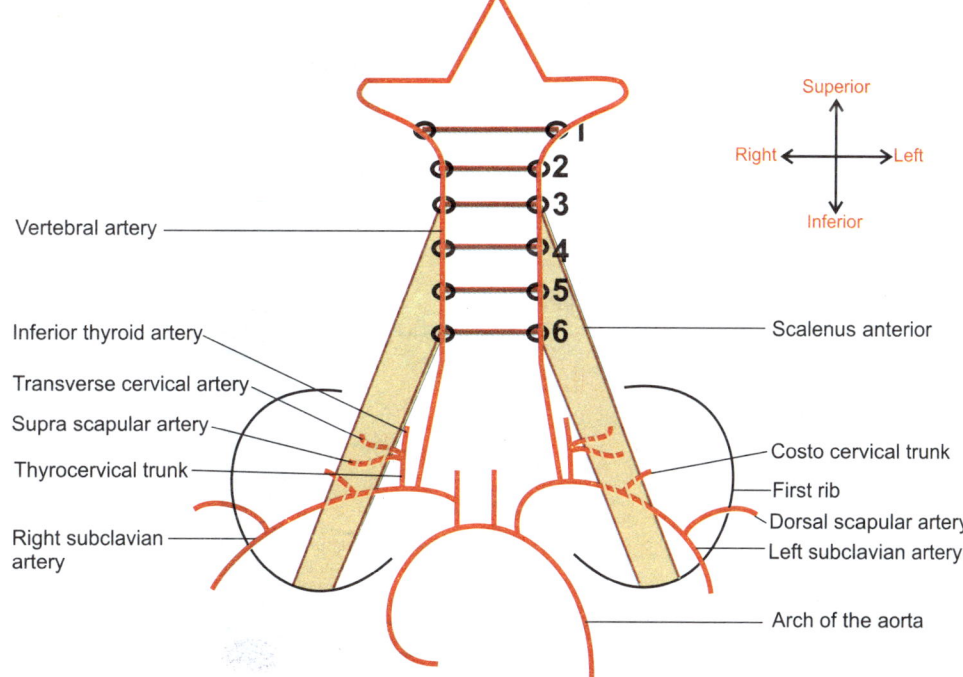

Fig. 3.71 : Subclavian artery and its branches.

First part of subclavian artery is medial, second part is posterior and third part is lateral to scalenus anterior muscle.

5. **Branches :** 🔑 **VIT C D**
    A. First part :
       a. **V**ertebral artery.
       b. **I**nternal thoracic artery.
       c. **T**hyrocervical trunk which divides into : 🔑 **SIT**
          I. **S**uprascapular.
          II. **I**nferior thyroid.
          III. **T**ransverse cervical.
    B. Second part : **C**ostocervical artery.
    C. Third part : **D**orsal scapular artery.

6. **Applied anatomy :** Subclavian steal syndrome takes place in obstruction of the subclavian artery proximal to the origin of vertebral artery. Some amount of blood is stolen from the brain through the vertebral artery of the opposite side in order to provide collateral circulation to the affected arm. This may result in ischaemic neurological symptoms.

SN-31   Internal jugular vein

It is direct continuation of sigmoid sinus.

1. **Extent :** It extends from jugular foramen to sternal end of clavicle. It joins the subclavian vein to form brachiocephalic vein.

2. **Tributaries :**
    A. Pharyngeal vein,
    B. Superior thyroid vein,
    C. Middle thyroid vein,
    D. Lingual vein,
    E. Common facial vein and
    F. Inferior petrosal sinus.

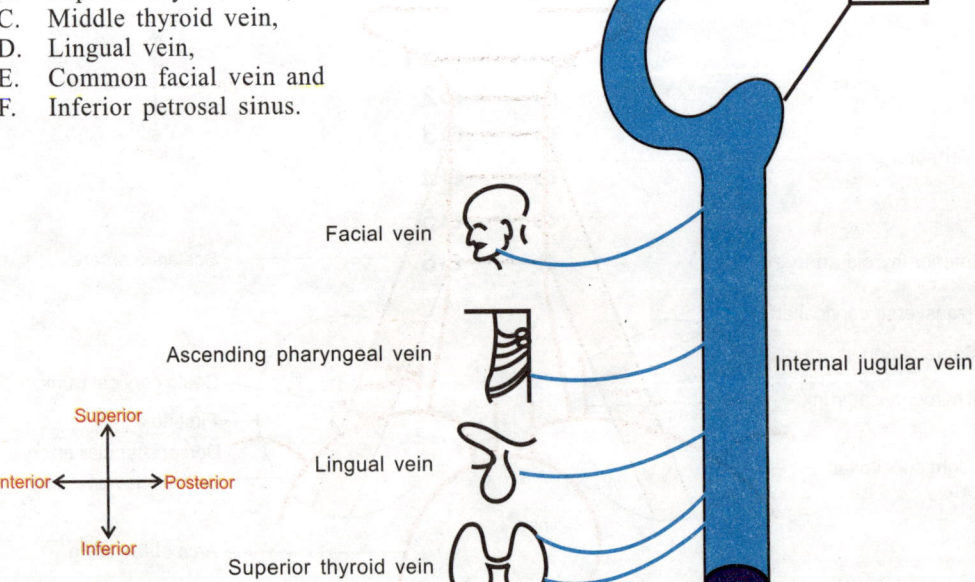

Fig. 3.72 : Internal jugular vein and its tributaries.

3. **Relations :**
   A. Posteriorly : The relation are from above downwards
      a. Rectus capitis lateralis.
      b. Transverse process of atlas.
      c. Levator scapulae.
      d. Scalenus medius and cervical plexus of nerves.
      e. Scalenus anterior and phrenic nerve.
      f. Thyrocervical trunk and first part of vertebral artery.
      g. First part of subclavian artery.
   B. Anterolaterally :
      a. It is crossed by superior belly of omohyoid and posterior belly of digastric.
      b. Below the omohyoid : Sternohyoid and sternothyroid.
   C. Medially :
      a. Common carotid artery.
      b. Vagus nerve.

4. **Applied anatomy :**
   A. The internal jugular vein is accessible deep to the supraclavicular fossa. This vein is used for recording venous pulse pressure.
   B. In the congestive cardiac failure the internal jugular vein is most dilated vein.
   C. The deep cervical lymph nodes lie on the internal jugular vein.

LAQ-25 | Describe glosso pharyngeal nerve under
1. **Functional components**   2. **Course and relations**
3. **Branches   and   4.   Applied anatomy.**

Glossopharyngeal nerve. [Cartico parotico tonsili tympani]
1. **Functional components :**

Table 3.22 : The table shows functional components & the functions of the glossopharyngeal nerve.

Functional components	Functions
A. General somatic afferent.	Pain, touch and temperature from posterior one-third of tongue, tonsil, soft palate & oral part of pharynx.
B. Special visceral afferent SVAd.	Taste sensations from the circumvallate papillae and posterior one-third part of tongue.
C. General visceral afferent sensation.	From baro-receptor and chemo-receptor of the carotid body and carotid sinus.
D. Branchial efferent (special visceral efferent). SaVE	Motor to stylopharyngeus.
E. General visceral efferent. GiVE Glands.	Secretomotor fibers to parotid gland.

2. **Course and relations :** The nerve arises by 3 to 4 filaments from postero lateral sulcus of medulla oblongata. The nerve leaves the skull by passing through middle part of jugular foramen, anterior to the 10th and 11th cranial nerves. It has a separate dural sheath.

Extraneural course :
A. The nerve descends between internal jugular vein and internal carotid artery.
B. It lies deep to styloid process and muscles attached to it.
C. It passes between external and internal carotid artery.
D. It lies on muscles of pharynx. Here it gives a pharyngeal branch. It enters the submandibular region deep to hyoglossus muscle where it breaks up into tonsillar and lingual branch.

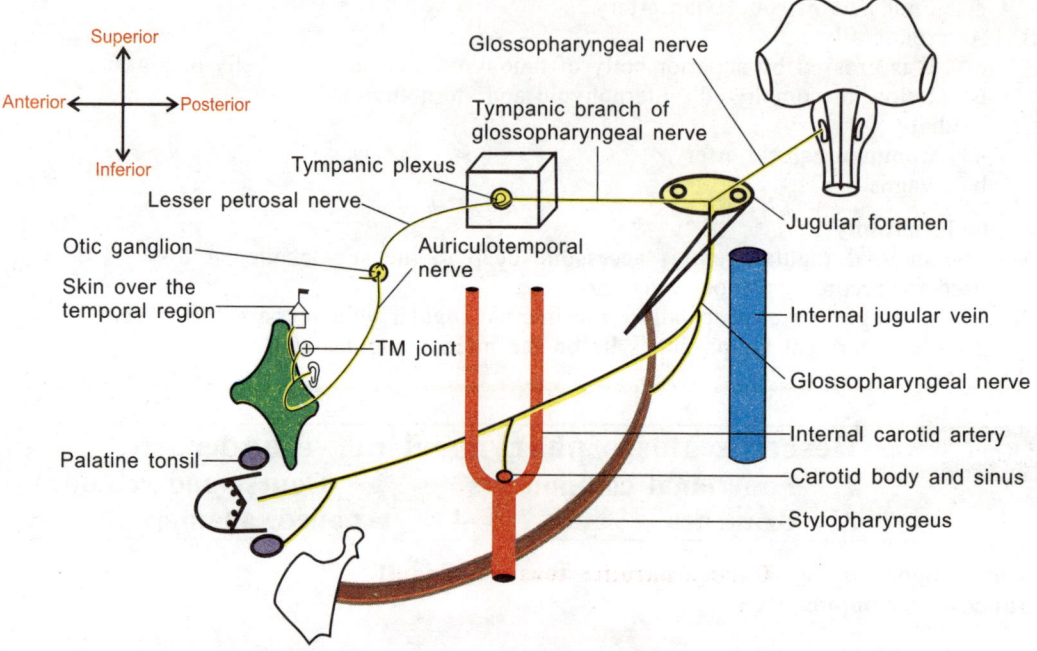

Fig. 3.73 : Course and distribution of glossopharyngeal nerve.

3. **Branches :** The word glossopharyngeal indicates *glosso* = tongue, *pharyngeal* = pharynx. It is sensory nerve of pharynx and tongue and motor nerve of muscle of pharynx i.e. stylopharyngeus. In addition to this the nerve is renamed as
🔑 **CAROTICO PAROTICO TONSILI TYMPANI**
meaning thereby it supplies carotid body and carotid sinus,
supplies parotid gland, tonsils and middle ear cavity (Tympanic branch) Dr. Kadasne
A. Carotid branch
    a. Carotid body and
    b. Carotid sinus.
B. Tympanic branch ⟶ tympanic plexus ⟶ lesser petrosal nerve ⟶ otic ganglion ⟶ auriculo temporal nerve ⟶ parotid gland.
C. Tonsiliar branch : Tonsil.
D. Tympanic branch : Middle ear cavity.
E. Lingual branch : Posterior one-third of tongue.
F. Muscular branch : Stylopharyngeus muscle.

4. **Applied anatomy :**
   A. The glossopharyngeal nerve is tested clinically by
      a. Tickling the posterior wall of pharynx. There is loss of reflex contraction of throat muscle in the lesion of glossopharyngeal nerve.
      b. Testing sensations from posterior one-third of tongue.
   B. Isolated lesion of glossopharyngeal nerve is almost unknown.

SN-32   **Recurrent laryngeal nerve**

1. **Origin :**
   A. *Right recurrent laryngeal nerve arises from vagus nerve in the neck.*
   B. *Left recurrent laryngeal nerve arises from the vagus nerve in the thorax.*

2. **Course and relations :** Is slightly different for the right and left recurrent laryngeal nerve.
   A. Right recurrent laryngeal nerve.
      a. *It is present in front of the subclavian artery and winds it.*
      b. It runs upwards and medially behind the subclavian and common carotid arteries and reach tracheo-oesophageal groove.
      c. In the upper part of groove, it is related to the inferior thyroid artery.

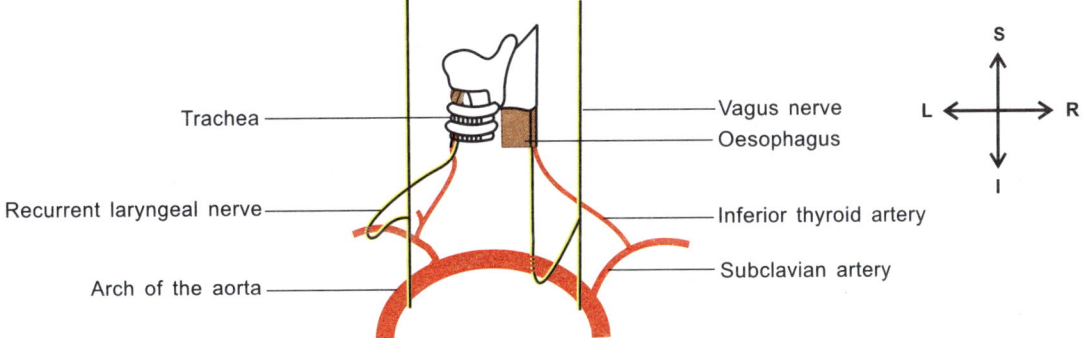

Fig. 3.74 : Course of recurrent laryngeal nerve.

      d. The nerve passes deep to lower border of inferior constrictor. It enters the larynx behind cricothyroid joint.
   B. Left recurrent laryngeal nerve.
      a. It crosses the left side of arch of the aorta.
      b. *It loops around the ligamentum arteriosum and reaches the tracheo-oesophageal groove.*
      c. It does not have to pass behind the subclavian and carotid arteries.

3. **Distribution :** It supplies
   A. All intrinsic muscles of larynx except cricothyroid.
   B. Sensory nerves of the larynx below the level of vocal cords.
   C. There are four cardiac branches from the right and left recurrent laryngeal nerve. These are two superior and two inferior. Out of the four cardiac branches the left inferior branch goes to superficial cardiac plexus. The three cardiac branches join the deep cardiac plexus.

D. Branches to trachea and oesophagus and

E. To the inferior constrictor.

4. Applied anatomy :

A. Irritation of the recurrent laryngeal nerve by enlarged lymph nodes in children may produce a persistent cough.

B. Recurrent laryngeal nerves may be injured in thyroid surgery or compressed by a growing tumor, aortic aneurysm or from other causes.

C. If only one recurrent laryngeal nerve is paralyzed, the affected vocal cord remains in the paramedian position and the vocal cord on the normal side compensates for phonation.

D. If both recurrent laryngeal nerves are paralyzed, the vocal cords remain in the paramedian position (in between abduction and adduction). This results in

a. Loss of phonation,

b. Dyspnoea (difficulty in breathing), and respiratory stridor.

LAQ-26 — Describe accessory nerve under
1. Functional components   2. Course and relations
3. Branches &   4. Applied anatomy.

1. Functional components : It has two roots, cranial and spinal.

A. Cranial root is special visceral efferent. It arises from nucleus ambiguus. It is distributed through pharyngeal plexus, to the

a. Muscles of palate,

b. Muscles of pharynx and

c. Muscles of larynx.

B. Spinal root is also special visceral efferent. It arises from spinal nucleus present in the anterior grey column of the spinal cord, extending from C_1 to C_5 segment. Its fibers supply

a. Sternocleido mastoid.

b. Trapezius.

2. Course and distribution :

A. Cranial root

a. It emerges by 4 to 5 rootlets, attached to posterolateral sulcus of the medulla.

b. It runs with ninth and tenth cranial nerve and the spinal accessory nerve and reaches the jugular foramen.

c. In the jugular foramen, the cranial root unites with the spinal root and again separates and passes out separately.

d. The cranial root, finally fuses with the vagus nerve and distributes to the muscles of pharynx and larynx.

B. Spinal root

a. It arises from upper five segment of spinal cord.

b. In the vertebral canal, the filaments unite to form a single trunk and enters the cranium through foramen magnum.

c. It runs along with cranial root of accessory and joins in the jugular foramen and again separates and comes out separately.

d. It descends vertically, between the internal jugular vein and internal carotid artery.

e. It reaches a point midway between the angle of the mandible and the mastoid process.

f. It runs downwards and backwards superficial to internal jugular vein and deep to sternomastoid.

g. It pierces the anterior border of sternomastoid at the junction of upper one-fourth with the lower three-fourth and emerges through the posterior border of sternomastoid a little above its middle.

h. It enters the posterior triangle and lies over the levator scapulae muscle.

i. It leaves the posterior triangle by passing deep to the anterior border of trapezius and ends by supplying it.

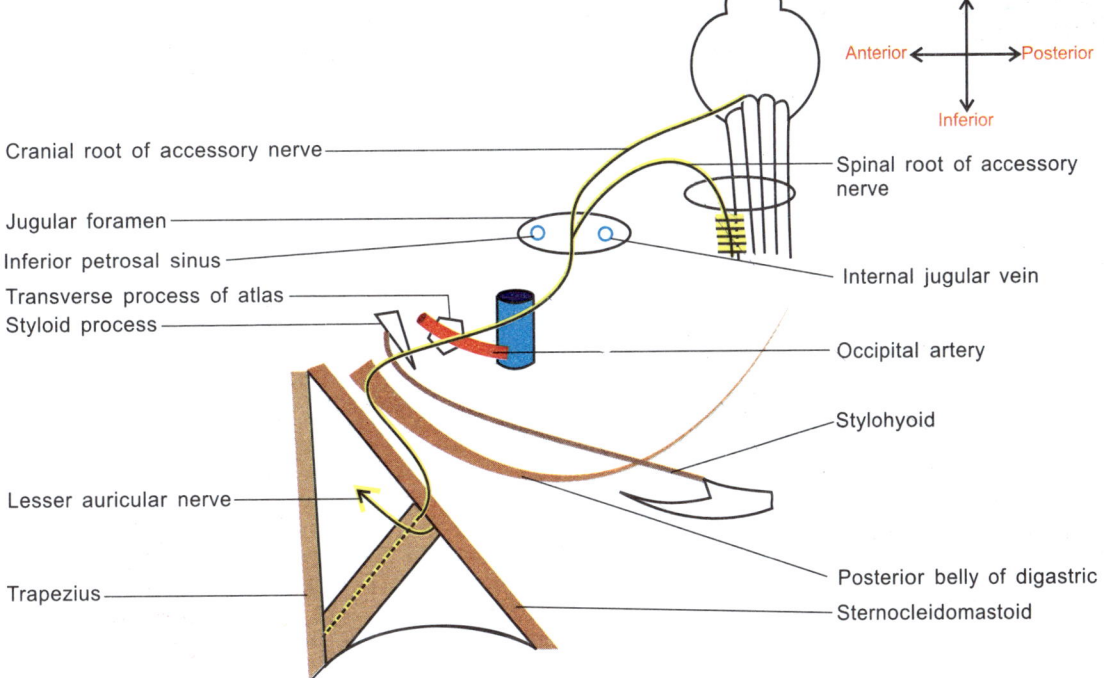

Fig. 3.75 : Course and distribution of accessory nerve.

3. **Branches :**
  A. Cranial root supplies :
    a. Muscles of palate,
    b. Muscles of pharynx and
    c. Muscles of larynx.
  B. Spinal root supplies :
    a. Sternocleido mastoid.
    b. Trapezius.

4. **Applied anatomy :**
  A. The accessory nerve is tested clinically :
    a. By asking the patient to shrug his shoulders (trapezius) against resistance and comparing the power on the two sides; and

b. By asking the patient to turn the face to the opposite side (sternomastoid) against resistance and again comparing the power on the two sides.
B. The effects of damage of the spinal part of accessory nerve.
   a. The face is turned towards the side of injury.
   b. There is an inability to shrug the shoulder towards the side of injury due to paralysis of trapezius muscle.
C. The pus accumulated near the posterior border is drained by taking incision across the sternomastoid, but not along the posterior border to avoid injury of the spinal part of accessory nerve.

LAQ-27 Describe hypoglossal nerve under
1. Functional components   2. Course and relations
3. Branches and distribution   4. Applied anatomy

1. **Functional components :** Somatic efferent supplies muscles of tongue.

2. **Course and relations :** It arises from anterolateral sulcus of medulla oblongata. The nerve leaves the skull through hypoglossal canal.
   Extracranial course :
   A. The nerve first lies deep to the internal jugular vein and descends between internal jugular vein and the internal carotid artery.
   B. It is present deep to the
      a. Parotid gland,
      b. The styloid process,
      c. The posterior belly of the digastric and

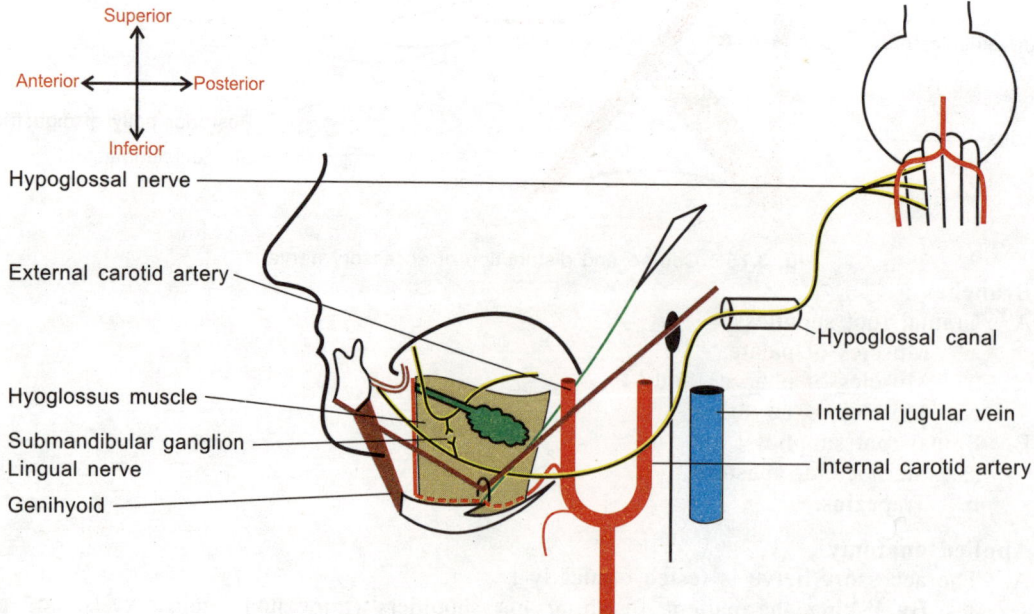

Fig. 3.76 : Course and distribution of hypoglossal nerve.

d.   Stylohyoid muscle.

C.   At the lower border of posterior belly of the digastric it curves forwards and crosses internal and external carotid artery and anterior to loop of lingual artery.

D.   The nerve then continues forwards on the hyoglossus and genioglossus muscle, deep to submandibular gland and mylohyoid muscle and enters the substance of the tongue to supply its muscles.

3.   Branches and distribution :

A.   *Muscular branches supply intrinsic and extrinsic muscles of the tongue except the palotoglossus, which is supplied by cranial root of accessory nerve.*   B. O t h e r branches containing C_1 nerve but through twelfth nerve.

a.   Meningeal branch.

b.   Ansa cervicalis.

c.   Branches to thyrohyoid and geniohyoid.

4.   Applied anatomy :

A.   Hypoglossal nerve is tested clinically by asking the patient to protrude his tongue.

B.   *Lesion of the hypoglossal nerve produces paralysis of the tongue to the side of lesion.* The position of the tongue indicate side of the lesion.

C.   If the lesion is infra nuclear there is gradual atrophy on the side of lesion.

SN-34   Inferior cervical sympathetic ganglion

1.   Introduction : It is a sympathetic ganglion present on the lateral side of vertebral column.

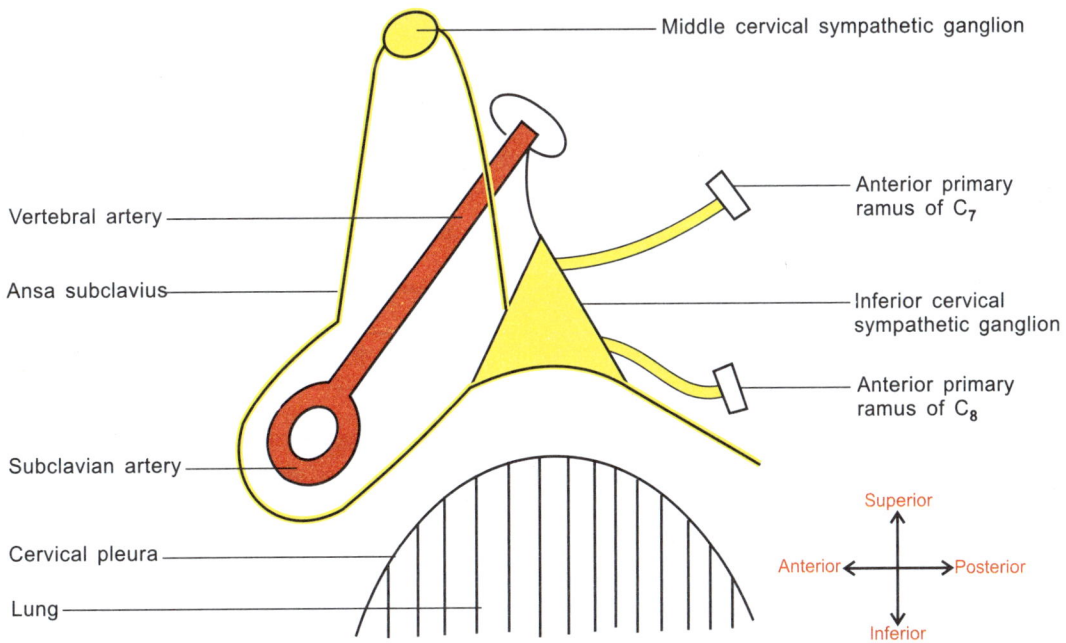

Fig. 3.77 : Inferior cervical sympathetic ganglion.

2. **Gross anatomy :**
   A. Situation : Cervical region in front of neck of first rib and transverse process of seventh cervical vertebra.
   B. Formation : By fusion of seventh and eighth cervical ganglia at C_7 vertebra. It forms stellate ganglion with T_1 ganglion.

3. **Relations :**
   A. Anterior : Eighth cervical spinal nerve.
   B. Posterior : Third part of vertebral artery.
4. **Branches :**
   A. Vascular branches :
      a. Vertebral artery and
      b. Subclavian artery.
   B. Visceral branches : To the heart by deep cardiac plexus.
   C. Other branches: Grey rami communicants are given to the ventral rami of nerves of C_7 and C_8.

5. **Applied anatomy :**

Horner's syndrome : It is due to involvement of sympathetic nerve, which is contributed by T_1. It usually occurs due to injury at the root of brachial plexus.

🗝️ HORNER. The letters of the word "Horner" give the information about clinical manifestations of Horner's syndrome.

1. **H**ypohydrosis (*hypo* less, *hydrosis* sweating) is due to involvement of sympathetic nerves, which arise from first thoracic nerve. These are secretomotor fibers supplying the sweat glands of the skin of the face and forehead.

2. **O**pening of eye is lost due to ptosis (drooping of the upper eyelid). It is caused by paralysis of Mullers muscle (smooth muscle of levator palpebrae superioris). In fact it is pseudo ptosis.

3. Argyll **R**obertson pupil [constricted pupil] due to paralysis of dilator pupillae(unopposed action of sphincter pupillae.

4. **N**arrowing of palpebral fissure.

5. **E**levation of lower eyelid.

6. **R**etraction of eyeball. (Sunken eyeball) - Enophthalmus is due to involvement of orbitalis muscle.

| SN-35 | **Phrenic nerve** |

1. **Origin :** It is mainly formed from C_4, with unimportant contribution from C_3 and C_5. It is one of the most important nerve in the body, the only motor supply to its own half of diaphragm. It also supplies peritoneum, pleura and pericardium.

2. **Course and relations :**
   A. The nerve is formed at the lateral border of scalenus anterior, at the level of upper border of thyroid cartilage.
   B. It runs vertically downwards on the anterior surface of scalenus anterior.

C.   The nerve lies deep to
   a.   Prevertebral fascia.
   b.   Inferior belly of omohyoid.
   c.   Transverse cervical artery.
   d.   Suprascapular artery.
   e.   Internal jugular vein.
D.   The nerve runs downward on the cervical pleura behind the commencement of brachiocephalic vein. It crosses the internal thoracic artery and enters the thorax.

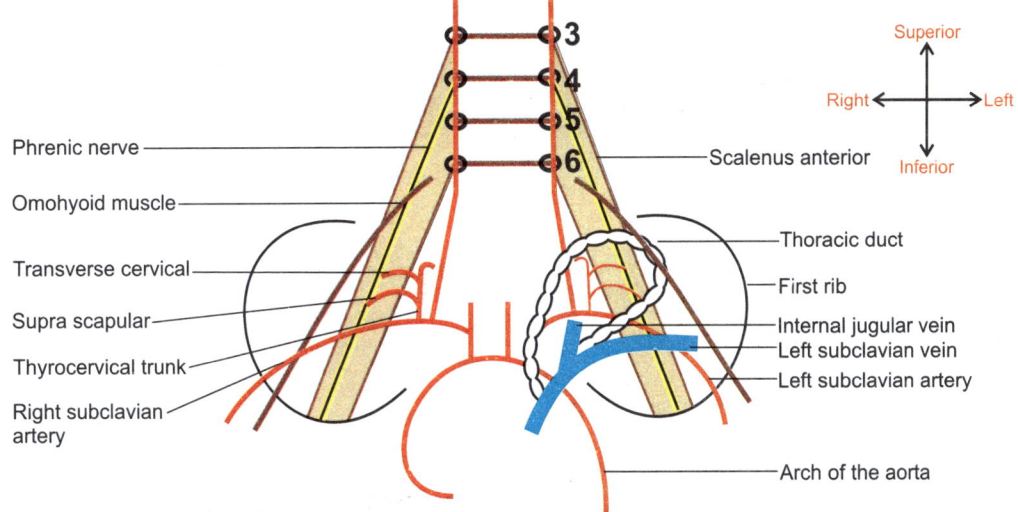

Fig. 3.78 : Phrenic nerve and its relations.

3.   **Branches :**
   A.   Motor branches
        Diaphragm: Phrenic nerve is a main motor nerve to the diaphragm.
   B.   Sensory branches
        a.   Central part of diaphragm.
        b.   Pleura,
        c.   Pericardium and
        d.   Peritoneum.

4.   **Applied anatomy :**
   A.   The phrenic nerve may be injured by penetrating wounds of the neck or damaged because of pressure from malignant tumors in the mediastinum.
   B.   *If phrenic nerve is damaged, the corresponding half of the diaphragm will be paralyzed. The paralyzed half of the diaphragm will be relaxed and pushed up into the thorax by the positive abdominal pressure. As a result, the lower lobe of the lung on that side may collapse.*

SN-36   **Scalenus anterior**

It is a deep muscle of side of neck.
1.   **Origin :** Anterior tubercles of transverse processes of typical cervical vertebrae (third, fourth, fifth and sixth cervical vertebrae).

2.   **Insertion :** Scalene tubercle present on the inner border of first rib.

3.   **Nerve supply :** Ventral rami of fourth, fifth and sixth cervical nerve.

4.   **Relations :** It is a key muscle of the lower part of neck because of its intimate relations to many important structures.
     A. Anterior :
         a.   Nerves
              I.   Phrenic nerve,
              II.   Descendens cervicalis.
         b.   Arteries
              I.   Transverse cervical,
              II.   Suprascapular and
              III. Ascending cervical.
         c.   Veins
              I.   Internal jugular vein and
              II.   Subclavian vein.
         d.   Muscles
              I.   Sternocleido mastoid and
              II.   Inferior belly of omohyoid.
         e.   Bone : Clavicle
     B. Posterior :
         a.   Brachial plexus (lower trunk).
         b.   Subclavian artery second part.
         c.   Deep cervical artery.
         d.   Superior intercostal artery.

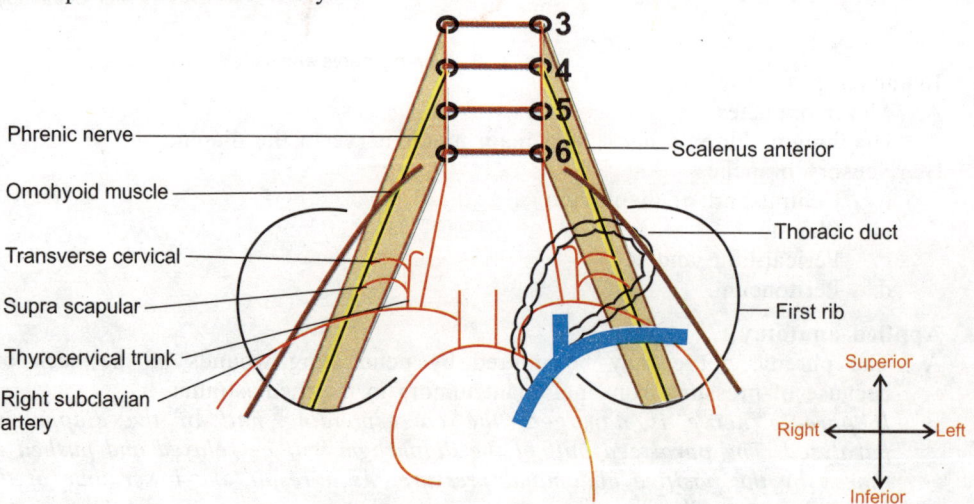

Fig. 3.79 : Scalenus anterior and its relations.

     C. Medially :
         a.   First part of subclavian artery.
         b.   Inferior thyroid artery.
         c.   Sympathetic trunk.
     D. Laterally :
         a.   Third part of subclavian artery.
         b.   Trunks of brachial plexus.

5. **Actions :**
   A. Anterolateral flexion of cervical spine.
   B. Rotation of cervical spine to opposite side.
   C. Elevation of first rib during inspiration.

6. **Applied anatomy :**
   A. Use of scalani muscles accompanied by laboured breathing is a sign of extreme respiratory distress as in asthma.
   B. Spasm of scalene muscles may compress subclavian artery and brachial plexus. This results into ischaemia of limb and pain along the distribution of affected nerves. This is called scalenus anticus syndrome.

SAQ-7   Anterior longitudinal ligament

1. **Attachment :** It is attached to upper and lower borders of anterior surface of bodies of all vertebrae.

2. **Extent :** It extends from anterior surface of upper sacral vertebra to anterior tubercle of second cervical vertebra.

3. **Variation in thickness :** It is triangular in shape, upper part is narrow, lower part is broad.

4. **Termination :** *It continues as anterior atlanto occipital membrane.*

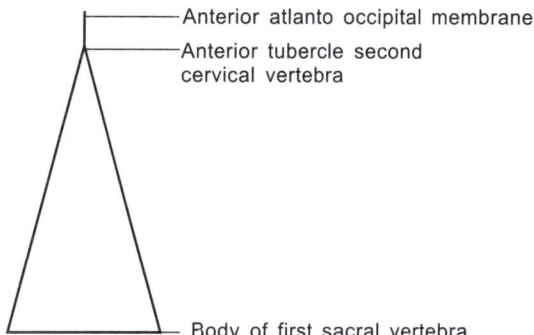

Anterior atlanto occipital membrane
Anterior tubercle second cervical vertebra
Body of first sacral vertebra

Fig. 3.80 : Anterior longitudinal ligament.

SAQ-8   Posterior longitudinal ligament

1. It is attached to the upper and lower border of the posterior surface of bodies of all vertebrae.

2. **Extent :** It extends from the body of first sacral to the lower border of body of second cervical vertebra.

3. **Termination :** *It continues as membrana tectoria above second cervical vertebra.*

4. **Relations :**
   A. Anterior : Basivertebral venous plexus,
   B. Posterior : Spinal cord with meninges.

5. **Variation thickness :** Upper part is broad and has uniform width, lower part is narrow.

6. **Types of fibers :**
   A. Superficial fibers : They join 3 to 4 vertebrae.
   B. Deep fibers : They merge with annulus fibrous.

LAQ-28   Describe atlanto-axial joints under
1. Articulating surface 2. Classification 3. Ligaments
4. Movements and muscles bringing movements &
5. Applied anatomy.

Table 3.23 : The table shows difference between median and lateral atlanto-axial joints.

	Median atlanto-axial joint	Lateral atlanto-axial joint
1. Articulating surface	A. Dens or odontoid process of the axis. B. Anterior arch of atlas.	a. Inferior articular facet of the lateral mass of atlas. b. Superior articular facet of the axis.
2. Classification of the joint	Pivot joint.	Plane synovial joint.

3. Ligaments (Refer Fig. of atlanto-occipital joint)	A. Transverse ligament of atlas: It extends between the two tubercles on the medial side of lateral masses of atlas.
	B. Apical ligaments : It connects the tip of the dens to the dorsal surface of basilar part of occipital bone.
	C. Alar ligament:
	  a. It extends form upper part of lateral surface of the dens to the medial surface of condyles.
	  b. These are strong ligaments.
	  c. They are stretched during flexion and relaxed during extension.
	  d. They check excessive rotation.
		Capsular ligament:
		a. They are loose. The laxity of the fibrous capsule permits forward or backward gliding movements during rotation of the atlas.
		b. They are attached to the peripheral margin of articular surface.
		c. Excessive stretching of the fibrous capsule is prevented by curvatures of articular surfaces.

4. **Movements and muscles bringing movements :** Movements at all three joints are rotatory movements and take place around a vertical axis. The dens forms a pivot around which the atlas rotates (carrying the skull with it). It is called NO movement.
   A. Ipsilateral :
     a. Obliqus capitis inferior.
     b. Rectus capitis posterior major and minor.
     c. Longissimus capitis.
     d. Splenius capitis.
   B. Contralateral : Sternocleidomastoid.

5. **Applied anatomy :**
   Death by hanging may be due to rupture of the transverse ligament of atlas or fracture of the dens of axis. As a result, the atlas is dislocated from the axis and compresses the spinal cord with fatal outcome.

LAQ-29 | **Describe atlanto-occipital joints under**
1.   Classification   2. Ligaments
3.   Movements and muscle bringing movements &
4.   Applied anatomy.

1. **Classification :**
    A. Structural : Simple, condylar, ellipsoid variety of synovial joint.
    B. Functional : Diarthrosis.
        There is no intervertebral disc at the atlanto-occipital joint, which accounts for the extensive range of flexion and extension.

2. **Ligaments :**
    A. Fibrous capsule :
        a.   Attached to peripheral margin of articular surface.
        b.   It is thick posterolaterally, thin and loose anteromedially.
    B. Synovial membrane : Internally it lines the fibrous capsule.
    C. Anterior atlanto-occipital membrane :
        a.   It connects the anterior arch of atlas with the anterior margin of foramen magnum.
        b.   Laterally it continues with the anterior part of capsular ligament.
        c.   Anteriorly it is strengthened by the anterior longitudinal ligament.
        d.   It prevents excessive movements.
    D. Posterior atlanto-occipital membrane :
        a.   It extends from posterior margin of foramen magnum to the posterior arch of atlas.
        b.   Laterally it continues as the posterior part of capsular ligament.

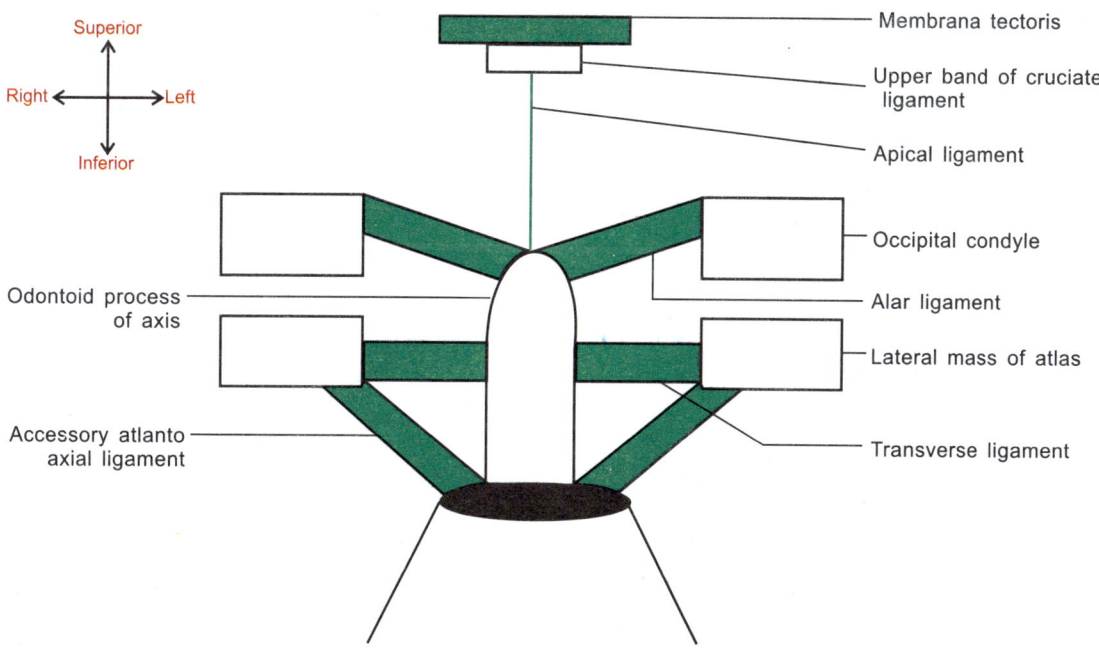

Fig. 3.81 : Ligaments of atlanto occipital and atlanto axial joint.

3. **Movements and muscles bringing movements :** Flexion and extension collectively called as <u>YES</u> movement.
   A. Flexion :
      a. Longus capitis.
      b. Rectus capitis anterior.
      c. Sternocleidomastoid.
   B. Extension :
      a. Rectus capitis posterior Major.
      b. Rectus capitis posterior Minor.
      c. Obliqus capitis.
      d. Semispinalis capitis.
      e. Splenius capitis.
      f. Longissimus capitis.
      g. Trapezius.
   C. Lateral flexion :
      a. Sternomastoid (Acting unilaterally).
      b. Obliqus capitis.

4. **Applied anatomy :**
   A. The atlantoaxial region of the cervical spine can be visualized in transoral anteroposterior radiographs.
   B. The transoral route is also utilized in surgical approaches to this region, with upward retraction of the soft palate and division of the posterior wall of the pharynx.

LAQ-30   **Describe muscles of soft palate under**
     1. Origin   2. Insertion
     3. Action &   4. Nerve supply.

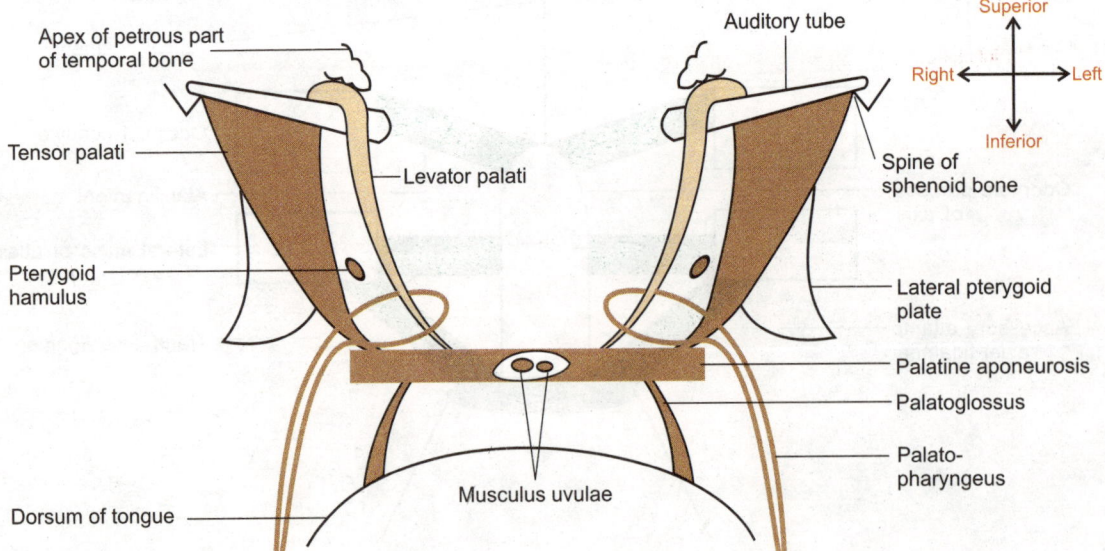

Fig. 3.82 : Muscles of soft palate.

Table 3.24 : The table shows origin, insertion and action of muscles of soft palate.

Muscles	Origin	Insertion	Action
A. Tensor palati	a. Lateral side of auditory tube. b. Adjoining part of the base of the skull (greater wing and scaphoid fossa of sphenoid bone)	Insertion is in the form of a aponeurosis, which is attached to: a. Posterior border of hard palate. b. Inferior surface of hard palate behind the palatine crest.	a. Tightens the soft palate, chiefly the anterior part. b. It dilates the auditory tube hence it is known as dilator tubae.
B. Levator palati	a. Inferior aspect of auditory tube. b. Adjoining part of inferior surface of petrous part of temporal bone.	Upper surface of palatine aponeurosis.	a. Elevates soft palate and closes the pharyngeal isthmus. b. Opens the auditory tube, like the tensor palati.
C. Musculus uvulae	a. Posterior nasal spine. b. Palatine aponeurosis.	Mucous membrane of uvula.	Pulls up the uvula.
D. Palatoglossus	Oral surface of palatine aponeurosis.	Side of the tongue at the junction of anterior two-third and posterior one-third.	Elevates the base of the tongue and closes the oro-pharyngeal isthmus.
E. Palatopharyngeus	a. Anterior fasciculus : From posterior border of hard palate b. Posterior fasciculus : From palatine aponeurosis.	a. Posterior border of the lamina of thyroid cartilage. b. Wall of the pharynx and its median raphe.	Pulls up the wall of the pharynx and shortens it during swallowing.

4. **Nerve supply :**
   A. *Motor nerves : All muscles of the soft palate are supplied by pharyngeal plexus except tensor palati, which is supplied by the mandibular nerve. The fibers of this plexus are derived from the cranial part of the accessory nerve (through the vagus).*
   B. General sensory nerves are derived from
      a. Lesser palatine nerves, which are branches of the maxillary nerve (through the pterygopalatine ganglion) and from the
      b. Glossopharyngeal nerve.
   C. Special sensory (gustatory) nerve : The fibers travel through the greater petrosal nerve - geniculate ganglion of the facial nerve - nucleus of the solitary tract.
   D. Secretomotor nerves : Lesser palatine nerves. They are derived from the superior salivatory nucleus and travel through the greater petrosal nerve.

SN-37   Waldeyer's ring   Imp

It is a ring of submucosal lymphoid tissue which surrounds the beginning of respiratory and gastro intestinal tract.

1. **Formation :**
   A. Infront and below : Lingual tonsil.
   B. On each side : Palatine tonsil.
   C. Above and on each side : Tubal tonsil.
   D. Above and behind : Nasopharyngeal tonsil.
   The internal ring of Waldeyer drains into precervical chain of lymph node and deep cervical lymph node which together constitute the "external ring of Waldeyer".

2. **Functions :**
   A. It filters tissue fluid coming from inner surface of oral cavity.
   B. It prevents the entry of organism from outside and thereby acting as a guard.
   C. It serves as the first line of defence & protects the body against ingested and inspired bacteria by producing antibodies against such invading organisms. When the tonsil itself becomes infected, it becomes a source for the spread of infection.

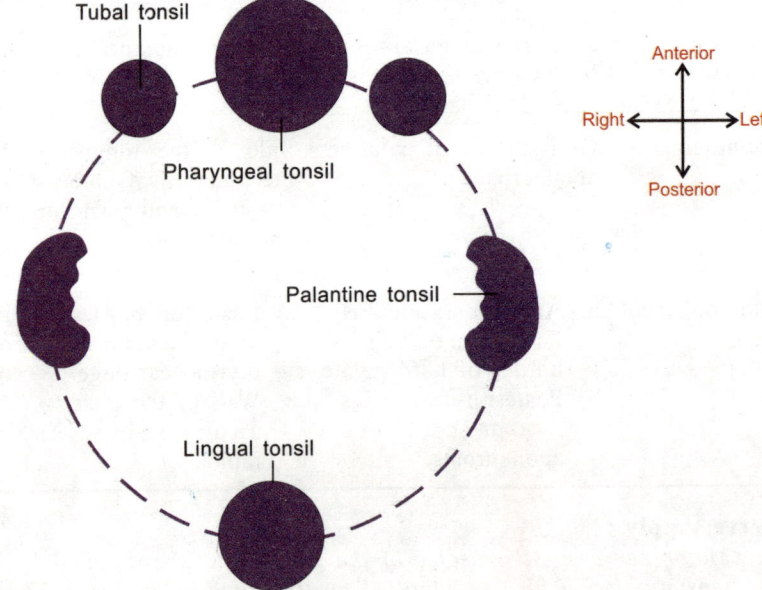

Fig. 3.83 : Waldeyer's ring.

3. **Applied anatomy :**
   A. Waldeyer's ring forms a strong defense system to prevent the spread of infection from the oral and nasal cavities into the lower respiratory tract consisting of larynx, trachea, bronchi and lungs.
   B. The lymphatic ring helps in defensive mechanism of the respiratory and alimentary systems by destroying the entry of microorganisms from the external environment.
   C. In preantibiotic era : Enlargement of the lymphoid follicle in the Waldeyer's ring used to block the respiratory tract.

SN-38 Palatine tonsil

1. **Gross :** Tonsils are collection of lymphoid tissue situated bilaterally in the lateral wall of oropharynx.
   A. Situation : Tonsillar sinus between palatoglossal and palatopharyngeal fold.
   B. Dimension : 2 cms.
   C. Capsule : Capsule is condensed connective tissue present on the lateral side. It can easily be separated from the pharyngeal muscular wall except at its antero-inferior part.
   D. Morphology :
      a. 2 surfaces : Medial and lateral.
      b. 2 borders : Anterior and posterior.
      c. 2 ends : Upper and lower.

2. **Relations :**
   A. Surface :
      a. Medial : Presence of 8 - 12 crypts.
      b. Lateral :
         I. Artery :
            i. Facial artery with its ascending palatine and tonsillar branches.
            ii. Ascending pharyngeal artery.
         II. Muscle :
            i. Styloglossus muscle.
            ii. Medial pterygoid muscle.
            iii. Posterior belly of digastric.
         III. Gland : Submandibular and parotid gland.
   B. Border :
      a. Anterior : Palatoglossus.
      b. Posterior : Palatopharyngeus.

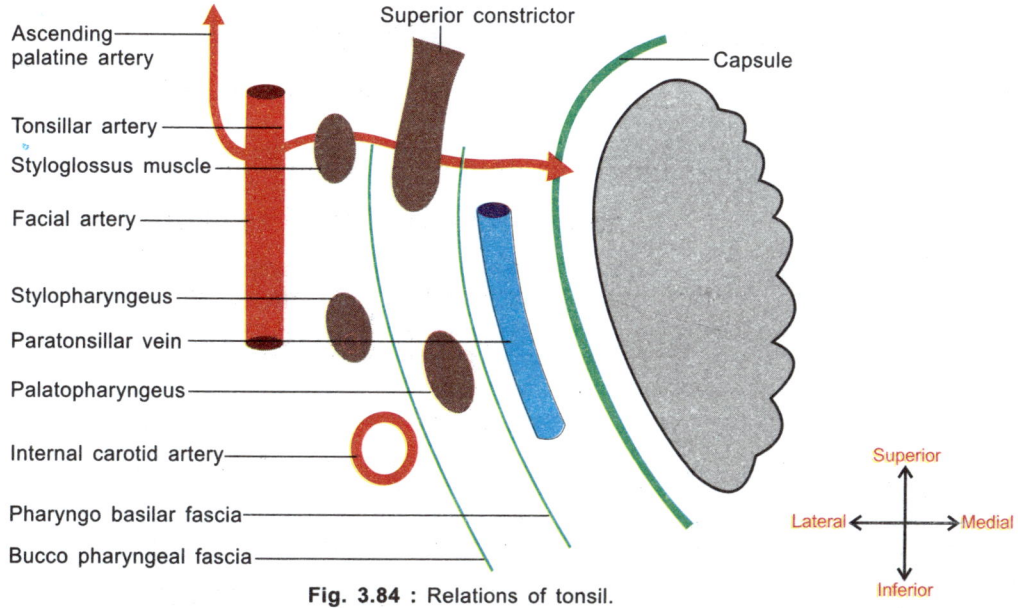

Fig. 3.84 : Relations of tonsil.

3. **Blood supply :**
   A. Arterial :
      a. *Main source : Inferior tonsillar branch of facial artery. It enters the tonsil from its lateral surface.*
      b. Additional sources :
         I. Anterior tonsillar, a branch of lingual artery.
         II. Posterior tonsillar, a branch of ascending palatine.
         III. Superior tonsillar, a branch of descending palatine.

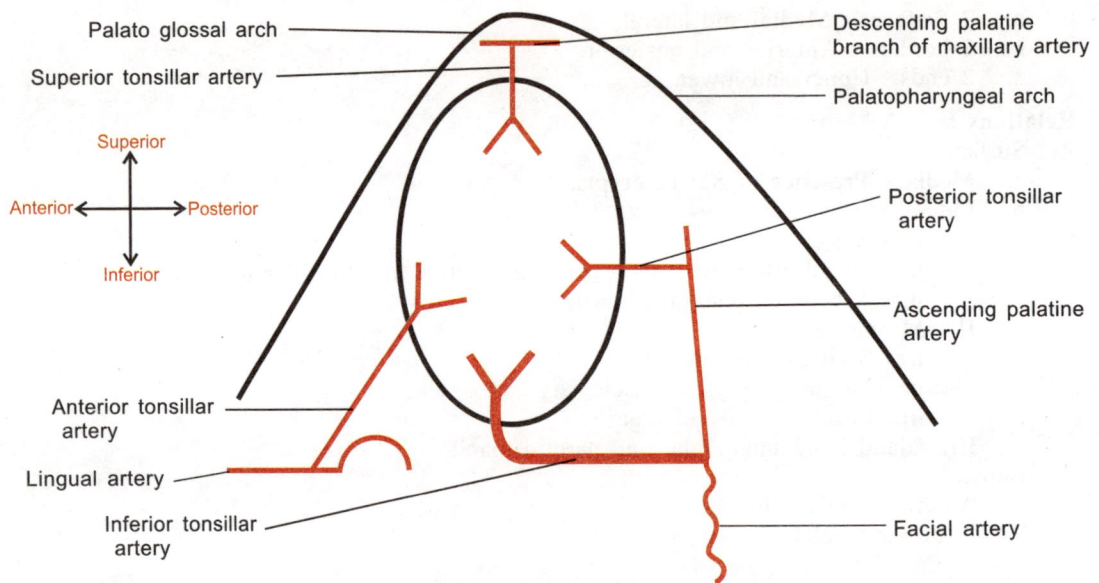

Fig. 3.85 : Arterial supply of tonsil.

   B. Venous drainage :
      a. Into the pharyngeal venous plexus.
      b. Principal drainage is by the tonsillar vein, tributary of the lingual vein.

4. **Nerve supply :** Glossopharyngeal nerve.

5. **Development :**
   A. Chronological age : It develops in the fourth week of intrauterine life.
   B. Germ layer : The epithelium develops from the endoderm of the second pharyngeal pouch and remaining structures from the local mesenchymal tissue.
   C. Source : It develops from ventral part of the second pharyngeal pouch. The endodermal cells proliferate outwards as solid buds which are subsequently canalized to form tonsillar pits and crypts. Lymphocytes either develop from mesoderm of adjoining arches or from circulating lymphocytes.
   D. Site : On the lateral side of adult oral cavity.

6. **Histology :** It is lymphoid organ consists of
   A. Stratified squamous non-keratinized epithelium,
   B. With crypts,

C. Fibrous capsule on the outer side and
D. Lymphoid tissue - (Diffuse and lymph nodule).

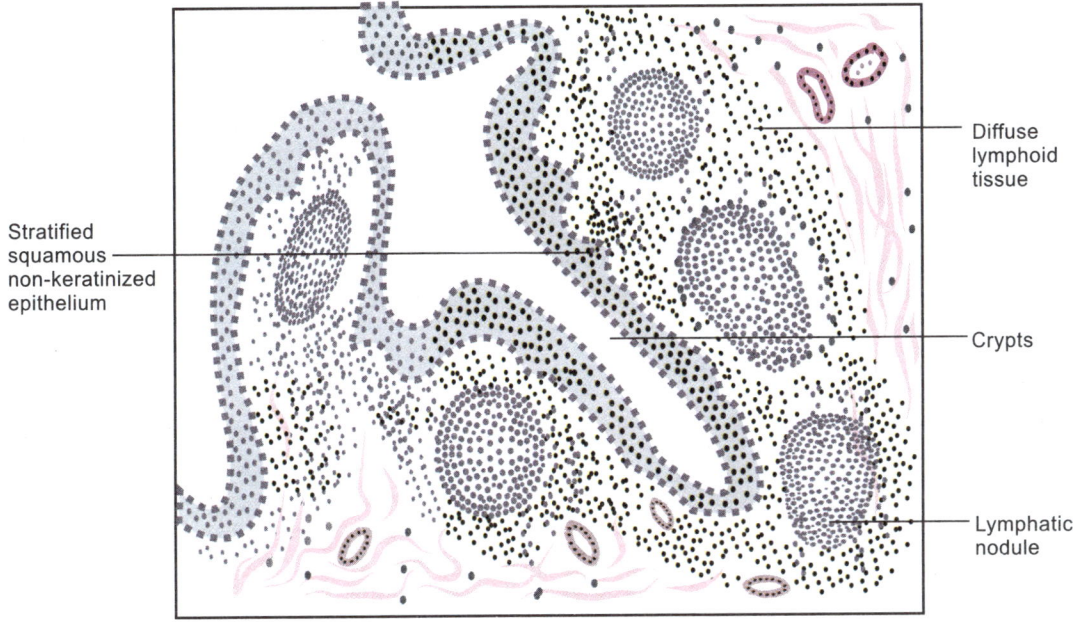

Fig. 3.86 : Histology of tonsil.

7. **Applied anatomy :**
    A. Referred pain from the infected tonsil extends to the middle ear, because both are supplied by the glossopharyngeal nerve.
    B. The capsule of the tonsil is removed during tonsillectomy, because it is attached to deep surface of the tonsil and extends to form septa which conducts nerves and vessels.
    C. After tonsillectomy all clots in the tonsillar fossa are removed to prevent the interference of retraction of blood vessels. Such removal of clots is also done in uterus after delivery to prevent post partum haemorrhage.
    D. Quinsy is peritonsillar abscess.

LAQ-31	**Describe pharynx under**
	1. **Parts** 2. **Structure of pharynx**
	3. **Muscles of pharynx** 4. **Blood supply**
	5. **Nerve supply and** 6. **Applied anatomy.**

1. **Parts :** It is a wide, muscular tube situated behind the nose, mouth and larynx. It is divided into three parts :
    A. Nasopharynx,
    B. Oropharynx and
    C. Laryngopharynx.

Table 3.25 : The table shows different parts of the pharynx.

Particulars	Nasopharynx	Oropharynx	Laryngopharynx
a. Situation :	Behind nose.	Behind oral cavity.	Behind larynx.
b. Extent :	Base of skull (body of sphenoid) to soft palate.	Soft palate to upper border of epiglottis.	Upper border of epiglottis to lower border of cricoid cartilage.
c. Communications :	Anteriorly with nose.	I. Anteriorly with oral cavity, II. Above with nasopharynx & III. Below with laryngopharynx.	Inferiorly with oesophagus.
d. Nerve supply	Pharyngeal branches of pterygopalatine ganglion.	Ninth and tenth nerve.	Ninth and tenth nerve.
e. Relations : a. Anterior	Posterior nasal aperature.	Oral cavity.	I. Inlet of larynx, II. Posterior surface of cricoid III. Arytenoid cartilage.
b. Posterior	Body of sphenoid bone.	Body of second and third cervical vertebrae.	Fourth and fifth cervical vertebrae.
c. Lateral wall	Opening of auditory tube.	Tonsillar fossa	Pyriform fossa
f. Lining epithelium :	Ciliated columnar epithelium.	Stratified squamous nonkeratinised epithelium.	Stratified squamous nonkeratinised epithelium.
g. Function :	Passage for air (Respiratory function).	Passage for air and food.	Passage for food.

2. **Structures of pharynx :**
   A. Mucosa.
   B. Submucosa.
   C. Pharyngobasilar fascia : Fibrous sheet filling the gap extending from base of skull to upper margin of superior constrictor muscle.
   D. Muscular coat :
       a. Outer circular muscle consists of
           I. Superior constrictor.
           II. Middle constrictor.
           III. Inferior constrictor.
       b. Inner longitudinal layer consists of
           I. Stylopharyngeus.
           II. Salphingopharyngeus.
           III. Palatopharyngeus.

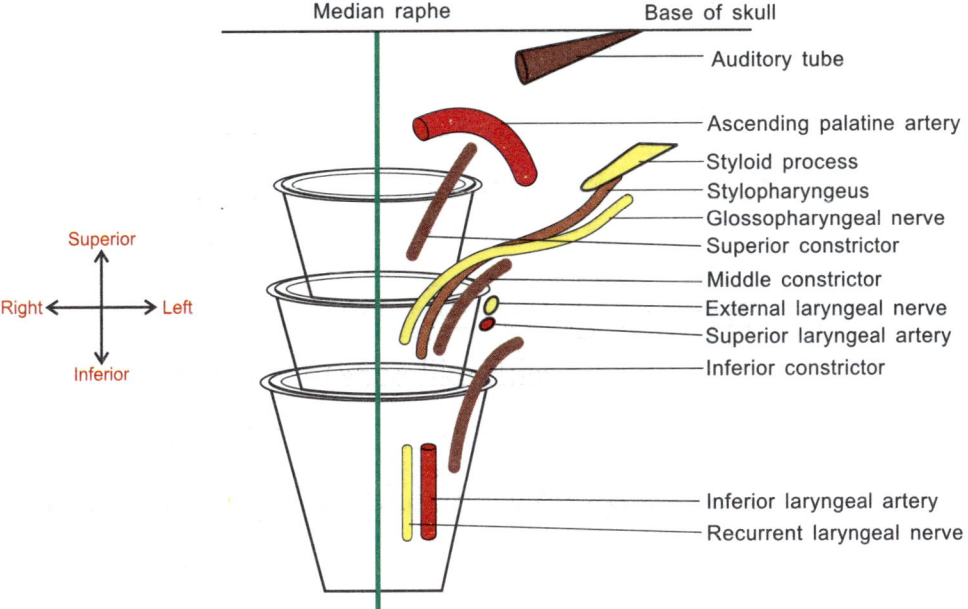

Fig. 3.87 : Pharynx opened from front showing constrictor muscles of pharynx and structures passing between them.

3.   **Muscles of pharynx** are described as inner longitudinal and outer circular.
   A.   The circular muscles of pharynx are described as follows:
      a.   Origin :
         I.   Superior constrictor :
            i.   Pterygopharyngeus :
               -   Posterior border of medial pterygoid plate and
               -   Pterygoid hamulus.
            ii. Bucco-pharyngeus : Pterygomandibular raphe.
            iii. Mylo-pharyngeus : Posterior end of mylohyoid line of mandible.
            iv. Glossopharyngeus : Side of tongue.
         II.   Middle constrictor :
            i.   Chondro-pharyngeus :
               -   Lower part of stylohyoid ligament and
               -   Lesser cornu of hyoid bone.
            ii. Ceratopharyngeus : Upper border of greater cornu of hyoid bone.
         III. Inferior constrictor :
            i.   Thyro-pharyngeus (propulsive part) :
               -   From oblique line of thyroid cartilage and
               -   The tendinous band across the cricothyroid muscle.
            ii. Crico-pharyngeus (sphincter part : from side of the cricoid)
      b.   Insertion :
         I.   Pharyngeal tubercle and
         II.   Median pharyngeal raphe.
   B.   Longitudinal muscles of pharynx are described in following table :

Table 3.26 : The table shows origin and insertion of longitudinal muscles of pharynx.

Muscles	Origin	Insertion
A. Stylopharyngeus	Arises from the medial surface of the base of styloid process.	Posterior border of lamina of thyroid cartilage.
B. Palatopharyngeus	I. Anterior fasciculus : From posterior border of hard palate. II. Posterior fasiculus : From palatine aponeurosis.	a. Posterior border of lamina of thyroid cartilage. b. Wall of pharynx and its median raphe.
C. Salphigophary-Ngeus	Anterior end of the cartilage of auditory tube.	Blends with palatopharyngeus

4. **Blood supply :**
   A. Arterial :
      a. Ascending pharyngeal branch of external carotid artery.
      b. Ascending palatine   } branch of facial.
      c. Tonsillar artery
      d. Dorsal lingual : Branch of lingual
      e. Greater palatine : Branch of maxillary.
   B. Venous drainage : Form a plexus which drains into internal jugular and facial vein.
   C. Lymphatic drainage :
      a. Retropharyngeal and
      b. Deep cervical group of lymph nodes.

5. **Nerve supply of pharynx :** Pharyngeal plexus which is formed by
   A. Sensory :
      a. General : Pharyngeal branch of glossopharyngeal nerve.
      b. Special : Taste fibres through internal laryngeal nerve, a branch of superior laryngeal nerve, branch of vagus nerve.
   B. Motor :
      a. Somatomotor : Pharyngeal branch of vagus - chiefly motor.
      b. Secretomotor : Fibres from greater petrosal nerve.
      c. Vasomotor : Pharyngeal branch of superior cervical sympathetic ganglion.

6. **Applied anatomy :**
   A. Dysphagia : Difficulty in swallowing.
   B. Killian's dehiscence.

SAQ-9   Killians dehiscence

Killian's dehiscence : Part of posterior wall of pharynx between lower part of vocal folds and cricopharyngeus is weak and is not covered by the muscle. This weak area is called Killians dehiscence.

Pharyngeal diverticula are formed by outpouching of the dehiscence. The anatomical contributing factor for this condition is the neuromuscular incoordination of the two parts of inferior constrictor. The propulsive thyropharyngeus is supplied by pharyngeal plexus and sphincteric cricopharyngeus by recurrent laryngeal nerve.

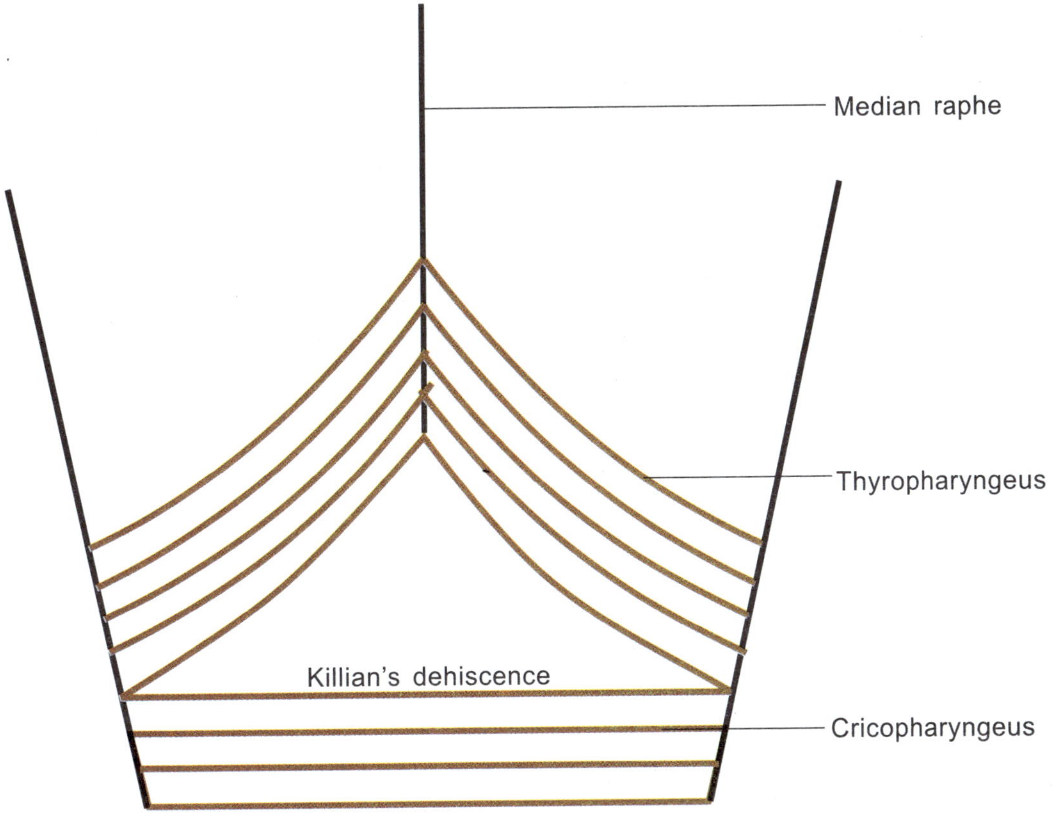

Median raphe

Thyropharyngeus

Killian's dehiscence

Cricopharyngeus

Fig. 3.88 : Killian's dehiscence.

Auditory Tube

1. **Introduction :** It is a funnel shaped tube which connects middle ear cavity to nasopharynx.

2. **Gross :**
   A. Length : 36 mm.

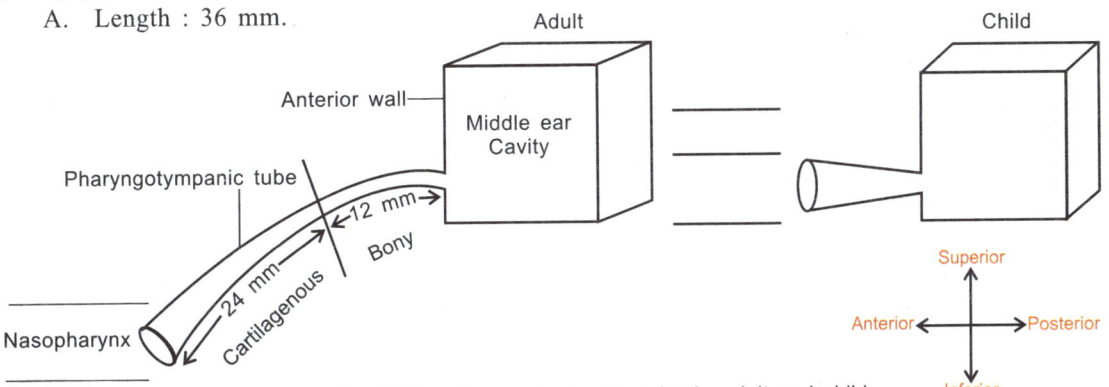

Adult

Child

Anterior wall

Middle ear Cavity

Pharyngotympanic tube

←12 mm→

Bony

24 mm

Cartilagenous

Nasopharynx

Superior

Anterior ←→ Posterior

Inferior

Fig. 3.89 : Pharyngotympanic tube in adult and child.

B.   Parts : 2 Parts.

Table 3.27 : The table shows bony and cartilagenous part of auditory tube.

Particulars	Bony	Cartilagenous
A. Site	Petrous parts of temporal bone.	Sulcus tubae
B. Length (in mm)	12 (1/3rd)	24 (2/3rd)
C. Formation	Bony	Cartilaginous
D. Opening	Middle ear	Pharynx
E. Relations	Below : Tympanic plate of temporal bone. Medially : Carotid canal.	Anterolaterally a. Spine of sphenoid. b. Middle meningeal artery. c. Mandibular nerve. d. Otic ganglion. e. Tensor veli palati. f. Chorda tympani.

3.   **Age difference :**

Table 3.28 : The table shows difference of auditory tube in child and adult.

Particulars	Child	Adult
A. Length (in mm)	18(½)	36
B. Position	Straight	Oblique
C. Bony part	Much shorter	One-third
D. Tubal elevation	Absent	Present

4.   **Blood supply :**
   A.   Middle meningeal artery (maxillary artery).
   B.   Ascending pharyngeal artery (external carotid artery).

5.   **Venous Drainage :** Pterygoid venous plexus.

6.   **Nerve supply :** Tympanic plexus formed
   A.   Tympanic branch of glossopharyngeal nerve, a sensory nerve.
   B.   Tympanic branches from plexus around internal carotid artery, a sympathetic nerve.

7.   **Functions :**
   A.   Maintains equilibrium of air pressure on either side of tympanic membrane for proper vibration of sounds.
   B.   Increased pressure in middle ear forces the auditory tube to open with a click.

8.   **Applied anatomy :**
   A.   In children, infection of oral cavity, nasal cavity or pharynx usually spreads to the middle ear because auditory tube is short in length and horizontal in position.
   B.   Sometimes tube is blocked due to inflammation of tubal tonsil.

LAQ-32	**Describe nasal septum under**

1.   Formation   2.   Blood supply
3.   Nerve supply &   4.   Applied anatomy.

It is usually deviated to one side and each nasal cavity somewhat asymmetrical.
1.   **Formation :** Partly by bones and partly by cartilage.
    A.   Bony part is
       a.   Mainly formed by
          I.   Vomer : Below and behind.
          II. Perpendicular plate of ethmoid.

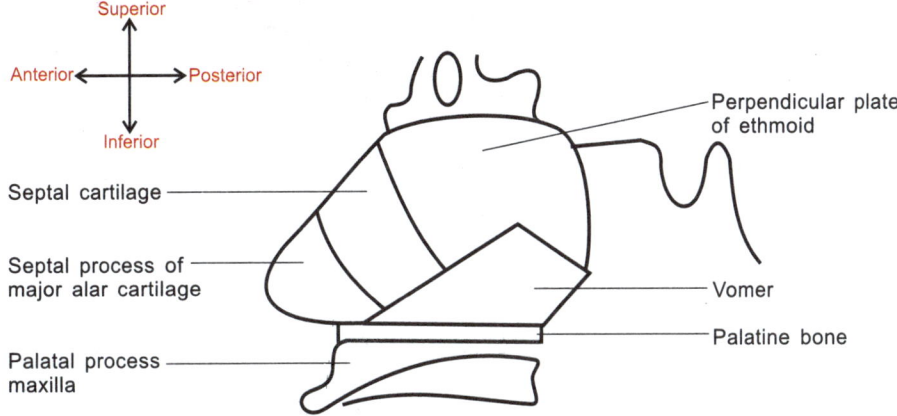

Fig. 3.90 : Bones forming nasal septum.

       b.   Accessory bones are :
          I.   Nasal spine of frontal.
          II. Crest and rostrum of sphenoid.
          III. Palatine process of maxilla.
          IV. Horizontal part of both palatine.
    B.   Cartilaginous part is formed by :
       a.   Septal cartilage.
       b.   Septal process of inferior nasal cartilage.
    C.   Cuticular part is formed by fibro fatty tissue.

2.   **Blood supply :**
    A.   Arterial supply :
       a.   Anterosuperior part by
          I.   Anterior ethmoidal artery, a branch of ophthalmic artery.
          II. Superior labial, a branch of facial artery.
       b.   Posteroinferior part by spheno - palatine artery.
    B.   Venous drainage :
       a.   Anterosuperior part drains by superior ophthalmic vein, which opens into cavernous sinus.
       b.   Posteroinferior part drains into pterygoid venous plexus.
       c.   Upper part of the septum drains into inferior cerebral vein.

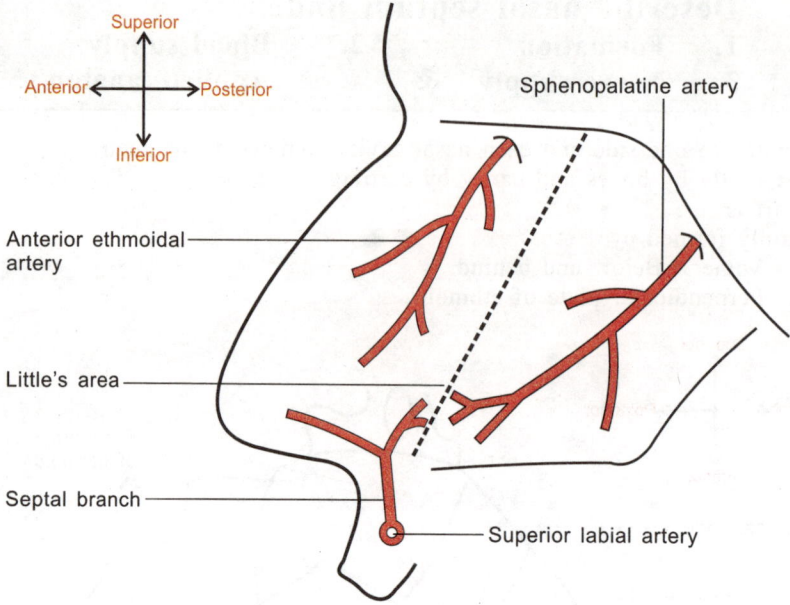

Fig. 3.91 : Arterial supply of nasal septum.

d. Lower mobile part of septum drains into facial vein which drains into internal jugular vein. An infection from this part may extend into cavernous sinus via
I.   Deep facial vein and
II. Pterygoid venous plexus.
This belongs to dangerous area of face.

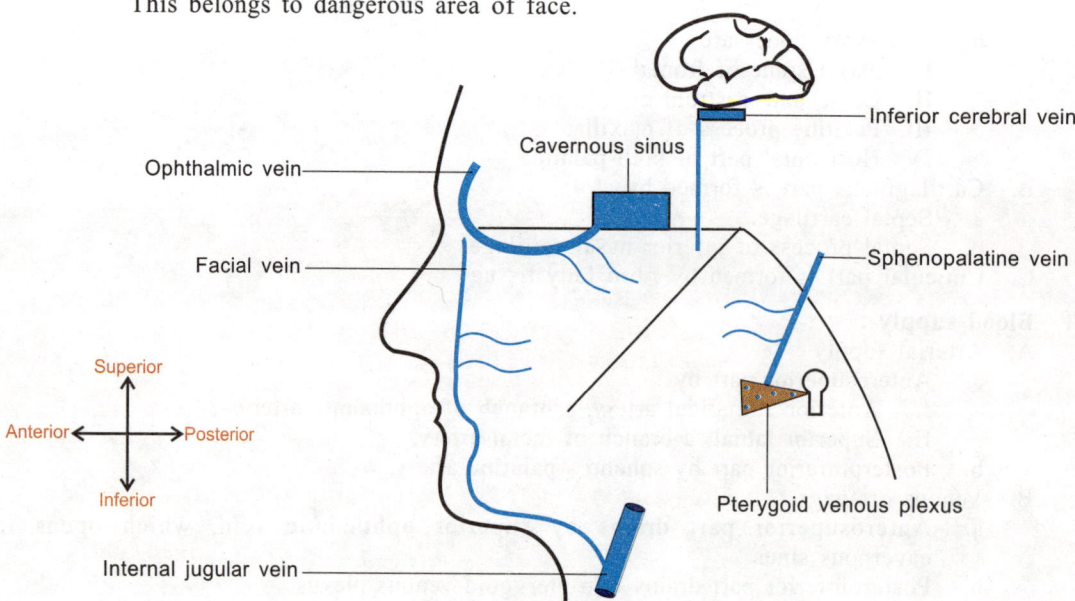

Fig. 3.92 : Venous drainage of nasal septum.

C. Lymphatic drainage :
    a.   Anterior half : To the submandibular nodes.
    b.   Posterior half : To the retropharyngeal and deep cervical nodes.

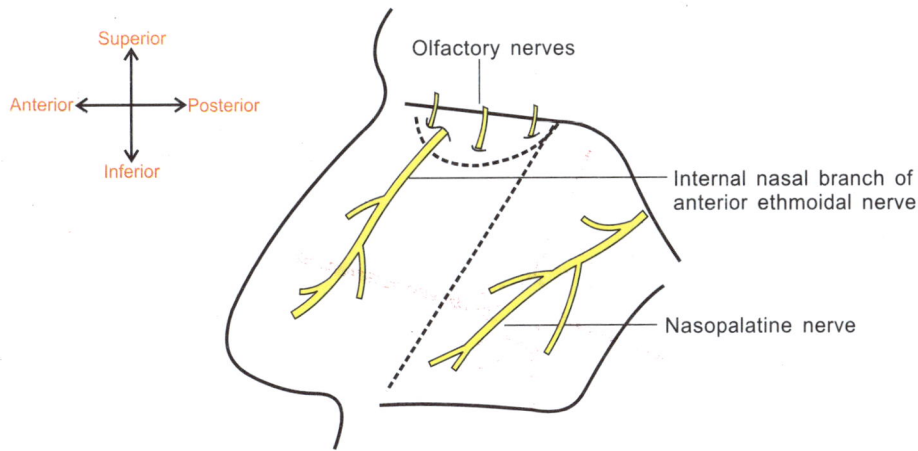

Fig. 3.93 : Nerve supply of nasal septum.

3. **Nerve supply :**
    A. General sensory nerves.
        a.   Anterosuperior : Anterior ethmoidal nerve a branch of ophthalmic nerve.
        b.   Posteroinferior part : Nasopalatine branch of pterygopalatine ganglion.
    B. Special sensory nerves are olfactory nerves.

4. **Applied anatomy :**
    A. Deviation of nasal septum may be due to cartilage or bone. It may be due to
        a.   Postnatal trauma (most common cause).
        b.   Congenital malformation.
    Excessive nasal deviation produces unilateral nasal obstruction and is treated by submucous resection of the septum (SMR).
    B. Little's area or Kiesselbach's area.

SAQ-10   Little's area OR Kiesselbach's area

Introduction : It is an area on antero inferior part of nasal septum. The nose bleeding is relatively common because nasal mucosa is highly vascular. The mild epistaxis results from nose pricking which tears the veins in the vestibule.

The profuse bleeding occurs due to rupture of one of the following arteries :
    A. Septal branch anterior ethmoidal (Ophthalmic).
    B. Septal branch of the superior labial artery, a branch of facial.
    C. Septal branch of sphenopalatine (Maxillary artery) and
    D. Septal branch of greater palatine (Maxillary artery).

The anastomosis formed by these arteries is called **"Kiesselbach's plexus"**. Even a small ulcer affecting this area can cause profuse bleeding.

Septal branch of sphenopalatine artery is longest and tortuous. It is also called as **"artery of nose bleeding"** or **"rhinologist's artery"**.

Sudden and severe nasal bleeding in elderly hypertensive patient may be due to rupture of the venous communication and thereby performs nature's safety procedure to reduce increased intracranial vascular pressure.

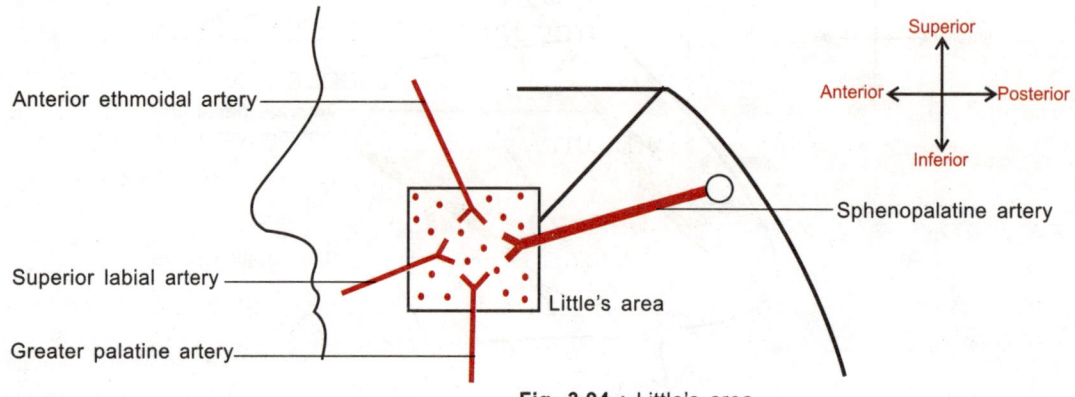

Fig. 3.94 : Little's area.

LAQ-33 Describe lateral wall of nose under
1. Formation 2. Features 3. Blood supply
4. Nerve supply & 5. Applied anatomy.

1. **Formation :**
   A. Bony part is formed by
      a. Nasal.
      b. Frontal process of maxilla.
      c. Lacrimal.
      d. Ethmoid: Superior concha and middle concha.
      e. Inferior nasal concha.
      f. Perpendicular plate of palatine bone.
      g. Medial pterygoid plate of sphenoid bone.

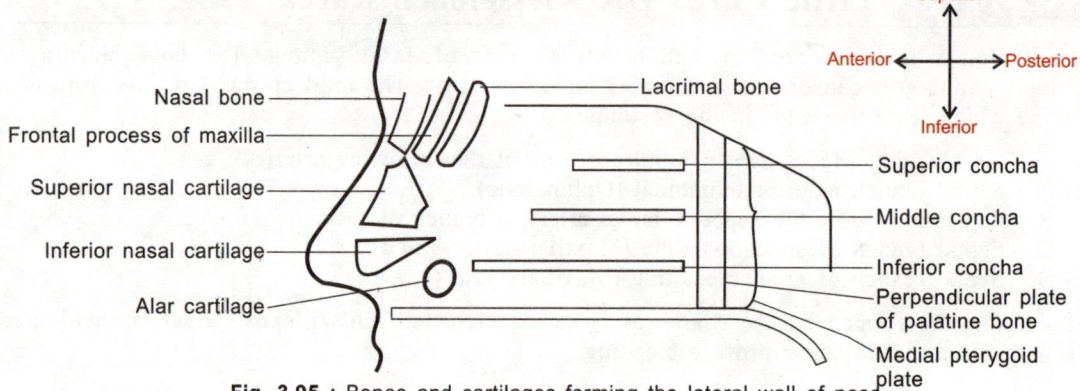

Fig. 3.95 : Bones and cartilages forming the lateral wall of nose.

B. Cartilaginous part is formed by
    a. Upper, lower nasal cartilage and
    b. Alar cartilage.
C. Cuticular part is formed by fibro-fatty tissue.

2. **Features :**
  A. The epithelium of lateral wall is as follows -
    a. Above superior concha : Olfactory epithelium.
    b. Below superior concha : Respiratory mucosa.
    c. Below inferior concha : Erectile tissue arteriovenous shunt.
  B. Lateral wall shows bony projections called nasal conchae. These are :
    a. Superior concha : A projection of ethmoid bone. This is smallest concha, situated above the middle concha. It encloses a space called superior meatus.
    b. Middle concha : A projection of ethmoid bone. It encloses middle meatus. Inferior concha is independent bone. It encloses inferior meatus.

Table 3.29 : The table shows important structures present in the lateral wall of nose.

Site	Structure
I. Sphenoethmoidal recess.	Sphenoidal air sinus.
II. Superior meatus.	Posterior ethmoidal air sinus.
III. Middle meatus. Ethmoidal bulla : Rounded elevation produced by upper margin of ethmoidal bulla. i. Hiatus semilunaris deep semicircular sulcus below the bulla. - At anterior end. - Middle part. - Posterior end.	Middle ethmoidal air sinus. Frontal air sinus. Anterior ethmoidal air sinus. Maxillary air sinus.
IV. Inferior meatus.	Naso lacrimal duct.

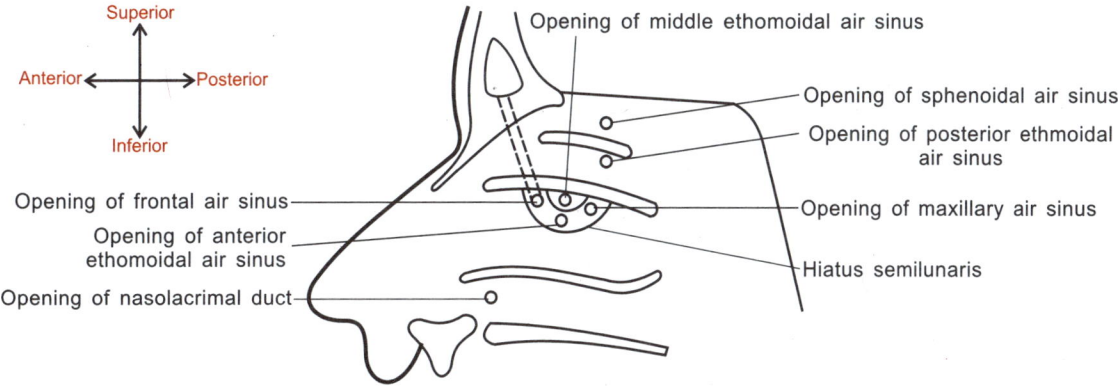

Fig. 3.96 : Openings in the lateral wall of nose.

3. **Blood supply :**
    A. Arterial :

Table 3.30 : The table shows arterial supply of lateral wall of nose.

Quadrant	Anterior	Posterior
a. Superior	Anterior ethmoidal artery (Ophthalimic artery).	Sphenopalatine artery (Maxillary artery).
b. Inferior	I. Alar branch of facial artery. II. Greater palatine artery (Maxillary artery).	Greater palatine artery (Maxillary artery).

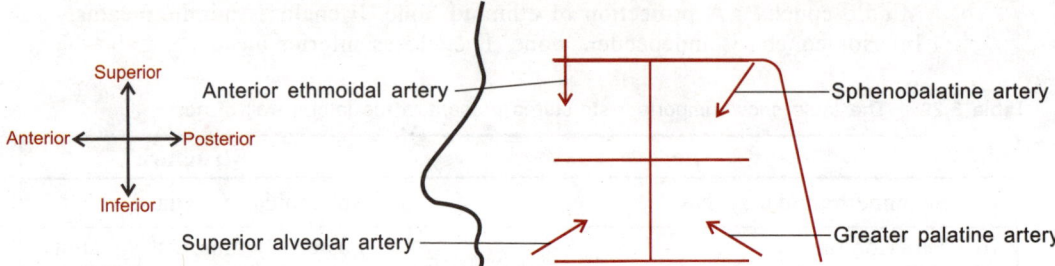

Fig. 3.97 : Arterial supply of lateral wall of nose.

B. **Venous drainage :**
    a. Anterior veins form a plexus and drains into facial vein.
    b. Posterior veins drain into pharyngeal plexus of veins.
    c. Middle part drains into pterygoid plexus of veins.

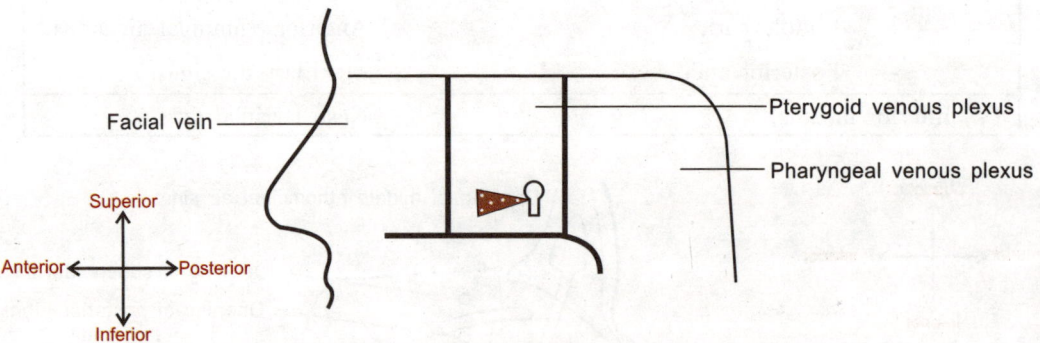

Fig. 3.98 : Venous drainage of lateral wall of nose.

C. **Lymphatic drainage :**
    a. Anterior half drains into submandibular lymph nodes.
    b. Posterior half drains into retropharyngeal and deep cervical lymph nodes.

4. **Nerve supply :**
    A. Special sensory nerve : Olfactory (I).
    B. General sensory : Trigeminal (V).

Table 3.31 : The table shows nerve supply of the lateral wall of the nose.

Quadrant	Anterior	Posterior
Superior	Anterior ethmoidal nerve (ophthalimic nerve) (V_1).	Posterior superior lateral nasal branches from pterygopalatine ganglion (maxillary nerve) V_2.
Inferior	Anterior superior alveolar nerve.	Anterior palatine branch from pterygopalatine ganglion.

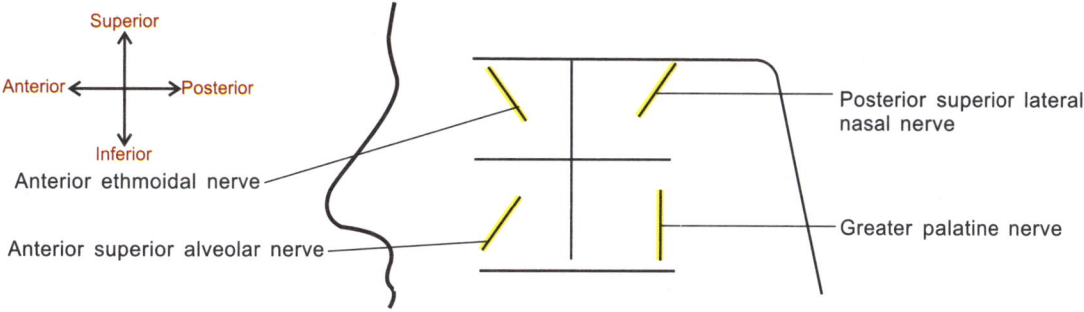

Fig. 3.99 : Nerve supply of lateral wall of nose.

5. **Applied anatomy :**
   A. Common cold is the commonest viral infection of nose.
   B. Paranasal air sinus may get infected from the infection of nose.
   C. Hypertrophy of mucosa over the inferior nasal concha is a common feature of allergic rhinitis presenting as sneezing, nasal blockage and excessive water discharge.

SN-40   Maxillary air sinus (antrum of Highmore)

1. **Introduction :** Largest and important paranasal air sinus present in maxilla, lined by ciliated epithelium.

2. **Importance :**
   A. It helps in conditioning of the air by adding humidity.
   B. It acts as resonating chamber for production of sounds.
   C. It increases the quality of voice (timber).
   D. It reduces the weight of the skull.

3. **Gross anatomy :**
   A. Shape is pyramidal.
       a. Base is formed by nasal surface of body of maxilla and forms lateral wall of nose.
       b. Apex : Towards the zygomatic bone.
   B. Boundaries :
       a. Superior wall or roof : Orbital surface of maxilla.
       b. Inferior wall or floor : Alveolar surface of maxilla.
       c. Anterior wall : Anterior surface of maxilla.
       d. Posterior wall : Posterior surface of maxilla.

C. Dimension :
    a. Vertical : 3.5 cm.
    c. Transverse : 2.5 cm
    c. Anteroposterior : 3.25 cm.
D. Opening is reduced by :
    a. Superiorly
        I.   Uncinate process of ethmoid bone.
        II. Descending part of lacrimal bone.
    b. Inferiorly : Inferior nasal concha.
    c. Posteriorly : Perpendicular plate of palatine bone.
    d. Thick mucosa lined by mucous gland.

4. **Opening :** It is present on the base, close to the roof of the oral cavity. Maxillary air sinus opens in the middle meatus by two openings.
    A. Upper opening is present in lower part of hiatus semilunaris. The opening is at higher level and is called antrum of Highmore (Dental surgeon).
    B. Lower opening is present at posterior end of hiatus.

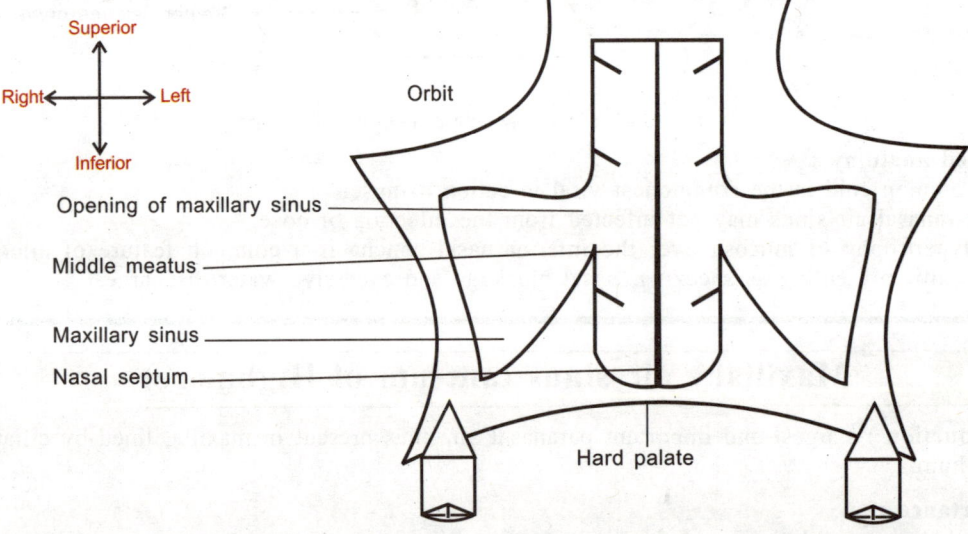

Fig. 3.100 : Maxillary air sinus.

5. **Development :** Developed from splitting of maxilla. It is first paranasal air sinus to develop. It develops in the fourth month of intra uterine life. It grows rapidly during 6-7 years and reach full size after the eruption of all permanent teeth.

6. **Blood supply :**
    A. Arterial supply :
        a. Infraorbital artery (Maxillary artery).
        b. Greater palatine artery (Maxillary artery).
        c. Posterior superior alveolar artery (Maxillary artery).
    B. Venous drainage :
        a. Infraorbital vein drains into angular vein.
        b. Greater palatine vein drains into pterygoid venous plexus.

7. **Nerve supply :**
    A. Infraorbital nerve (continuation of maxillary nerve).
    B. Greater palatine nerve (pterygopalatine ganglion).

8. **Lymphatic drainage :** By submandibular lymph node.

9. **Applied anatomy :**
    A. Sinusitis: Inflamation of maxillary air sinus presents by headache, which is maximum at 12:00 noon. At 12:00 noon there is maximum expansion of the air which is not accommodated in the maxillary air sinus, hence passes to the frontal air sinus.
    B. It can be visualised by taking X-rays of maxilla.
    C. Abscess of maxillary air sinus is drained by antral puncture.
    D. The maxillary sinus is most commonly infected probably because its opening in the nasal cavity is located much higher than the floor, a poor location for its natural drainage. Maxillary sinus becomes infected either from the nasal cavity or from caries of the upper molar teeth.
    E. The maxillary sinus is sometimes called the 'secondary reservoir' of the frontal air sinus. The frontal sinus drains into the hiatus semilunaris in the middle meatus, via infundibulum, close to the opening of maxillary sinus.
    F. The mucus or pus from maxillary sinus cannot be drained into the nasal cavity when the head is erect, until it is filled up to the top.
    G. In severe cases drainage of maxillary sinus may require a surgical intervention. The 'antral puncture' is done by passing a trocar and cannula through the nasal cavity in an outward and backward direction below the inferior nasal concha, thus producing a hole in the lower part of the lateral wall of the nasal cavity.
        For more adequate drainage a portion of medial wall of the sinus below the inferior nasal concha is removed or the sinus is fenestrated in the region of gingivolabial fold (Caldwell-Luc operation).

SN-41 Pterygopalatine ganglion

1. **Introduction :** It is a largest peripheral parasympathetic ganglion It is a collection of cell bodies present on parasympathetic nerve situated in the peripheral part of cranium.
    A. Topographically it is related to maxillary nerve and
    B. Functionally it is related to greater petrosal nerve (facial nerve).

2. **Gross :**
    A. Situation : Pterygopalatine fossa.
    B. Relations :
        a. Medially : Pharyngeal artery.
        b. Laterally : Artery of pterygoid canal.
        c. Superior : Maxillary nerve.
        d. Posteriorly : Pterygoid canal.

3. **Connections :**
    A. Parasympathetic (motor root).
        a. Preganglionic fibres arises from lacrimatory nucleus (pons) - facial nerve (VII) - geniculate ganglion - greater petrosal nerve + deep petrosal nerve (plexus around internal carotid artery) - nerve to pterygoid canal - pterygopalatine ganglion - relay.

    b.   Postganglionic fibers - maxillary nerve - zygomatic branch - zygomaticotemporal branch - communicating branch to lacrimal nerve.

B. Sensory : From maxillary nerve passes through pterygopalatine ganglion without interruption.

C. Sympathetic :
    a.   Preganglion fibres - spinal nerve - superior cervical sympathetic ganglion.
    b.   Postganglionic fibres - plexus around internal carotid artery (deep petrosal nerve) passes without interruption.

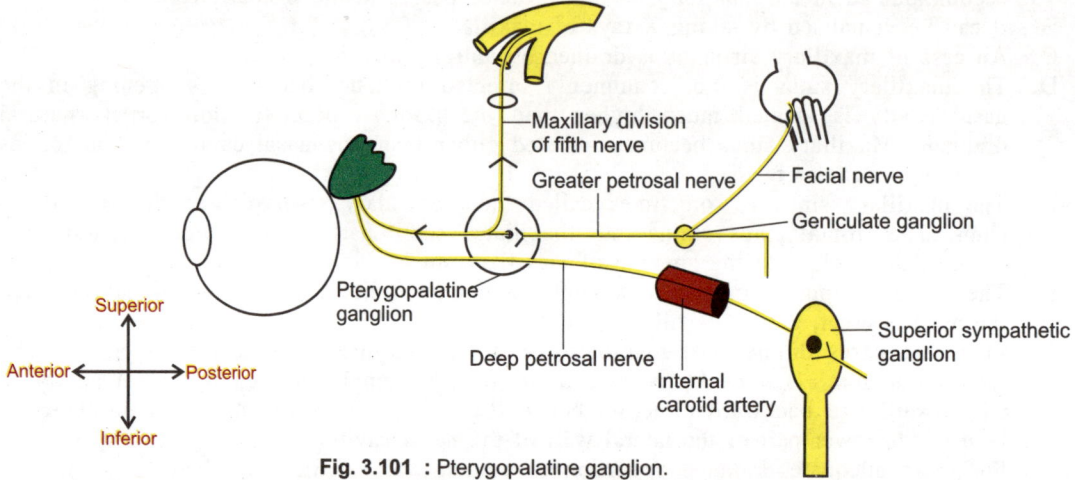

Fig. 3.101 : Pterygopalatine ganglion.

4. **Branches :** They are virtually derived from maxillary nerve.
    A. Orbital branch supplies :
        a.   Orbitalis muscle,
        b.   Mucous membrane of sphenoid and
        c.   Mucous membrane of posterior ethmoidal sinus.
    B. Palatine :
        a.   Greater palatine nerve which supplies mucous membrane of lateral wall of nose.
        b.   Lesser petrosal nerve - mucous membrane of soft palate and palatine tonsil.
    C. Nasal branches :
        a.   Posterior superior lateral nasal.
        b.   Medial nasal.

5. **Applied anatomy :**
    A. It is called ganglion of hay fever and produces running of nose and eyes.
    B. Injection of alcohol is occasionally employed in intractable cases of allergic rhinitis.

LAQ-34   Describe larynx under
1. Formation   2. Intrinsic muscles 3. Actions of muscles 4. Nerve supply &   5. Applied anatomy.

1. **Formation :** Larynx is formed by paired and unpaired cartilages. They are
    A. Unpaired : Thyroid, cricoid, epiglottis.
    B. Paired : Arytenoid, corniculate, cuneiform cartilages.

2. **Intrinsic muscles :** Muscles of larynx are divided into extrinsic and intrinsic muscles.
   A. Extrinsic muscles take origin outside and get inserted inside the organ. They are sternothyroid, thyrohyoid, omohyoid, digastric.
   B. Intrinsic muscles take origin and get inserted in the same organ. They are described as follows :

Table 3.32 : The table shows origin and insertion of muscles of larynx.

Muscle	Origin	Insertion
a. Posterior cricoarytenoid	Posterior surface of cricoid cartilage.	Muscular process of arytenoid cartilage.
b. Lateral cricoarytenoid	Upper border of lateral surface of cricoid cartilage.	Muscular process of arytenoid cartilage.
c. Cricothyroid	Arch of cricoid cartilage.	Inferior horn of thyroid cartilage.
d. Thyroarytenoid	Deep surface of thyroid cartilage.	Lateral surface of arytenoid cartilage.
e. Thyroepiglotticus	Thyroarytenoid cartilage.	Epiglottis.
f. Oblique arytenoid	Muscular process of one arytenoid cartilage.	Apex of other arytenoid cartilage.
g. Vocalis	Posterior surface of thyroid cartilage in midline.	Vocal process of arytenoid cartilage.
h. Transverse arytenoid	Posterior surface of arytenoid cartilage of one side.	Posterior surface of other side.
i. Aryepigloticus	Muscular process of arytenoid cartilage.	Epiglottis

3. **Actions of muscles :**
   A. Acting on the vocal cords
      a. Abductor : Posterior cricoarytenoid, abductor of vocal cords.

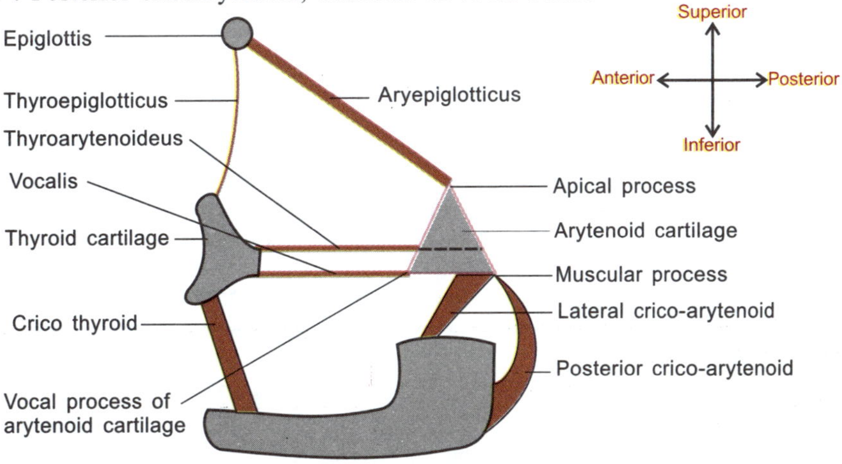

Fig. 3.102 : Muscles of larynx.

    b. Adductor :
        I.   Lateral cricoarytenoid,
        II. Thyroarytenoid and
        III. Oblique arytenoid.
    c. Tensor of the vocal folds : Cricothyroid.
    d. Relaxor of the vocal fold : Vocalis.
  B. Acting on the inlet of larynx
    a. Closing of the inlet : Aryepiglotticus.
    b. Opening of the inlet of larynx : Thyroepiglotticus.

4. **Nerve supply :**
  A. Sensory (sensation).
    a. Above vocal fold : Internal laryngeal nerve (superior laryngeal nerve, a branch of vagus nerve)
    b. Below the vocal fold : Recurrent laryngeal nerve.
  B. Motor (muscle) : All muscles of larynx are supplied by recurrent laryngeal nerve, a branch of vagus except cricothyroid, which is supplied, by external laryngeal nerve a branch of superior laryngeal nerve, a branch of vagus nerve.
    a. Embryological correlation:
        I.   Cricothyroid develops from fourth pharyngeal arch therefore supplied by nerve of fourth arch i.e. external laryngeal nerve, branch of superior laryngeal.
        II. Remaining muscles developed from sixth arch and hence supplied by nerve of sixth pharyngeal arch i.e. recurrent laryngeal nerve.
    b. Functional correlation :
        The cricothyroid muscle acts as a tuning fork. It first, receives impulses and starts vibrating. The remaining muscles receive impulses, which help in producing voice.

5. **Applied anatomy :**
  A. Examination of larynx is called laryngoscopy.
  B. Laryngitis is inflammation of larynx, occurs in common cold. The swelling of vocal cords is rare in acute laryngitis.
    The laryngitis is the inflammation of the mucous membrane of the larynx. The vocal cords do not swell due to following reasons :
    a. The vocal cords are lined by stratified squamous epithelium (remember that rest of the larynx is line by pseudostratified ciliated columnar epithelium).
    b. The mucous membrane is firmly attached to the vocal ligaments.
    c. There is no submucous tissue and glands over the vocal cords.
        For the same reason the vocal cords appear pearly white in color.
  C. Damage to internal laryngeal nerve produces anaesthesia (loss of sensation in supraglottic part of larynx). Therefore foreign body can easily enter. Foreign bodies can readily enter the larynx if internal laryngeal nerve is damaged.
  D. Damage to external laryngeal nerve causes paralysis of cricothyroid muscle. It results into weakness of phonation.
  E. When both recurrent laryngeal nerves are injured vocal cords lie in cadaveric position.

| SN-42 | **Rima glottis** |

1. **Introduction :** Narrowest anteroposterior cleft, or space of laryngeal cavity, lined by a stratified squamous nonkeratinized epithelium (without submucous coat).

2. **Attachment :**
   A. Anteriorly : The middle of angle of thyroid cartilage.
   B. Posteriorly : Vocal process of arytenoid cartilage.
   Limited - Posteriorly by an interarytenoid fold of mucous membrane.
      - Shape & size of rima glottis is changed by movements of vocal cords.

Table 3.33 : The table shows difference between inter membranous and inter cartilaginous part of rima glottis.

Particulars	Inter membranous	Inter cartilaginous
Contribution	3/5	2/5
Phase		
a. Quiet breathing	Triangular	Quadrangular
b. Forced inspiration	Triangular	Triangular
c. Phonation: Speech	Chink	Chink
d. Whispering	Closed	Widely open

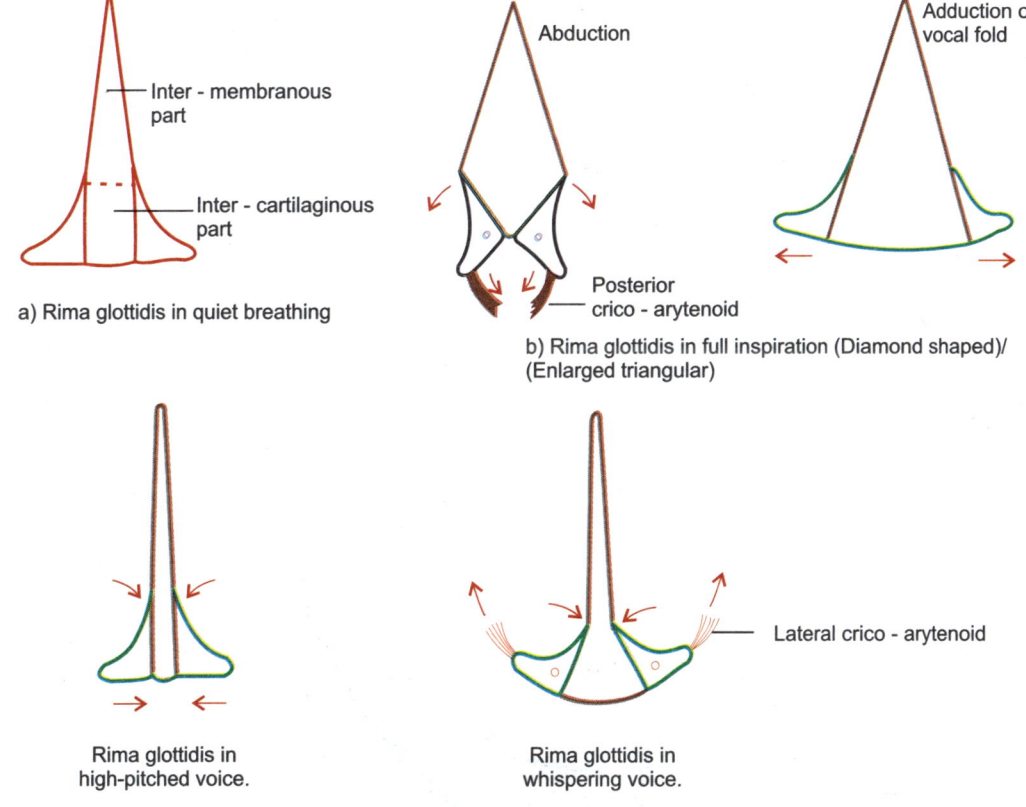

a) Rima glottidis in quiet breathing

b) Rima glottidis in full inspiration (Diamond shaped)/ (Enlarged triangular)

Rima glottidis in high-pitched voice.

Rima glottidis in whispering voice.

Fig. 3.103 : Extrinsic muscles of tongue.

4. **Nerve Supply :** All muscles of larynx are supplied by recurrent laryngeal nerve (vagus nerve) except cricothyroid, which is supplied, by external laryngeal nerve.(superior laryngeal, branch of vagus nerve).

LAQ-35   **Describe tongue under**   V. V. Imp.
            1. **Muscles of tongue**   2. **Blood supply**
            3. **Lymphatic drainage**   4. **Nerve supply**
            5. **Papillae of tongue**   6. **Development and**
            7. **Applied anatomy.**

1. **Muscles of tongue :** These are grouped into intrinsic and extrinsic muscles.
   A. Intrinsic muscles : They alter the shape and size of tongue and are described in the table no. 3.34.

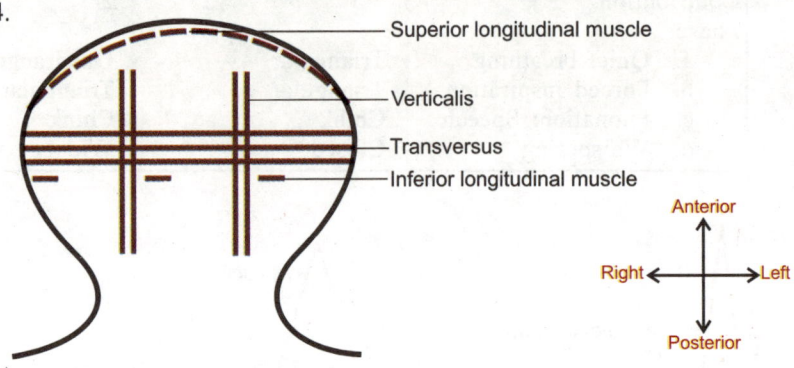

Fig. 3.104 : Intrinsic muscles of tongue.

Table 3.34 : The table shows origin and insertion of intrinsic muscles of tongue.

Muscle	Origin	Insertion	Action
a. Superior longitudinal	Posterior part of median fibrous septum.	Sides of tongue.	Reduces the length of tongue.
b. Inferior longitudinal	Posterior part of side of tongue.	Anterior part of median fibrous septum.	Shortens the tongue.
c. Transversus	Median fibrous septum.	Side of tongue.	Reduces the width.
d. Verticalis	Lamina propria of dorsum of tongue.	Sides of tongue.	Reduces the thickness of tongue.

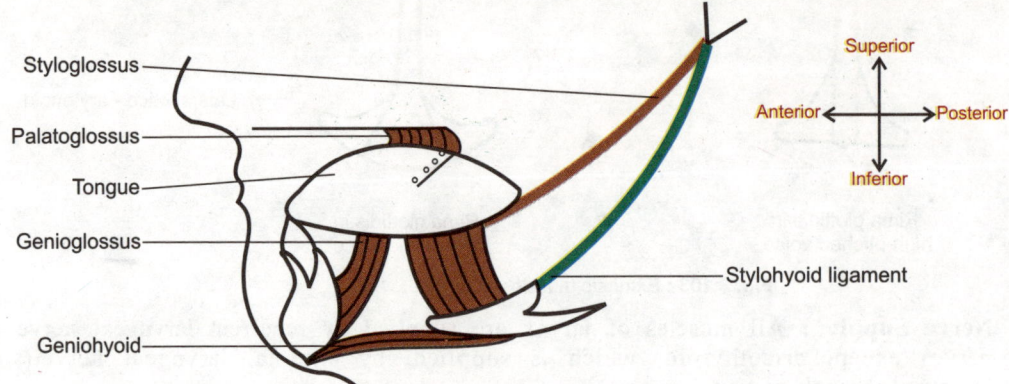

Fig. 3.105 : Extrinsic muscles of tongue.

B. Extrinsic muscles of tongue :

Table 3.35 : The table shows origin, insertion and action of extrinsic muscles of tongue.

Muscle	Origin	Insertion	Action
a. Genioglossus: Fan shaped.	I. Superior genial tubercle. II. Symphysis menti present on the inner surface of mandible	i. Upper fibers: Root to apex of the tongue. ii. Middle fibers: Mixes with constrictor of pharynx. iii. Lower fibers: Body of hyoid bone.	i. Protrusion of tongue. ii. Safety muscle of tongue. iii. Saves the life by preventing the backward fall.
b. Hyoglossus: Quadrilateral.	I. Upper surface of greater cornu of hyoid bone. II. Body of hyoid bone	Side of the tongue between styloglossus laterally and inferior longitudinal muscle medially.	Makes dorsum of the tongue convex. It retracts the protruded tongue.
c. Chondroglossus: Detached part of the hyoglossus	I. Lesser cornu of hyoid bone. II. Part of body of hyoid bone.	Side of tongue.	Depression of tongue.
d. Styloglossus:	Tip of styloid process and stylomandibular ligament.	Side of tongue.	Retraction of tongue
e. Palatoglossus	Under surface of palatine aponeurosis.	Side of tongue.	Elevation of tongue.

2. **Blood supply** :
   A. Arterial supply :
      a. Lingual artery (chief artery of tongue), branch of external carotid artery supplies tongue through
         I. Profunda lingual artery : It supplies oral part of tongue.
         II. Dorsal lingual artery : It supplies pharyngeal part of tongue.
      b. Facial artery through.
         I. Ascending palatine.
         II. Tonsilar branch.
      c. Ascending pharyngeal branch of external carotid artery.
   B. Venous drainage : Veins are arranged in two sets.

Table 3.36 : The table shows superficial and deep veins of tongue.

Particulars	Superficial	Deep
a. Location	Superficial to hyoglossus.	Deep to hyoglossus.
b. Distribution	Tip and under surface of tongue.	Dorsum of tongue.
c. Structures accompanied	Hypoglossal nerve (XII).	Lingual artery.
d. Drains into	Internal jugular vein.	Internal jugular vein.

3. **Lymphatic drainage :**
   A. Peculiarities :
      a. Do not accompany the blood vessels.
      b. Tip of the tongue presents richest lymph drainage and drains bilaterally.
      c. Lymphatic in the posterior one third of tongue drains bilaterally.
      d. Lymphatic of the tongue ultimately drains into jugulo omohyoid nodes, hence they are called lymph nodes of tongue.
         Lymphatic of tongue consists of following sets :

Table 3.37 : The table shows lymphatic drainage of the tongue.

Lymph node	Afferent (Receiving)	Efferent (Draining)
I. Apical	i. Tip ii. Frenulum	- Submental (major lymphnode)
II. Marginal	Side of tongue in front of sulcus terminalis	- Submandibular node - Jugulodigastric
III. Central	Anterior 2/3rd lymphatics of tongue in front of vallate papillae.	- Jugulo omohyoid
IV. Dorsal	Posterior 1/3rd	- Bilaterally into jugular and diagastric (major part) - Jugulo omohyoid lymph nodes.

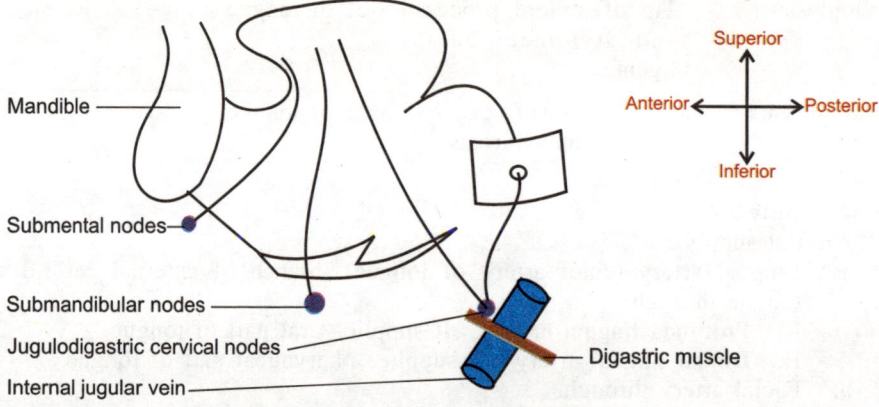

Fig. 3.106 : Lymphatic drainage of tongue.

B. Applied anatomy of lymphatic :
   a. Malignancy in the tip and posterior one third of tongue is more dangerous since it drains bilaterally.
   b. Lymph vessels piercing mylohyoid are often closely related to the periosteum of mandible accounting early spread to the bone.

4. **Nerve supply of tongue :**
   A. Motor :
      a. Somatomotor : All the extrinsic & intrinsic muscles of tongue are supplied by hypoglossal nerve (nerve of occipital myotome) except palatoglossus which is supplied by pharyngeal plexus.

b. Secretomotor fibres are derived from superior salivary nucleus - facial nerve - chorda tympani - lingual nerve - submandibular ganglion - lingual glands.

c. Vasomotor nerve arises from spinal cord - superior sympathetic ganglion - plexus around external carotid artery (plexus around lingual artery).

B. Sensory :

Table 3.38 : The table shows sensory nerve supply of tongue.

Particulars	Anterior two-thrid	Posterior one-third	Most posterior part
a. General sensation: Touch, pain and temperature.	Lingual branch of mandibular (trigeminal): Nerve of first pharyngeal arch.	Glossopharyngeal (IX) nerve, a nerve of third pharyngeal arch.	Vagus (nerve of fourth and sixth arch).
b. Special sensation: Taste.	Chorda tympani (facial) pretrematic nerve (of second pharyngeal arch) to first arch.	Glossopharyngeal (IX) nerve, a nerve of third pharyngeal arch.	Vagus (nerve of fourth and sixth arch).
c. Papillae : I. Circumvallate	Glossopharyngeal nerve, nerve of third pharyngeal arch:		
II. Fungiform, filiform and foliate.	Lingual nerve (branch of mandibular nerve).		

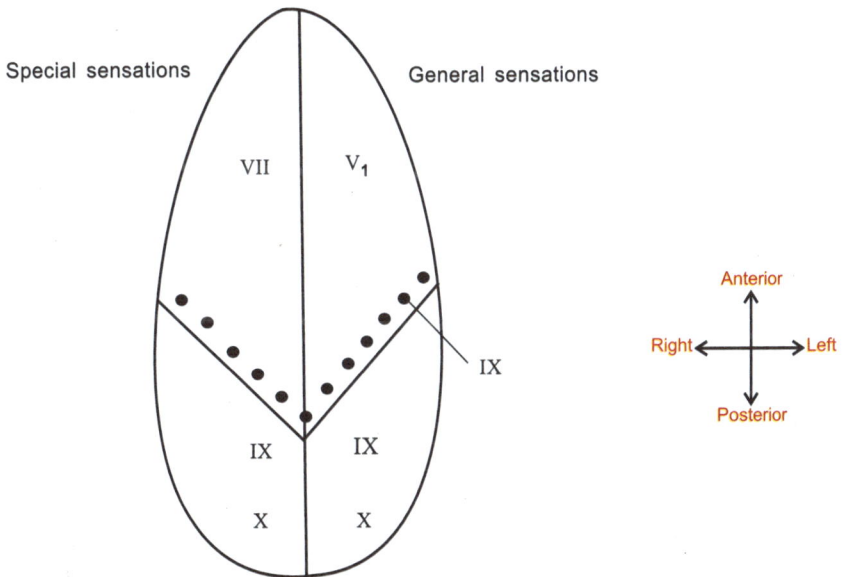

Fig. 3.107 : Sensory nerve supply of tongue.

5. **Papillae of tongue** - Projection of epithelium caused by projections of subepithelial connective tissue (dermal core). Tongue shows following papillae :

A. Circumvallate papillae.

B. Filiform and fungiform papillae are described as follows :

Table 3.39 : The table shows details of filiform and fungiform papillae.

Particulars	Filiform	Fungiform
a. Number	Numerous	Few
b. Arrangement	Uniform	Irregular
c. Distribution	All over tongue	Tip and sides
d. Shape	Thread like pointed	Club shaped
e. Taste buds	Absent	Few

6. **Development of the tongue :**
   A. Chronological age : It develops in the fourth week of intrauterine life.
   B. Germ layer :
      a. Epithelium is developed from endoderm of the first, second, third, fourth and sixth pharyngeal arch.
      b. Muscles are developed from occipital myotome.
   C. Site : Floor of the pharynx just cranial to median thyroid diverticulum.
   D. Sources :
      a. Muscles: All the muscles of tongue are developed from occipital myotome except palatoglossus. The nerve of the occipital myotome is hypoglossal (twelfth cranial nerve). Hence all the muscles are supplied by hypoglossal nerve.
      b. Mucous membrane: It is developed from endoderm of the floor of pharynx and is subdivided into
         I. Anterior two third is developed from :
            i. Fusion of a pair of lingual swelling arising from pouch of the first branchial arch and
            ii. Tuberculum impar (*impar* unpaired) a midline swelling arises from first pouch and gives a very little contribution. The post trematic nerve of first arch is lingual nerve and pre-trematic nerve of second arch is chorda tympani nerve.
         II. Posterior one third is developed from cranial part of hypobranchial eminence, which is formed by fusion of third and fourth brachial arches only. The eminence is divided by a transverse groove into cranial and caudal part. The nerve of third arch is glossopharyngeal nerve, nerve of fourth arch is superior laryngeal nerve and the nerve of the sixth arch is recurrent laryngeal nerve.
      c. Fibrous Stroma : Blood vessels and lymphatics are developed from mesoderm of the adjacent arches.
      d. Papillae :
         I. Formed by thickening of epithelium of dorsum of tongue.
         II. Fungiform and filiform papillae develop in anterior two-third of tongue.
         III. Circumvallate papillae develop in posterior one-third from second arch. It gets submerged by the overgrowth of third arch and these papillae occupy the anterior wall of sulcus terminalis. Hence they are supplied by glossopharyngeal nerve (IXth nerve).
   E. Anomalies :
      a. Ankyloglossia :
         I. Ankyloglossia superior : Tongue is adherent to palate.

    II.   Ankyloglossia inferior or tongue-tie : Tongue is adherent to floor of the mouth.
b. Microglossia : Too small tongue.
c. Aglossia : Absence of tongue. This is due to complete agenesis of the tongue.
d. Hemiglossia : Supression of one of the lingual swelling.
e. Macroglossia : Too large tongue.

7. Applied anatomy :
  A. Injury to the hypoglossal nerve produces paralysis of the muscles of the tongue on the side of the lesion. Infranuclear lesion shows ipsilateral hemiatrophy of the tongue. Supra nuclear lesion produces paralysis without wasting.
  B. In unconscious patient, the mouth may fall back and obstruct the air passage. This can be prevented by keeping the tongue on one side or pulling the tongue.
  C. Carcinoma of the tongue is quite common. It is better treated by radio therapy than by surgery.

SAQ-11   Circumvallate papillae

1. Papillae surrounded by trench.

2. **Size :** 2 mm pinhead size.

3. **Number :** About 10 to 12.

4. **Situation :** Single row in front of sulcus terminalis.

5. It contains taste buds, present on lateral wall of papillae.

6. **Taste buds :** They contain three types of cells.
  A. Gustatory cell or bipolar cells.
  B. Sustentacular or supporting cells.
  C. Basal cells.

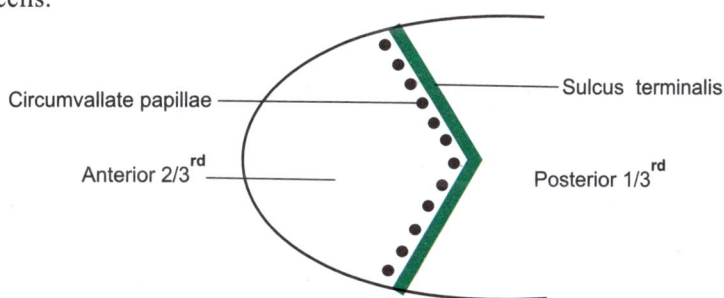

Fig. 3.108 : Circumvallate papillae.

SN-43   Tympanic membrane

1. **Gross features :** It is a thin, translucent partition between the external and the middle ear. It is oval in shape, measuring 9 x 10 mm. It is placed obliquely at an angle of 55° with the floor of the meatus. It has outer and inner surface.
  A. Outer surface : Covered by thin skin.
  B. Inner surface : Provides attachment to the handle of malleus. The point of maximus convexity lies at the level of tip is called umbo.

The membrane is thick at its circumference, which is fixed to the tympanic sulcus. Superiorly, the sulcus is deficient. Here the membrane is attached to the tympanic notch. Greater part of the tympanic membrane is tightly stretched and is called pars tensa. The part between the two malleolar fold is loose and is called pars flaccida. *The part flaccida is crossed by the chorda tympani, which passes between middle fibrous layer and inner mucous layer.*

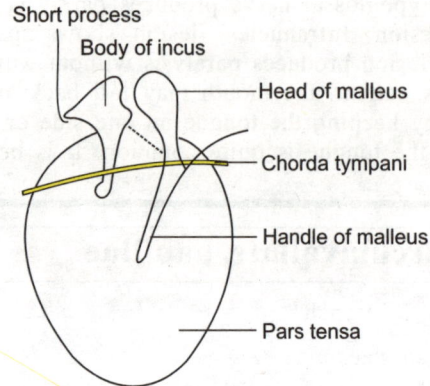

Fig. 3.109 : Tympanic membrane.

2. **Structure :** Composed of three layers.
   A. Outer cuticular layer.
   B. Middle fibrous layer made up of superficial radiating fibers and deep circular fibers. The circular fibers are sparse at the center and maximum at the periphery.
   C. Inner mucous layer is lined by low ciliated columnar epithelium.

Table 3.40 : The table shows blood supply and lymphatic nerve supply of tympanic membrane.

Particulars	Outer surface	Inner surface
3. Blood supply: A. Arterial supply:	Deep auricular branch of maxillary artery.	a. Anterior tympanic branch of maxillary artery. b. Posterior tympanic branch of stylomastoid branch of posterior auricular artery.
B. Venous drainage:	External jugular vein.	a. Transverse sinus. b. Venous plexus around auditory tube.
C. Lymphatic:	Preauricular lymph nodes.	Retropharyngeal.
4. Nerve supply:	Auriculotemporal nerve.	Tympanic branch of glossopharyngeal nerve.

5. **Applied anatomy :**
   A. The otoscopic examination reveals the redness, bulging, perforation or retraction of the tympanic membrane.
   B. The membrane is incised to drain pus present in the mid layer. The incision is called myringotomy. *It is usually made in the postero inferior quadrant of the membrane. In giving an incision, it has to be remembered that the chorda tympani nerve runs downwards and forwards across the inner surface of membrane, lateral to the long process of incus, but medial to the neck of mandible.*

LAQ-36   **Describe middle ear under**
1. Gross anatomy   **2. Contents**   **3. Blood supply**
4. Nerve supply &   **5. Applied anatomy.**

1. Gross anatomy :

  A. Introduction : Narrow space situated between external and internal ear present in the petrous part of temporal bone.

  B. Dimensions : It is biconcave in shape.
     a. Vertical : 15 mm.
     b. Anteroposterior : 15 mm.
     c. Transverse
         I.   Roof : 6 mm.
         II. Centre : 2 mm.
         III. Floor : 4 mm.

  C. Communication :
     a. Anteriorly : Nasopharynx through auditory tube.
     b. Posteriorly : Mastoid antrum and air cells through aditus to antrum.

  D. Boundaries :
     a. Roof or tegmental wall : Separates ear from middle cranial fossa.
     b. Floor or jugular wall :
         I.   Separates middle ear from superior bulb of internal jugular vein.
         II. Formed by jugular fossa of temporal bone.
     c. Anterior wall or carotid wall :
         I.   It is constricted.
         II. Consists of three parts :
             i.   Upper part forms : Canal for tensor tympani.
             ii. Middle part forms : Opening of auditory tube.
             iii. Lower part forms : The posterior wall of carotid canal.

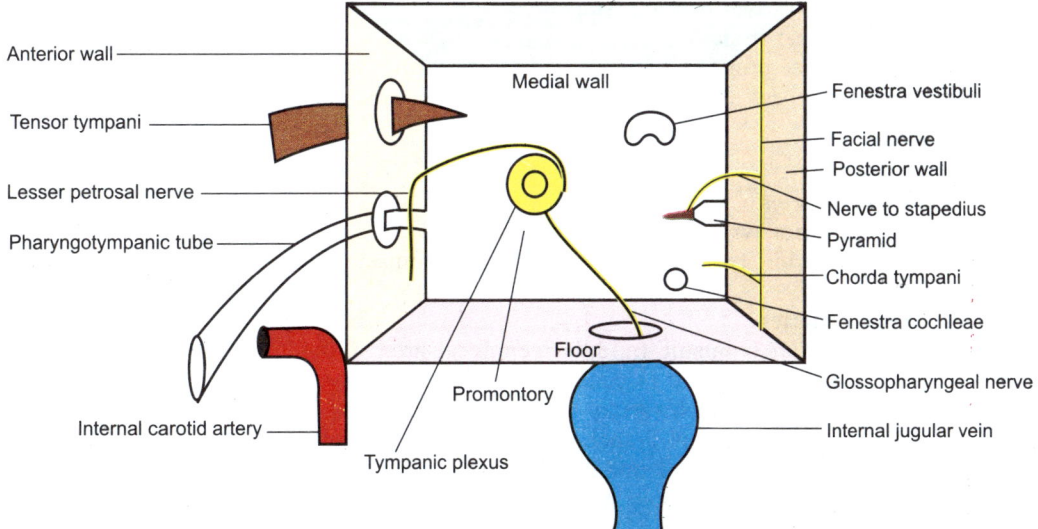

Fig. 3.110 : Middle ear showing roof, floor, anterior, posterior and medial wall

    III. There is a septum between canal for tensor tympani and canal for auditory tube.

d. Posterior wall or mastoid wall : Represents following features from above downwards :
  I. Superiorly : Aditus to mastoid antrum.
  II. Fossa incudis : Depression for incus.
  III. Pyramid (projection) : Apex of pyramid presents an opening for tendon of stapedius.
  IV. Lateral to pyramid : Posterior canaliculus for chorda tympani.

e. Lateral or membranous wall.
  I. Separates middle ear from external ear.
  II. Formed mainly by:
    i. Tympanic membrane.
    ii. Partly by squamous part of temporal bone.
  III. Near the tympanic notch there are two aperatures -
    i. Petrotympanic fissure.
    ii. Anterior canaliculus for chorda tympani.

f. Medial or labyrinthine wall : It separates middle ear from internal ear. It presents following features :
  I. Promontory produced by first turn of cochlea.
  II. Fenestra vestibuli : Oval opening leads to vestibule of internal ear.
  III. Prominence of facial canal.
  IV. Fenestra cochlea ends in scala tympani and closed by secondary tympanic membrane.
  V. Sinus tympani depression behind promontory.

2. **Contents :**
A. Air.
B. Bone : Ear ossicles namely malleus, incus and stapes.
C. Vessels, which supply and drain middle ear.
D. Muscles : Tensor tympani and stapedius.
E. Ligaments of ear ossicle.
F. Tympanic cavity proper : Lies opposite to tympanic membrane.
G. Epitympanic recess above tympanic membrane.

3. **Blood supply :**
A. Arterial supply :
  a. Large arteries
    I. Anterior tympanic (branch of maxillary).
    II. Posterior tympanic branch from stylomastoid, branch of posterior auricular artery.
  b. Small arteries
    I. Superior tympanic (middle meningeal artery).
    II. Inferior tympanic (ascending pharyngeal).
    III. Tympanic branch (artery of pterygoid canal).
    IV. Caroticotympanic branch of ICA.
    V. Petrosal branch of middle meningeal artery.
B. Venous drainage : Veins from middle ear drain into:
  a. Superior petrosal sinus.
  b. Pterygoid plexus of vein.

4. **Nerve supply :** Tympanic plexus formed by
    A. Tympanic branch of glossopharyngeal nerve.
    B. Caroticotympanic nerve (plexus around ICA).

5. **Applied anatomy :** Throat infections commonly spread to the middle ear through auditory tube, which are more common in children. In children the tube is small and horizontal. The pus may be discharged into one of the following courses.
    A. May be in the external ear following rupture of tympanic membrane.
    B. May erode the roof and results in meningitis.
    C. May erode the floor & spread downward and causes thrombosis of internal jugular vein.
    D. May cause mastoid abscess.
    E. Fracture of middle cranial fossa can cause bleeding through the ear.

SN-44   Spiral organ of Corti

1. **Introduction :** End organ for hearing.

2. **Gross :** It is located on basilar membrane of cochlear duct.

3. **Microscopic structure :** Consists of following parts:
    A. **Basilar membrane :** Extends from osseous spiral lamina to the outer cochlear wall, It consists of collagen fibres.

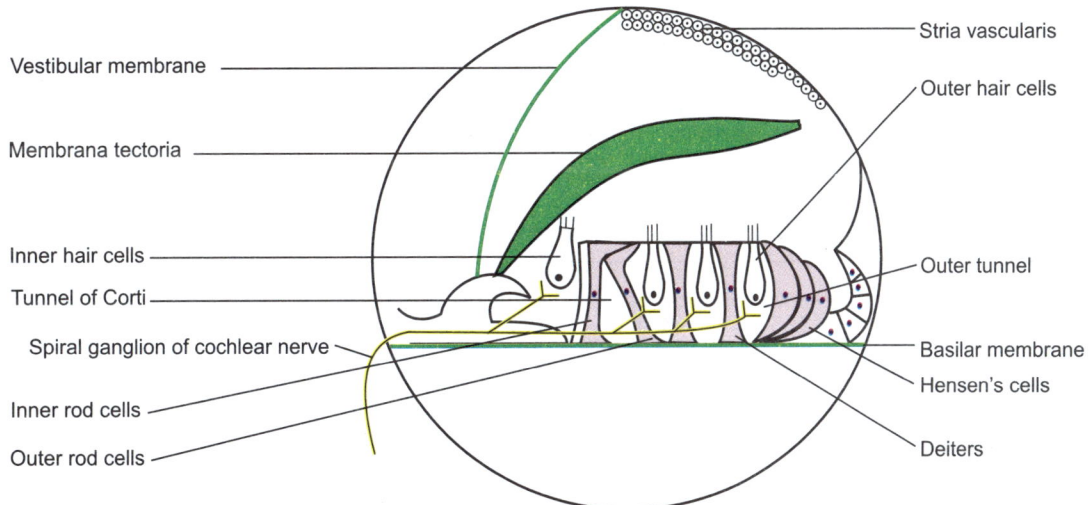

Fig. 3.111 : Structure of spiral organ of Corti.

B. Rods of Corti : Enclose tunnel of Corti. The details of rods is as follows

Table 3.41 : The table shows details of inner and outer rods.

Particulars	Inner rods (pillar)	Outer rods (pillar)
Row	Single	Single
Number	6000	4000

C. Hair cells are essential components of organ of Corti. It bears stereocilia.
   Functions :
   a. Detects the movements of endolymph.
   b. Detects the vibrations of basilar membrane.
   c. Transfers vibration into nerve impulse going to cochlear nerve.
      The hair cells are divided into inner and outer hair cells.

Table 3.42 : The table shows details of inner and outer hair cells.

Particular	Inner hair cells	Outer hair cells
Situation	Medial to inner rod of Corti	Outer to outer rod of Corti
Rows	Single	Three to four
Number	3500	12000
Shape	Pear	Cylindrical
Type	Predominantly afferent	Afferent as well as efferent
Nerve supply	Type I Neuron	Type II, unmyelinated Efferent from contralateral Superior olivary nucleus
Function	Auditory sensation	Auditory discrimination

These inner hair cells are supported by phalangeal supporting cells.
Outer supporting cells of Hensen.
Membrana tectoria : Gelatinous membrane for protection of hair cells.
Tonotopic localisation :
      High tones : Lower part of organ of Corti.
      Low tones : Upper part of organ of Corti.

SN-45   Cochlea

1. **Cochlea :** Shell of snail. Shape : conical; $2^{3/4}$ turns.

2. **Location :** Anterior to the vestibule.
   A. Apex is towards anterosuperior part of the medial wall of middle ear.
   B. Base is at the floor of internal acoustic meatus perforated by cochlear nerve.

3. **Dimension :**
   A. From base to apex 5 mm.
   B. Width 9 mm (at base).

4. **Structure :**
   A. Central bony axis : Modiolus (= axis of wheel) with spiral bony canal around. The bony canal is divided into three channels which are spirally arranged.
      a. Scala media (cochlear duct) : Triangular, bounded by
         I. Basilar membrane attached to osseous spiral lamina.
         II. Vestibular or Reissner's membrane.
         III. Outer wall of cochlea lies between basilar and vestibular membrane.
         IV. The apex of the cochlea is blind. It contains endolymph.

V. Spiral organ of Corti lies on basilar membrane.
b. Scala vestibuli:
   I. Canal above scala media.
   II. Communicates with
       i. Bony vestibule at base;
       ii. With scala tympani at apex of cochlea through helicotrema (spiral opening).
c. Scala tympani : Canal below scala media separated from the middle ear cavity by secondary tympanic membrane. Both scala vestibuli and scala tympani are filled with perilymph.
d. Modiolus : It is broad at the base, narrow at the apex, contains blood vessels and spiral ganglion. It gives out osseous spiral lamina which is attached to basilar membrane.

5. **Openings at basal turn of bony cochlea :**
   A. Oval window : Occupied by foot plate of stapes.
   B. Round window : Closed by secondary tympanic membrane.
   C. Cochlear canaliculus : Communicates scala tympani with subarchnoid space.

Short notes on Embryology

SN-46   **First pharyngeal**

First pharyngeal arch is also called mandibular arch.

Table 3.43 : The table shows derivatives of first pharyngeal arch.

Muscles	Skeletal element	Ligament	Nerve & Artery
1. **Temporalis** 2. **Lateral pterygoid** 3. **Medial pterygoid** } Muscles of mastication. 4. **Masseter** 5. **Mylohyoid** 6. **Anterior belly of digastric** 7. **Tensor tympani** 8. **Tensor palati**	A. Dorsal end forms maxillary process. a. Premaxilla. b. Maxilla. c. Zygomatic. d. Temporal (partly). B. Ventral part forms Meckel's cartilage It has: a. Ventral end forms mandible surrounding Meckel's cartilage. b. Dorsal end forms malleus and incus.	a. Anterior ligament of malleus. b. Spheno-mandibular ligament.	**Nerve** of first pharyngeal arch is mandibular nerve, a branch of trigeminal nerve (fifth cranial nerve). **Artery** of the first pharyngeal arch mostly disappears, part of this artery forms maxillary artery.

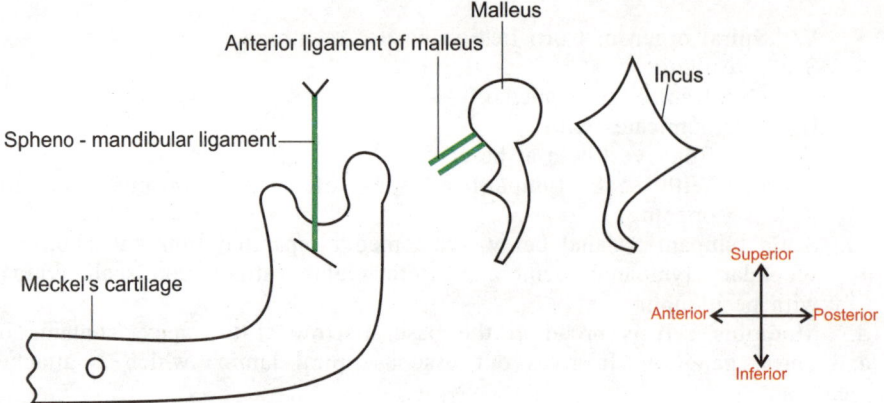

Fig. 3.112 : Skeletal elements and ligaments developed from first pharyngeal arch.

SN-47　Second pharyngeal arch

🔑 The word "second" and the derivatives of the second pharyngeal arch begins with the letter "**S**"

Table 3.44 : The table shows derivatives of second pharyngeal arch.

Muscles	Skeletal element	Ligament	Nerve and artery
1. **S**tapedius. 2. **S**tylohyoid. 3. Posterior belly of digastric. 4. Occipito frontalis. 5. Muscles of ear. 6. Muscles of facial expression. 7. Platysma.	A. **S**tapes. B. **S**tyloid process of temporal bone. C. **S**maller cornu of hyoid bone. D. **S**uperior surface of body of hyoid bone	**S**tylohyoid ligament.	**Nerve** of second pharyngeal arch is facial nerve (seventh cranial nerve). **Artery** of second pharyngeal arch mostly regresses except for dorsal part which forms **s**tapedial artery.

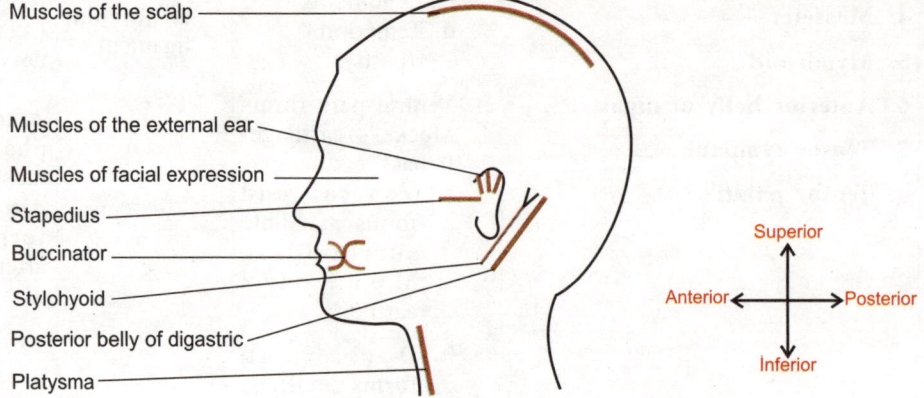

Fig. 3.113 : Muscles developed from first pharyngeal arch.

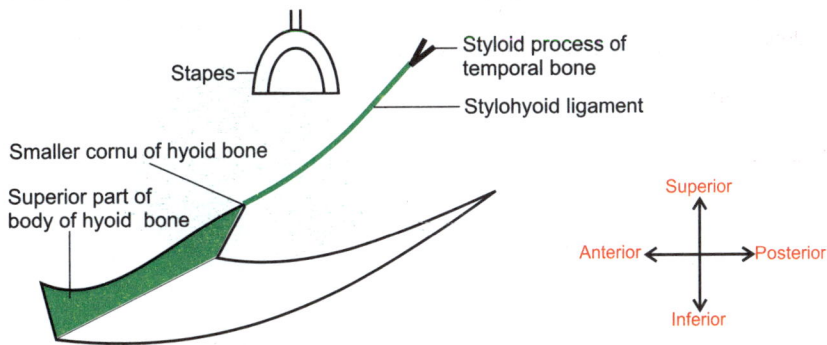

Fig. 3.114 : Skeletal elements and ligaments of second pharyngeal arch.

SN-48   Pharyngeal pouches

Endoderm of each pharyngeal arch is called pharyngeal pouch. Following are the structures given by the respective pouches.

Table 3.45 : The table shows derivatives of pharyngeal pouches.

Arch	Ventral end	Dorsal end
First	Tongue	Dorsal end of first and second arches combine and form pharyngotympanic recess which gives rise to :
Second	Tonsil	1. Proximal part : Pharyngo tympanic tube and 2. Distal part : Middle ear cavity.
Third	a. Inferior parathyroid gland. b. Thymus.	
Fourth	a. Superior parathyroid gland. b. Thyroid gland.	

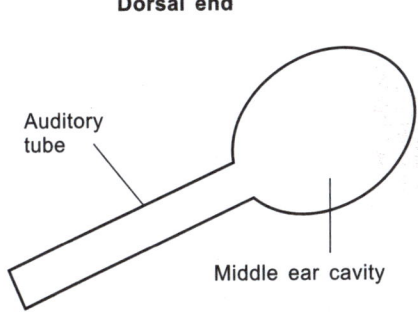

Fig. 3.115 : Tubotympanic recess (I & II).

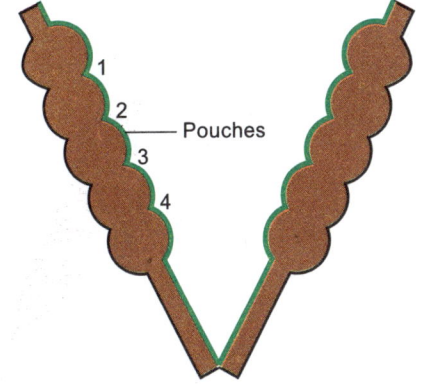

Fig. 3.116 : Pharyngeal pouches.

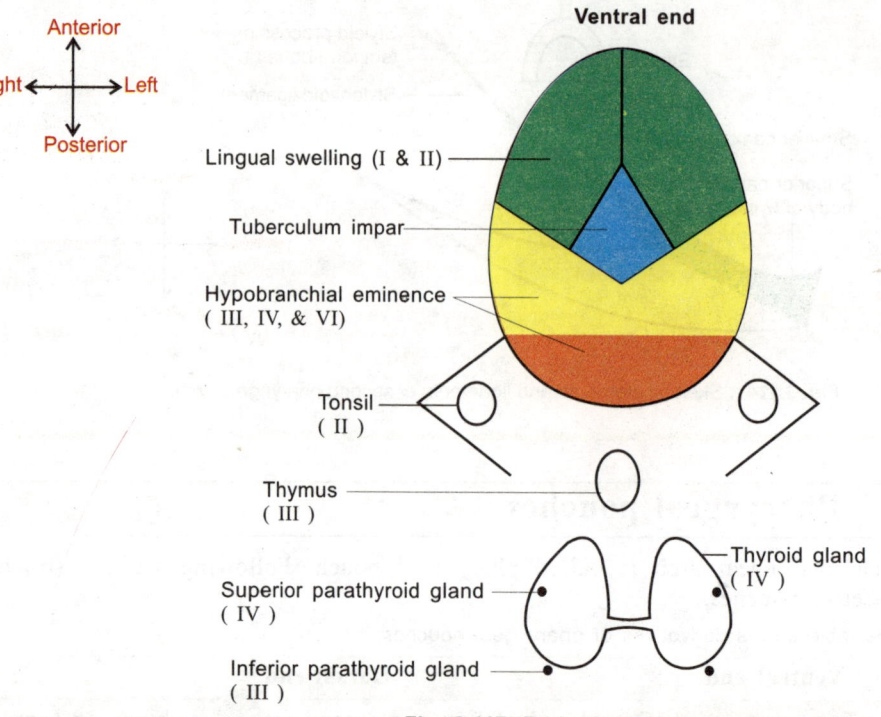

Fig. 3.117 : Derivatives of pharyngeal pouches.

SN-49   Pharyngeal cleft

Ectoderm of pharyngeal arch is called cleft.

First cleft - gives rise to external acoustic meatus.

Swellings appear on the first and second arches are called as hillocks, which give rise to pinna of ear.

Second arch develops faster than the remaining arches and overhangs the third, fourth and sixth arches.

A space is created in between over hanging second, third, fourth and sixth arches, which is called as cervical sinus. Subsequently the lower overhanging borders of second arch fuses with tissues caudal to the arches and the smooth part of side of neck are formed.

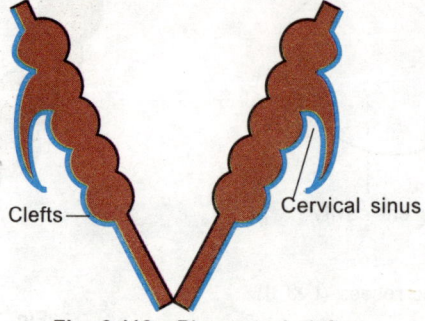

Fig. 3.118 : Pharyngeal clefts.

SN-50   Meckel's cartilage

1. **Definition :** Skeletal element of the first pharyngeal arch (mandibular arch) is called as Meckel's cartilage.

2. **Extend :** It extends from the developing otic capsule to mandibular prominence.

3. **Derivatives :** Following are the structures given by different parts of Meckel's cartilage.

Table 3.46 : The table shows derivatives of Meckel's cartilage.

Parts	Structures
Dorsal	A. Incus and malleus.
Intermediate	A. Anterior ligament of malleus. B. Sphenomandibular ligament.
Ventral	A. Body of mandible and B. Mental ossicle.

SN-51   Fourth and sixth pharyngeal arch

1. **Muscles:**
   A. Cricothyroid.
   B. Constrictor of pharynx.
   C. Intrinsic muscles of larynx.
   D. Striated muscle of oesophagus.
2. **Skeletal element:** The fourth and sixth pharyngeal arches fuse together and give following cartilages:
   A. Thyroid,
   B. Cricoid,
   C. Arytenoid,
   D. Corniculate and
   E. Cuneiform.
3. **Nerves :**
   A. Nerve of the fourth pharyngeal arch is superior laryngeal nerve, a branch of vagus nerve.
   B. Nerve of the sixth pharyngeal arch is recurrent laryngeal nerve, a branch of vagus nerve.
4. **Artery :**
   A. Fourth arch.
      a. Right side : Forms the proximal part of right subclavian artery.
      b. Left side : Arch of the aorta.
   B. Sixth arch.
      a. Ventral part : Forms pulmonary artery.
      b. Dorsal part :
      Right side : Ductus arteriosus which degenerates and forms ligamentum arteriosum.

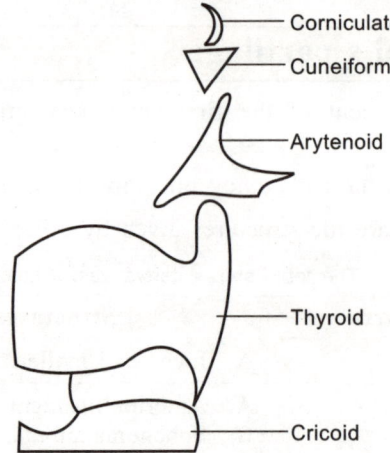

Fig. 3.119 : Skeletal elements developed from IV & VI th pharyngeal arches.

| SN-52 | **Development of palate** |

1. **Chronological age :** Eighth week of intrauterine life.

2. **Germ layer :** Mesoderm of pharyngeal arches.

3. **Site :** At the primitive oral cavity.

4. **Sources :** It consists of two parts
    A. Primitive palate is an area in front of incisive fossa. It is developed by fusion of medial nasal process & maxillary process.
    B. Permanent palate lies behind primitive palate and is developed from fusion of palatine process of both maxillae in midline. The fusion between the primitive and permanent palates take place in a 'Y' shaped manner. The fusion extends from before backwards.

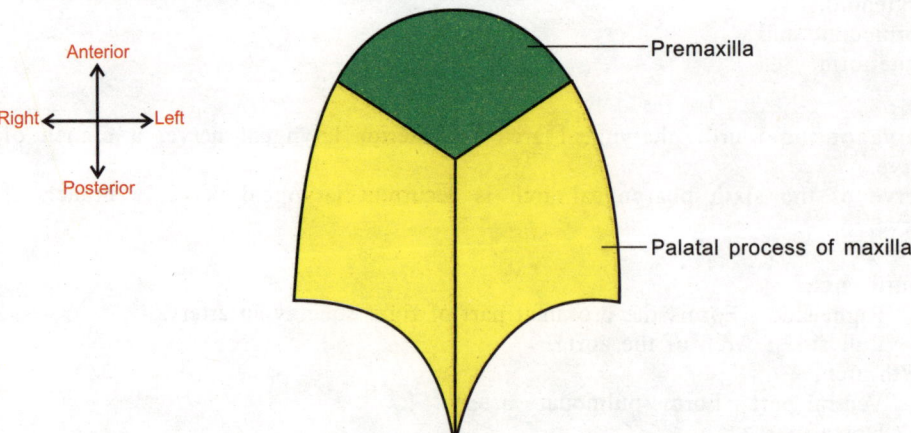

Fig. 3.120 : Development of the palate.

C. Anterior three-fourth of permanent palate : Ossifies & fuses with nasal septum.

D. Posterior one-fourth of the permanent palate does not fuse with lower edge of nasal septum and hangs as soft palate.

5. **Anomalies :**

A. Cleft palate.

B. Cleft lip.

Cleft palate

Introduction : Cleft palate: Failure of fusion of primitive and permanent palate is called cleft palate and varies in degree of severity.

1. **First degree :** Bifid uvula.

2. **Second degree :** Ununited palatal process.

3. **Third degree :** Ununited palatal process & a cleft of one side of premaxilla.

4. **Fourth degree :** Is rare. Ununited palatal process and cleft on both sides of premaxilla.

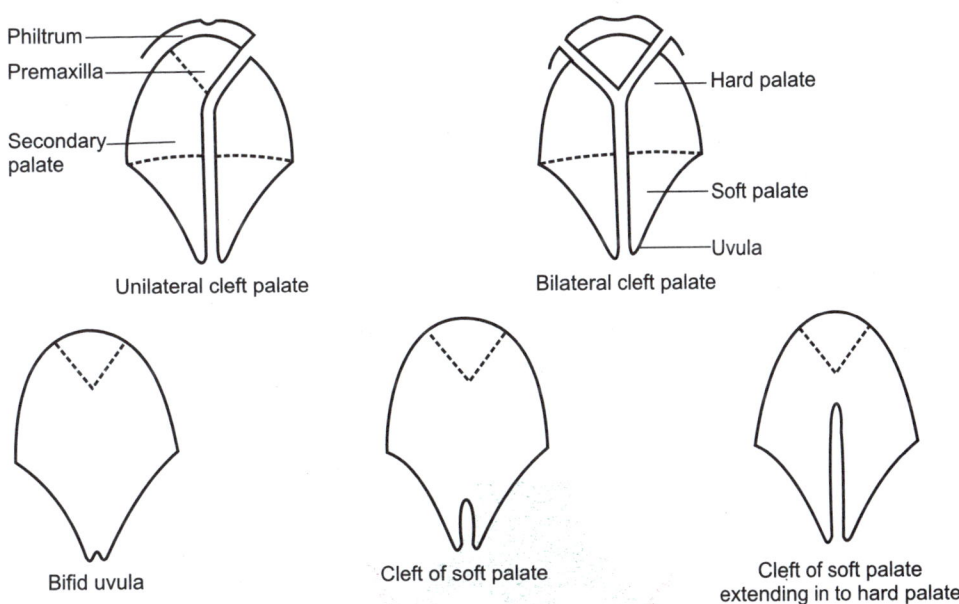

Fig. 3.121 : Typs of the cleft palate.

Cleft lip

Cleft lip : Due to failure or union of the globular processes of the medial nasal fold of the frontonasal process with the maxillary process of the mandibular arch. It may be unilateral or bilateral.

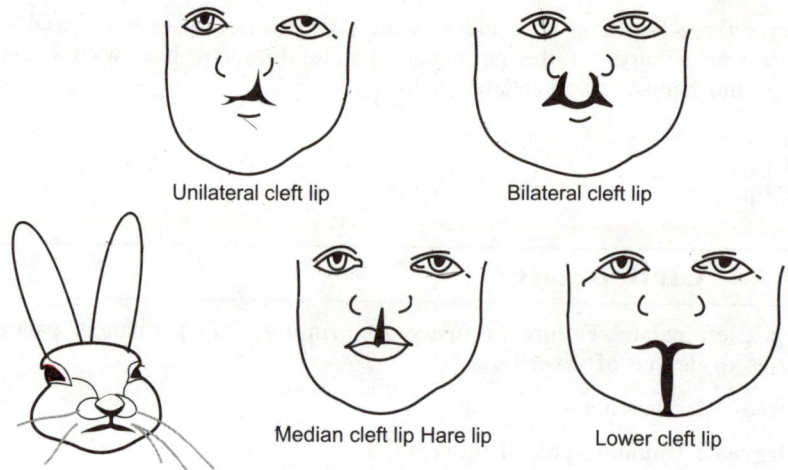

Unilateral cleft lip   Bilateral cleft lip

Median cleft lip Hare lip   Lower cleft lip

Fig. 3.122 : Development of face.

SN-53   Development of face

1. **Chronological age :** Fifth month of intrauterine life by
2. **Germ layer :**
   A. Upper lip : Ectoderm and mesoderm.
   B. Lower lip : Ectoderm and mesoderm.
   C. Cheek and vestibule of mouth: Ectoderm of alveolabial process.

3. **Sources :** It develops from five processes
   A. Unpaired frontonasal process which again forms medial and lateral nasal process.
   B. Paired maxillary processes.
   C. Paired mandibular processes.
      Above processes contribute for the formation of following structures :
        a. Lateral part of maxillary process give to lateral part of upper lip.
        b. Median nasal process give rise to philtrum of upper lip.

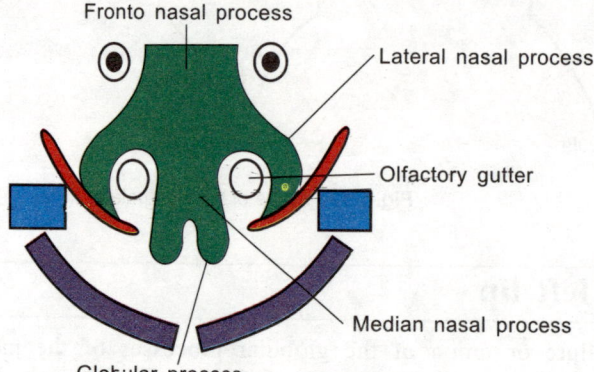

Fronto nasal process

Lateral nasal process

Olfactory gutter

Median nasal process

Globular process

Fig. 3.123 : Development of face.

    c.   Mandibular process give rise to lower lip.

4.   **Anomalies :** Most of the anomalies of the face are due to failure of union of different processes, which forms face.

   A.   Facial cleft or nasolabial furrow : It is due to failure of fusion between lateral nasal process and the maxillary process. It may be unilateral or bilateral. Nasolacrimal duct is absent in this anomaly.

   B.   Harelip (usually upper harelip) it may be median or lateral. Lateral harelip may be unilateral or bilateral.

      a.   Median harelip is due to failure of fusion of right and left medial process of frontonasal process.

      b.   Lateral harelip : It is very common and due to failure of fusion of medial nasal process and maxillary process.

      c.   Very rarely there may be failure of fusion of mandibular arches & results into split lower lip.

   C.   Macrostoma or wide opening of the mouth. It is due to failure or lesser degree of fusion between mandibular and maxillary process.

   D.   Microstoma (small oral fissure) - It occurs due to excessive fusion of maxillary and mandibular processes.

   E.   Other rare anomalies area of nose may be absent.

      a.   Proboscis : A cylindrical projection of nose below the forehead.

      b.   Cyclops : Fusion of two eyeballs.

SN-54   Development of thymus

1.   **Chronological age :** Sixth week of intrauterine life.

   Age changes

   A.   It is larger at birth.

   B.   It continuously increases till puberty.

   C.   After puberty it undergoes atrophy.

2.   **Germ layer :**

   A.   Hassal's corpuscle : is developed from the ventral part of the third pharyngeal pouch.

   B.   Lymphoid tissue is developed from mesoderm of the third pharyngeal arch.

3.   **Site :** Primitive pharynx.

4.   **Sources :** It is very closely associated with the inferior parathyroid gland. It gets separated from the inferior parathyroid gland as the thymic rudiment. This is divided into

   A.   Thinner portion which forms the cervical part of the thymus.

   B.   Broader portion is divided into two parts, which enters into thorax and forms thoracic part.

   These two parts unite with each other by means of connective tissue and the thymus is formed.

5.   **Anomalies :**

   A.   Abnormal site is the commonest anomalies of thymus. It may remain along the course of development.

   B.   Cervical part of the thymus may get fragmented & give rise to accessory thymic tissue.

SN-55   Development of eye

1. **Eye :** The components of the eye and its parts are derived as follows :
    A. Forebrain vesicle gives rise to :
        a. Retina and
        b. Optic nerve.
    B. Surface ectoderm gives rise to :
        a. The epidermis of the eyelids.
        b. Lacrimal gland and ducts.
        c. Conjunctival sac.
        d. Canaliculi and sac.
        e. Corneal epithelium.
        f. The lens.
    C. Neurectoderm gives rise to:
        a. Substantia propria of cornea.
        b. Sclera.
        c. Choroid.
        d. Ciliary body.
        e. Iris.

2. **Anomalies :**
    A. Coloboma (defect) : Defective closure of optic fissure, site ventromedial segment.
    B. The causes of congenital cataract may be :
        a. Hereditary or by
        b. Infection of rubella virus.
    C. Astigmatism : Faulty curvature of cornea or lens produces astigmatism.
    D. Rare anomalies are
        a. Aphakia : Absence of lens.
        b. Anophthalmus : Absence of eye.
        c. Cyclopia : Median eye.
        d. Aniridia : Absence of iris.
        e. Synophthalmia : Fusion of eyes.
        f. Microophthalmus too small eye.

Short notes on Histology

SN-56   Cornea

1. It forms anterior one-sixth of the outer coat of eyeball. Cornea is transparent because of following reasons.
    A. Regular arrangement of fibers.
    B. Refractive index of ground substance and fibers is same.
    C. Thickness of each fibril is less than wave length of light.
    D. Critical level of water is maintained by active absorption of water by endothelium.

2. **Peculiarities :** Cornea has
    A. No blood vessels,
    B. No lymphatics and
    C. Rich nerve supply. Nerves are non-myelinated.

3. **Layers :** There are five layers of the cornea. 🔑 **A B C D E**

A. **A**nterior Epithelium : (External Epithelial layer), stratified, squamous nonkeratinised epithelium).
  a. The deeper cells are columnar and have rod shaped nuclei.
  b. The superficial cells are squamous and have flat nuclei.
  c. The cells rest on linear basement membrane.
  d. The cells never keratinise.
  e. It contains numerous free nerve endings, hence this layer is extremely sensitive.

B. **B**owman's membrane (anterior limiting membrane) :
  a. Epithelium rests on this layer.
  b. It is structureless, transparent and homogenous membrane.
  c. It contains collagen fibers which are produced by substantia propria.

C. **C**onnective tissue proper : (substantia propria)
  a. This is the main substance of cornea.
  b. It is present deep to Bowman's membrane.
  c. It is a modified, transparent, flattened connective tissue.
  d. The connective tissue contains dens collagen fibers containing corneal spaces.
  e. It contains 200 - 250 lamellae and about 2000 fibers, embeded in ground substance containing sulphated glycosamino glycans.
  f. The collagen fibers are of Type II (diameters 20 n.m.).
  g. Arrangement of fibers is very regular.
  h. Fibers within one lamellae are parallel to one another and are at obtuse angle to those of fibers of adjacent lamellae.
  i. It contains fibroblast which are stellate or flat. They are also called as keratocytes or corneal corpuscles or corneocytes.

D. **D**escemet's membrane : (True basement membrane).
  a. It is formed by homogeneous material.
  b. Membrane breaks at the margin of the cornea into fibres which form inner wall of sinus venous sclera.
  c. The spaces between these trabecuale are called the spaces of iridocorneal angle.

E. **E**ndothelium of anterior chamber :
  a. It is bathed by aqueous humor. Hence, it is not a true endothelium as named.
  b. It is lined by low cuboidal epithelium.
  c. It is adapted for transport of ions.

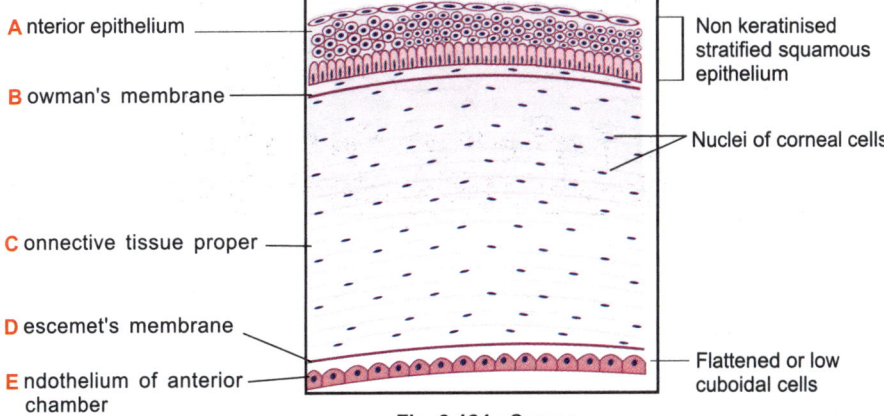

Anterior epithelium — Non keratinised stratified squamous epithelium

Bowman's membrane —

Nuclei of corneal cells

Connective tissue proper —

Descemet's membrane —

Endothelium of anterior chamber — Flattened or low cuboidal cells

Fig. 3.124 : Cornea.

SN-57   Retina

It has ten layers :

1. **Pigment cell layer :** It is single layer of cuboidal cells. The cells have rounded nuclei and the apical cytoplasm contains melanin granules.

2. **Layer of rods and cones :**
   A. Rods and cones are light receptors of the eye.
   B. The cones respond to 🔑 **ABC**
      a. **A**cuity of vision.
      b. **B**rightness of vision.
      c. **C**olor vision.
      Rods respond to dim light.

3. **Outer limiting membrane :** Contains lateral process of radial fibers of nuclear cells.

4. **Outer nuclear layer :** Contains cell bodies of rods and cones which contain photosensitive process of neurons.

5. **Outer plexiform layer :** Contains axonal process of rods and cones, dendrites of bipolar

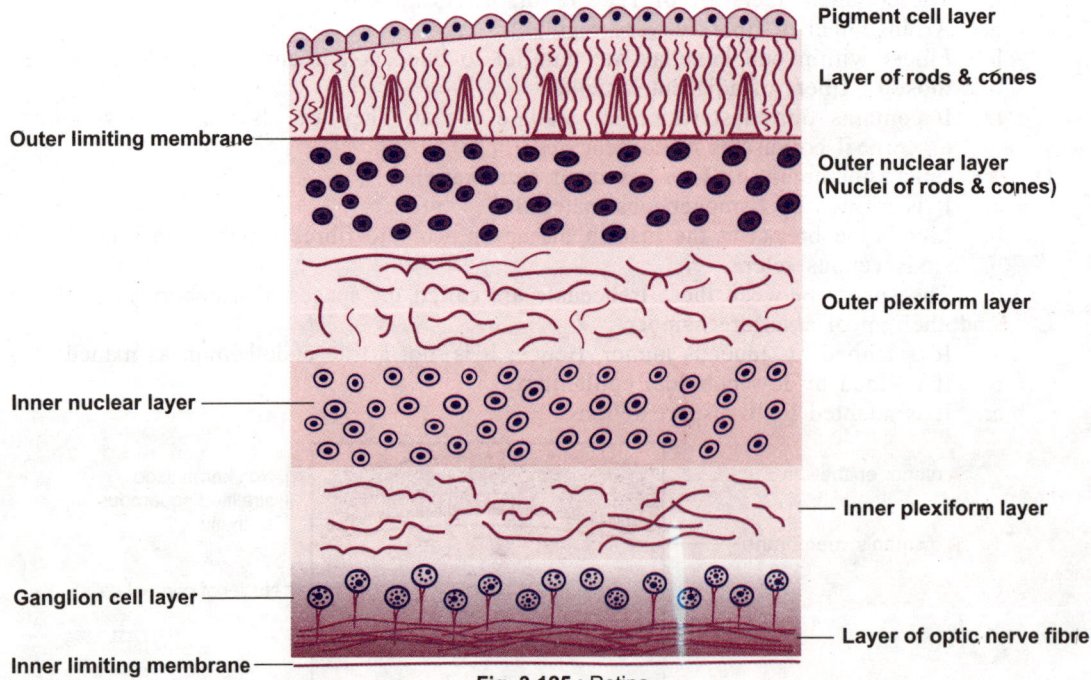

Fig. 3.125 : Retina.

Pigment cell layer
Layer of rods & cones
Outer limiting membrane
Outer nuclear layer (Nuclei of rods & cones)
Outer plexiform layer
Inner nuclear layer
Inner plexiform layer
Ganglion cell layer
Layer of optic nerve fibre
Inner limiting membrane

6. **Inner nuclear layer :** It contains
   A. Cell bodies and nuclei of bipolar neurons (second order neurons of visual pathway).
   B. Association neurons
      a. Horizontal cells
      b. Amacrine cells
   C. Supporting cells (Muller's cells)

7. **Inner plexiform layer :** Contains synapse between axons of bipolar cells and also process of association cells or amacrine cells.

8. **Ganglion cell layer :** Contains cell bodies of ganglion cells. These are large multipolar cells with prominent nissel granules. The axons of ganglion layer form the optic nerve.

9. **Optic nerve layer :** Contains optic nerve fibers and Muller's fibers.

10. **Inner limiting membrane :** The surface facing next layer is thrown into processes which insinuate between rods and cones. It prevents diffusion of light. It is innermost layer of retina and represent a basal lamina formed by the expanded inner ends of Muller cells.

SN-58   Eyelid

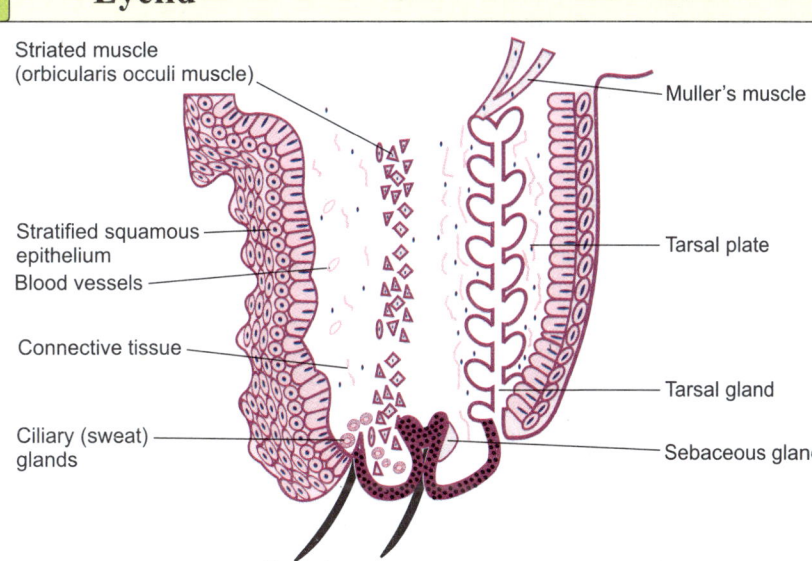

Fig. 3.126 : Eyelid.

Features :
1. Both the surfaces of the eyelid are lined by epithelium.
   A. Skin of the eyelid is lined by stratified squamous keratinised epithelium.
   B. Mucous membrane of the eyelid is lined by stratified columnar epithelium.

2. Skeleton is formed by a mass of fibrous tissue called tarsus or tarsal plate.

3. Fat cells are absent in the subepithelial connective tissue.

4. Arrector pilorum muscle is absent in the hair follicle.

5. Accessory lacrimal glands are present. They are also called glands of Wolfring or Krauses gland. They are serous in nature.

6. Tarsal glands (Meibomian gland) : It is a modified sebaceous gland.

7. Moll's gland : These are modified sweat glands.

8. Glands of Zeiss : These are sebaceous glands present in the eyelashes.

SN-59   Sclero corneal junction

1. **It is junction of transparent cornea and opaque sclera.**
    A. At the junction :
        a. There is change of epithelium to that of conjunctiva.
            I.   The epithelium of the palpebral conjunctiva is typically two layered :
                i.   Superficial columnar cells and
                ii. Deep flattened cells.
            II. At the sclera & fornix, epithelium is three layered :
                i.   Superficial columnar,
                ii. Middle polygonal and
                iii. Deep flattened cells.
            III. At sclera corneal junction : Stratified squamous epithelium.
            IV. At cornea epithelium stratified squamous.
        b. Bowman's membrane changes into subepithelial layer of connective tissue
        c. Collagenous bundles of the sclera continue directly into those of cornea where they become parallel with each other and the tissue becomes homogenous and transparent.
        d. Posterior lip forms a projecting ridge in which the ciliary body is fastened.
        e. Descents membrane terminate into trabecular meshwork enclosing small spaces known as
            I.   Spaces of Fontana which are lined by attenuated epithelium.
            II. These spaces communicate with the anterior chamber of eye.
            III. There are several small epithelial lined cavities, which are anterior and lateral to trabecular meshwork. These cavities are the cross sections of a circular canal known as the canal of Schlemn which are parallel to the border of cornea. This canal communicates with the venous spaces and is usually filled with clear aqueous humor.

Table 3.47 :   The table shows sclero corneal junction.

Particulars	Spaces of Fontana	Canal of Schlemn
Shape	Irregular	Circular
Position	At the termination of Descemet's membrane at the sclero - corneal junction	At anterior & lateral to the trabecular network
Lining	Attenuated epithelium	Living epithelium
Number	Less	More
Size	Small	Small
Communication with	Anterior chamber	Venous spaces.
Content		Clear aqueous humor

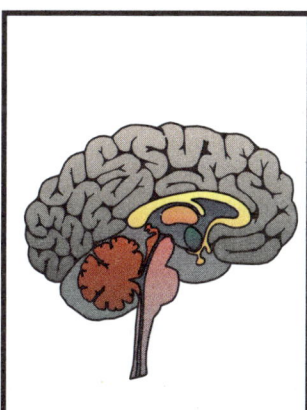

INDEX

SN-1 Neuroglia

Definition : These are non-excitable, supporting cells of nervous system. They are described in following table :

Table 4.1 : The table shows types of neuroglia, their situation, functions and development.

Type	Site	Function	Development

1. Macroglia
A. Oligodendrocyte
  (few processes)
  a. Intra-fascicular
	Myelinated tract	They give support & form myelin sheath.	Ectoderm

b. Perineuronal	Surface of the body of neurons		
B. Astrocyte (star shaped) a. Protoplasmic, thick and symmetrical processes	Grey matter		
b. Fibrous, thin and asymmetrical processes	White matter		
2. Microglia, small, flattened cell body with short processes	More in grey than white matter, near capillaries	Phagocytosis	Mesoderm
3. Ependymal cell	Ventricle of the brain and spinal cord.	Secrets CSF	Ectoderm
4. Satellite or capsular Companion	Sensory or autonomic ganglion	Supports & protects the neuron	Ectoderm
5. Schwann cell	Peripheral nerve	Myelin sheath	Ectoderm

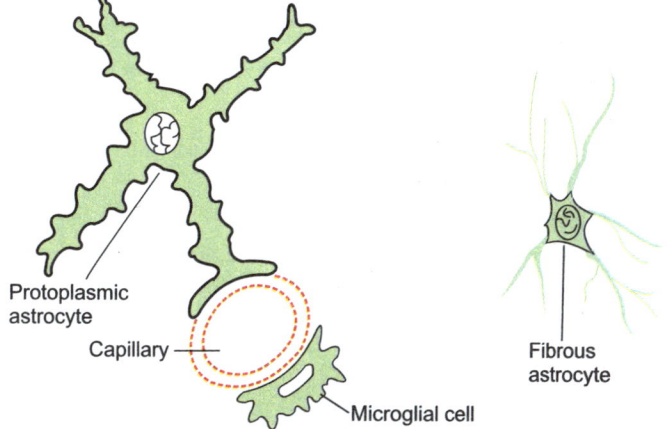

Protoplasmic astrocyte

Capillary

Microglial cell

Fibrous astrocyte

Fig. 4.1 : Protoplasmic and fibrous astrocyte.

SN-2   Cerebrospinal fluid

1. **The CSF** is modified tissue fluid. It is present in
    A. Ventricles of brain.
    B. Subarchnoid space around brain and spinal cord.

2. **Formation :**
    A. The bulk of the CSF is formed by choroid plexus of lateral ventricle.
    B. Small amount is formed by choroid plexus of third and fourth ventricle.
    C. The total quantity : About 150 ml.
    D. Rate of formation : 200 ml. / day.
    E. Normal pressure : 60 to 100 mm. of water.

3. **Circulation :**

    Foramen of Monro.   Cerebral aqueduct

    Lateral ventricle ⟶ Third ventricle ⟶

    Median and lateral apertures.

    Fourth ventricle ⟶ Subarchonoid space.

4. **Absorption :** Chiefly absorbed through
    A. Arachnoid villi.
    B. Arachnoid granulation.
    C. It is also absorbed partly by
        a. Perineural lymphatics around the first, second, seventh and eight cranial nerve.
        b. Veins related to spinal nerves.

5. **Functions :**
    A. Protection.
    B. Nutrition.
    C. Removal of waste products.

6. **Applied anatomy :**
    A. CSF can be obtained by
        a. Lumbar puncture.
        b. Cisternal puncture.
        c. Ventricular puncture.
    B. Biochemical analysis of CSF is of diagnostic value in various disease.
    C. Obstruction to the flow of CSF in the ventricular system leads to hydrocephalus in children and raised intracranial pressure in adult.

LAQ-1   Draw and label a transverse section of spinal cord showing main ascending and descending tracts.

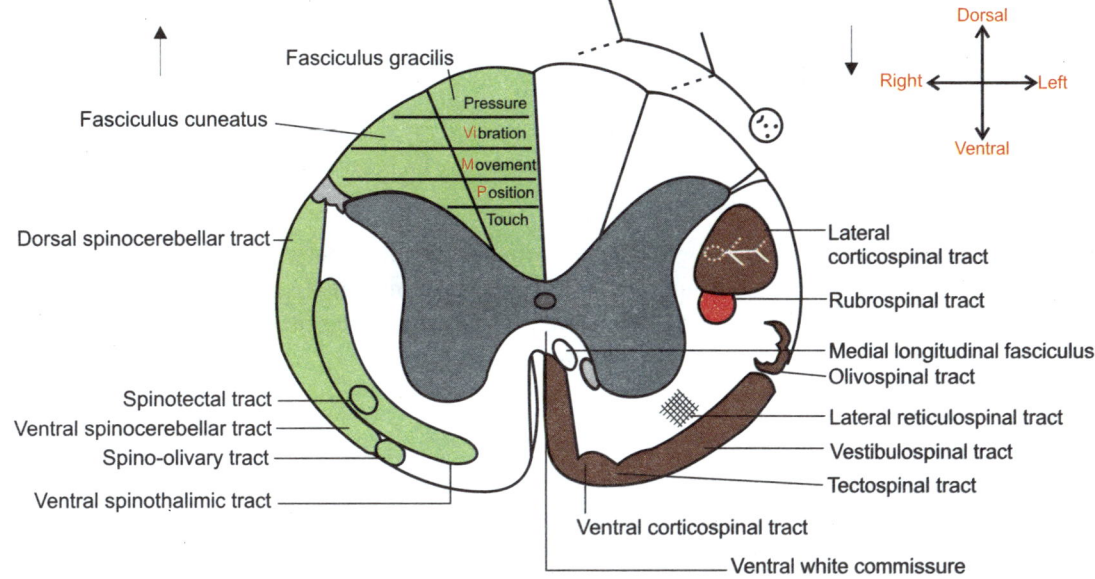

Fig. 4.2 : T. S. of spinal cord showing ascending and descending tracts.

LAQ-2   Draw and label ventral surface of the brainstem

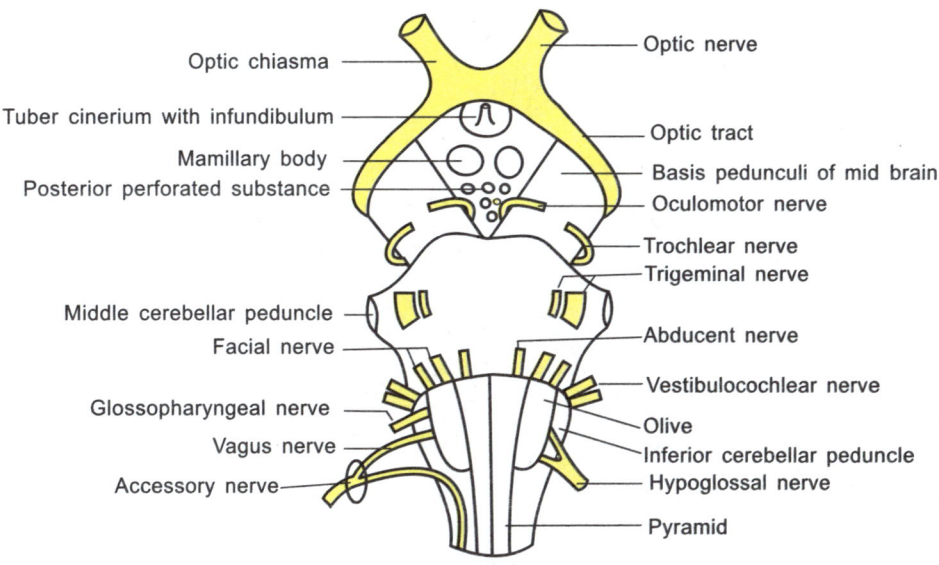

Fig. 4.3 : Brain stem (viewed from ventral surface).

SN-3   Pyramidal decussation

1. **Introduction :** It is a crossing of corticospinal fibers at the level of medulla oblongata.

2. **Origin :** Corticospinal fibers arise from the area no. 4, 6, 8 of precentral gyrus and from area no. 3, 1, 2 of postcentral gyrus.

3. **Location :** On the anterior surface of upper part of medulla, the corticospinal fibers start decussating. The decussating fibers form a bulging, which resembles a pyramid. Hence it is called pyramidal dicussation.

4. **Termination :** Most of the fibers of the corticospinal tract decussate and continue in the opposite side in the lateral column as lateral corticospinal tract. These fibers terminate in the laminae IV to VII of spinal grey matter. They are connected to the alpha and gamma motor neurons of the lamina IX through the interneurons.

5. **Applied anatomy :** Lesions of the corticospinal tract is called the upper motor neuron lesion.
    A. The lesion above the level of pyramidal decussation results in paralysis of the muscles of the upper limb and lower limb on opposite side of the body.
    B. The lesion below the level of pyramidal decussation results in the paralysis of the muscles on the same side of body.

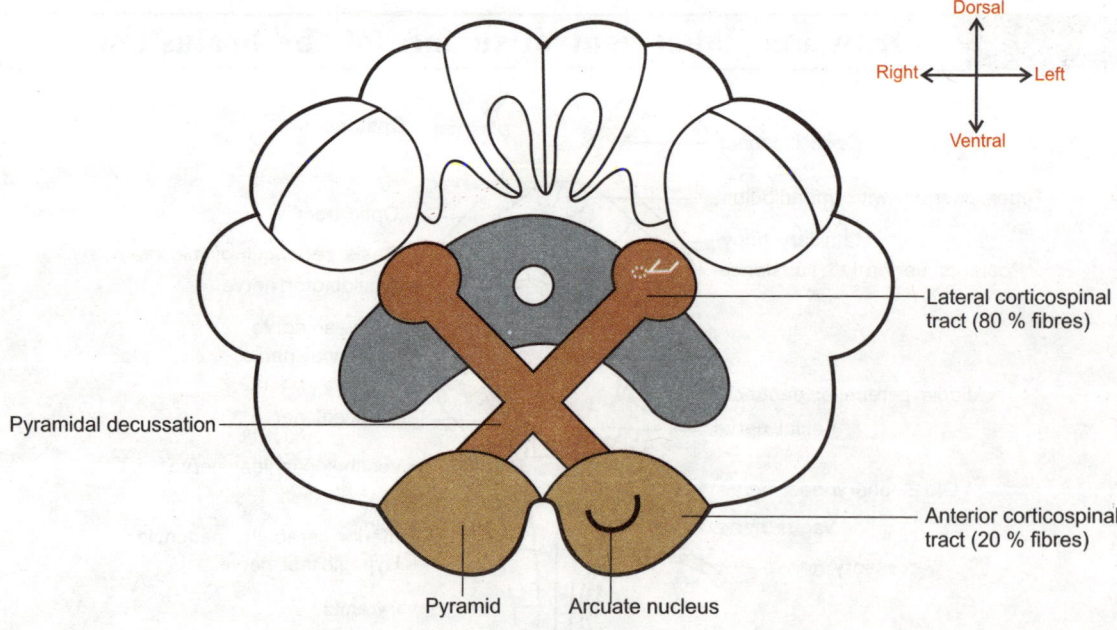

Fig. 4.4 : Pyramidal decussation.

LAQ-3 Draw and label a transverse section of medulla oblongata at the level of pyramidal decussation

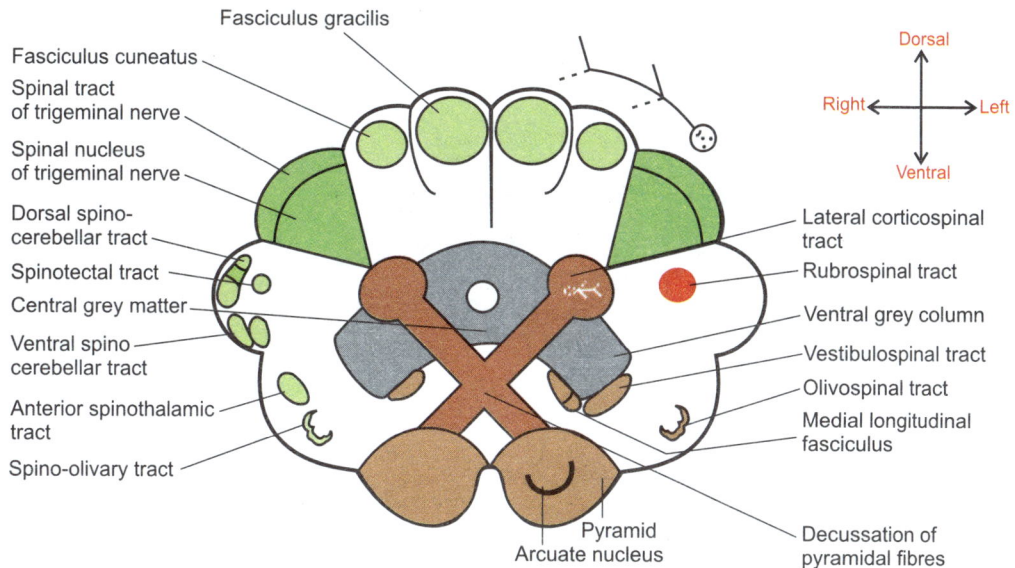

Fasciculus gracilis

Fasciculus cuneatus

Spinal tract of trigeminal nerve

Spinal nucleus of trigeminal nerve

Dorsal spino-cerebellar tract

Spinotectal tract

Central grey matter

Ventral spino cerebellar tract

Anterior spinothalamic tract

Spino-olivary tract

Dorsal

Right ←→ Left

Ventral

Lateral corticospinal tract

Rubrospinal tract

Ventral grey column

Vestibulospinal tract

Olivospinal tract

Medial longitudinal fasciculus

Decussation of pyramidal fibres

Pyramid
Arcuate nucleus

Fig. 4.5 : T. S. of medulla at the level of pyramidal decussation.

SN-4 Arcuate fibers

1. **Introduction** : The axons of various nuclei are arranged like the arc.

2. **Types :** These are
   A. Internal arcuate fibers -
      a. These are second order neurons arising from gracilis and cuneatus nuclei. These are situated on dorsal side of medulla.
      b. These fibers cross to the opposite side and forms medial lemniscus.
   B. External arcuate fibers : These are of following types
      a. Anterior external arcuate fibers
         I. These fibers arise from arcuate nuclei and reach the nuclei of the cerebellum on the same side.
         II. Function : They convey information from cerebrum to cerebellum.
      b. Posterior external arcuate fibers (Cuneocerebellar) :-
         I. These fibers arise from accessory cuneate nucleus and reach the nuclei of cerebellum on the same side.
         II. Function : These are homologous of posterior spino cerebellar tract in upper limb and carries unconscious proprioceptive sensations from upper limb.
      a. Before decussation :
         I. The fibers of lower limb are medially.
         II. The fibers of upper limb are laterally.
      b. After decussation :

I.   The fibers of the lower limb are anteriorly.
II.   The fibers of the upper limb are posteriorly.

3.   **Applied :**
A.   Before decussation : Loss of sensation of touch and pain on the same side.
B.   After decussation : Loss of touch and pain on the opposite side.

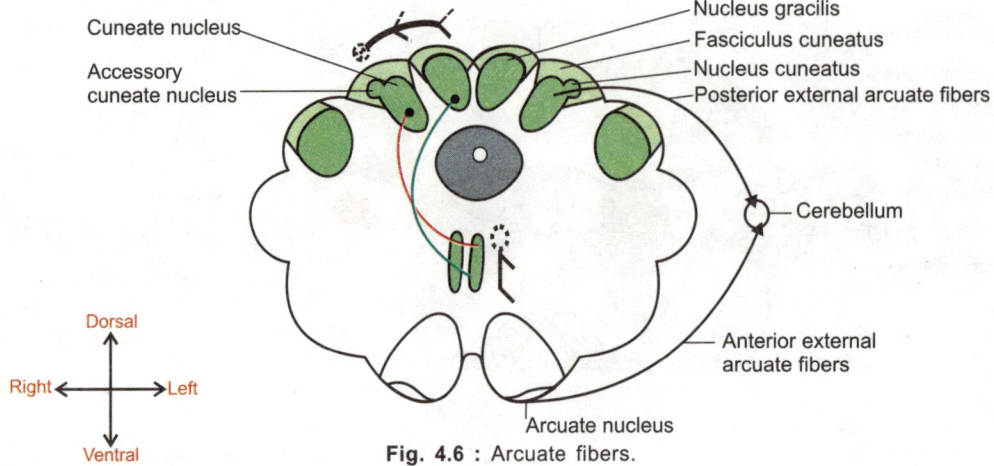

Fig. 4.6 : Arcuate fibers.

LAQ-4   **Draw and label a transverse section of medulla oblongata at the level of sensory decussation**

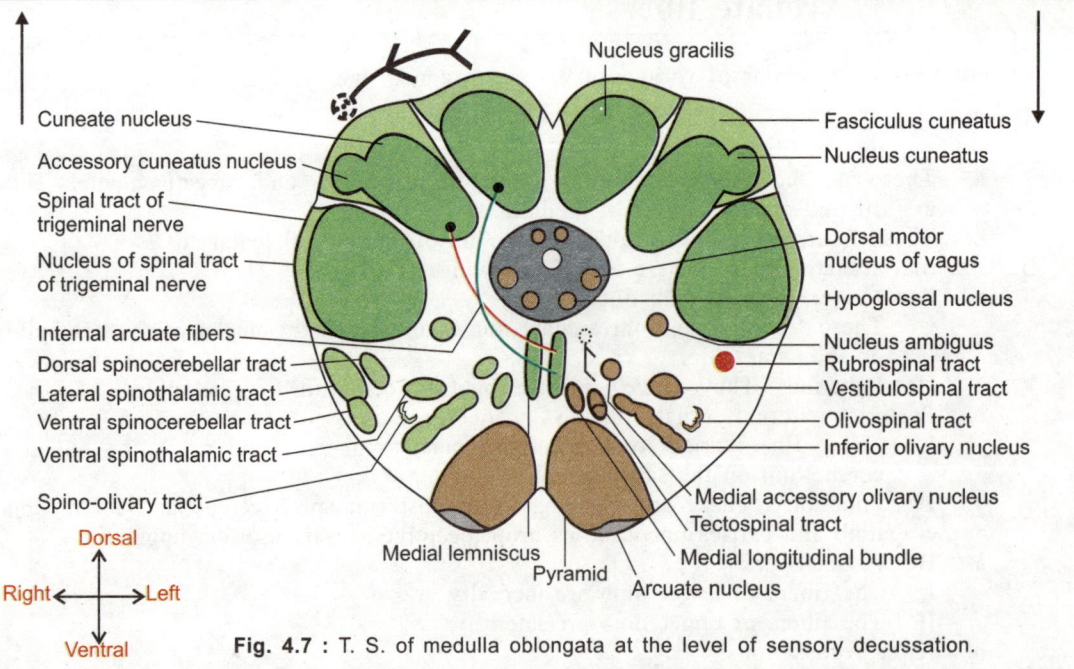

Fig. 4.7 : T. S. of medulla oblongata at the level of sensory decussation.

SN-5 Medial lemniscus

1. **Introduction** : It is a bigger bundle of the axons, which arises from gracile and cuneate nuclei. It consists of second order sensory neurons.

2. **Course** : Their axons run ventrally and medially as internal arcuate fibers to cross the mid line. The crossing fibers of the two sides constitute the sensory decussation.

3. **Formation** : It is formed by
   A. The fibers of the second order neurons of posterior column and
   B. The fibers of the anterior spinothalamic tract.

4. **Location** : It is formed in the middle of the medulla oblongata.

5. **Representation** :
   A. Somatotopic representation :
      a. Before formation of medial lemniscus :
         I. The fibers of the lower limb are placed medially.
         II. The fibers of the upper limb are placed laterally.
      b. After formation of medial lemniscus :
         I. The fibers of the lower limb are placed anteriorly.
         II. The fibers of the upper limb are placed posteriorly.

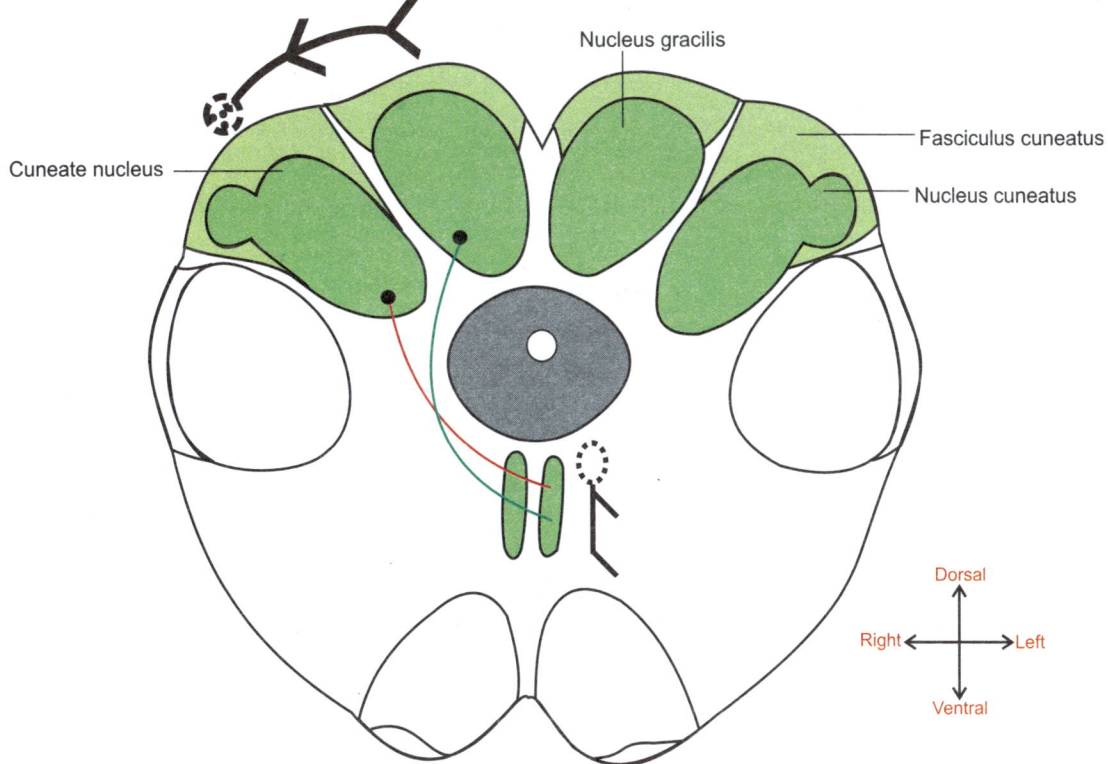

Fig. 4.8 : Formation of medial lemniscus.

B. Modality representation : The fibers arranged from dorsal to ventral in the posterior
    column are as follows :   ⚷━   **P Vi MP**
    a. **P**ressure.
    b. **V**ibration.
    c. **M**ovement.
    d. **P**osition.
    e. **T**ouch.
        I.   Tactile localization
        II.   Tactile discrimination
        III. Sterognosis

6. **Position of medial lemniscus at different levels :**
    A. In the upper part of medulla oblongata : Most medially and dorsally.
    B. In the pons : Tegmental part of pons.
    C. Midbrain : Tegmental part of the midbrain.
    D. Thalamus : **V**entro**p**osterio-**l**ateral nucleus of thalamus   ⚷━   **VPL**.

7. **Applied anatomy :**
    A. Lesion before formation of medial lemniscus : Loss of conscious proprioceptive
        sensations on the same side.
    B. Lesion after formation of medial lemniscus : Loss of conscious proprioceptive
        sensations of the opposite side.

SN-6   Medial longitudinal bundle (fasciculus)

1. **Introduction** : It is vertical running bundle of axons, present in the midline of
    brainstem.

2. **Extent :** It extends from upper border of midbrain to the upper cervical part of spinal
    cord.

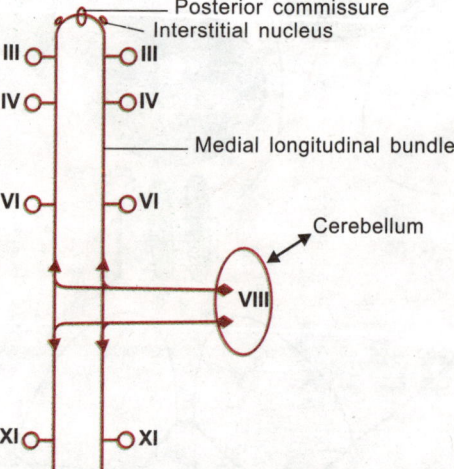

Fig. 4.9 : Fibers forming the medial longitudinal bundle.

3. **Formation :** It connects the nuclei of the following cranial nerves :
    A. Vestibular - VIII th cranial nerve.
    B. Oculomotor - III rd cranial nerve.
    C. Trochlear - IV th cranial nerve.
    D. Abducent - VI th cranial nerve.
    E. Spinal accessory - XI th cranial nerve.
    F. Reticular nuclei.

4. **Functions :**
    A. Coordination of conjugate movements of eyeball.
    B. The movements of head and neck in response to audio and visual reflexes.

5. **Location :** Just in front of (central canal/aqueduct of 4th ventricle) cavity.

LAQ-5 **Draw and label a transverse section of medulla oblongata at the level of inferior olivary nucleus or pontomedullary junction.**

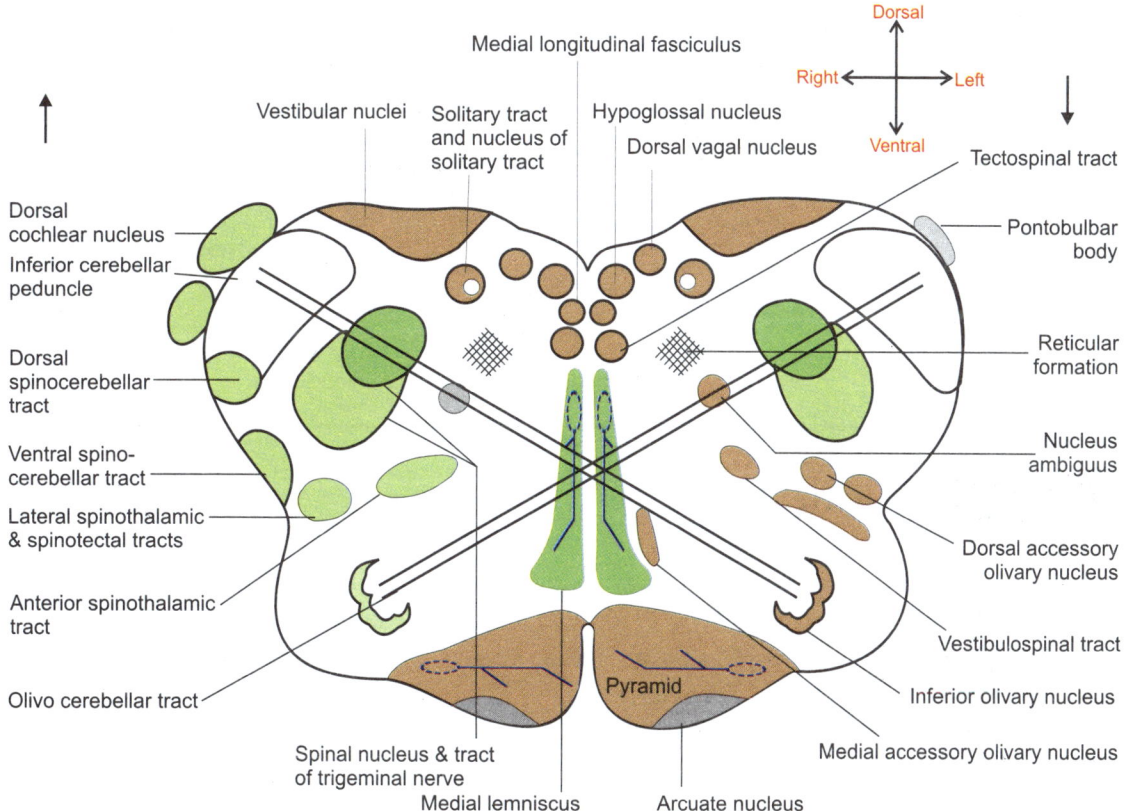

Fig. 4.10 : T. S. of medulla oblongata at the level of inferior olivary nucleus or pontomedullary junction.

LAQ-6 Draw and label a transverse section of pons at the level of facial colliculus

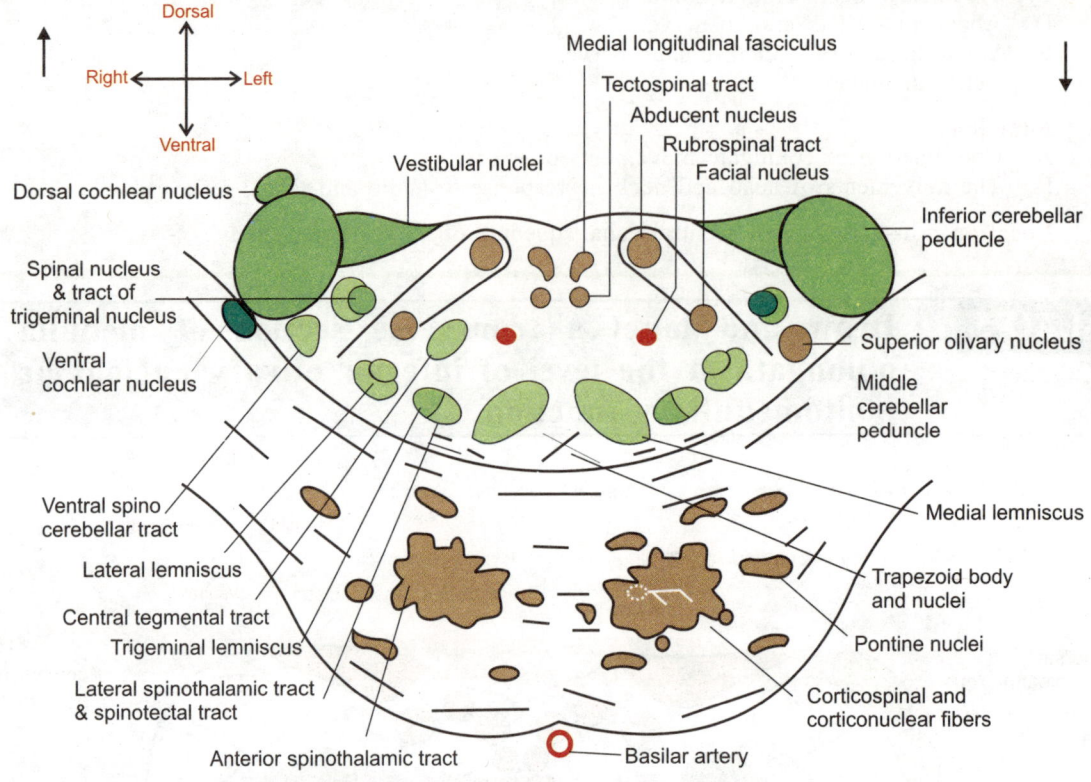

Fig. 4.11 : T. S. of pons at the level of facial colliculus.

SAQ-1 Stria medullaris

1. **Introduction :** These are transversely running glistening white fibers present in the floor of fourth ventricle.

2. **Origin :** They arise from arcuate nuclei present on the ventral surface of medulla oblongata.

3. **Course :** They run medial to medial lemniscus, traverse through the substance of medulla oblongata. They emerge from the medial sulcus and run transversely into the inferior peduncle. They terminate into dented nucleus of cerebellum. They divide the floor of fourth ventricle into upper and lower region.

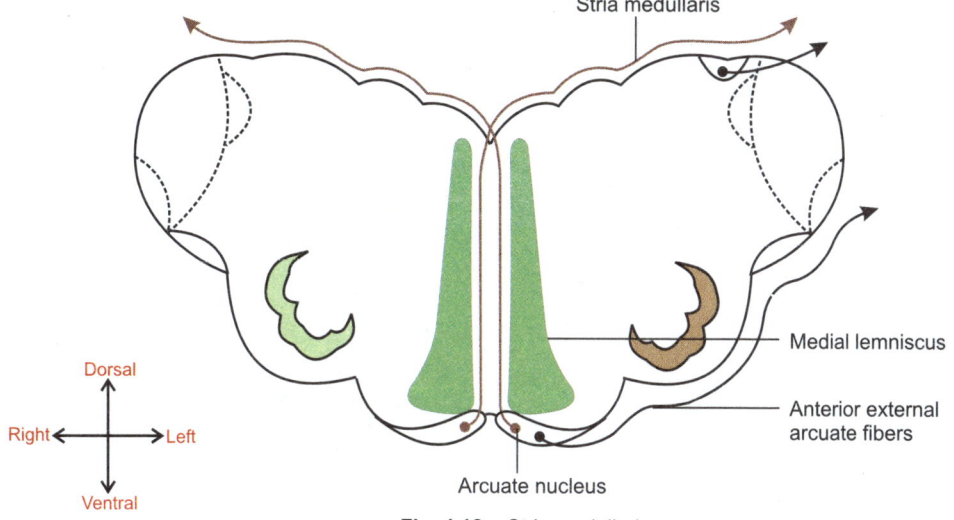

Fig. 4.12 : Stria medullaris.

Draw and label a transverse section at upper level of pons.

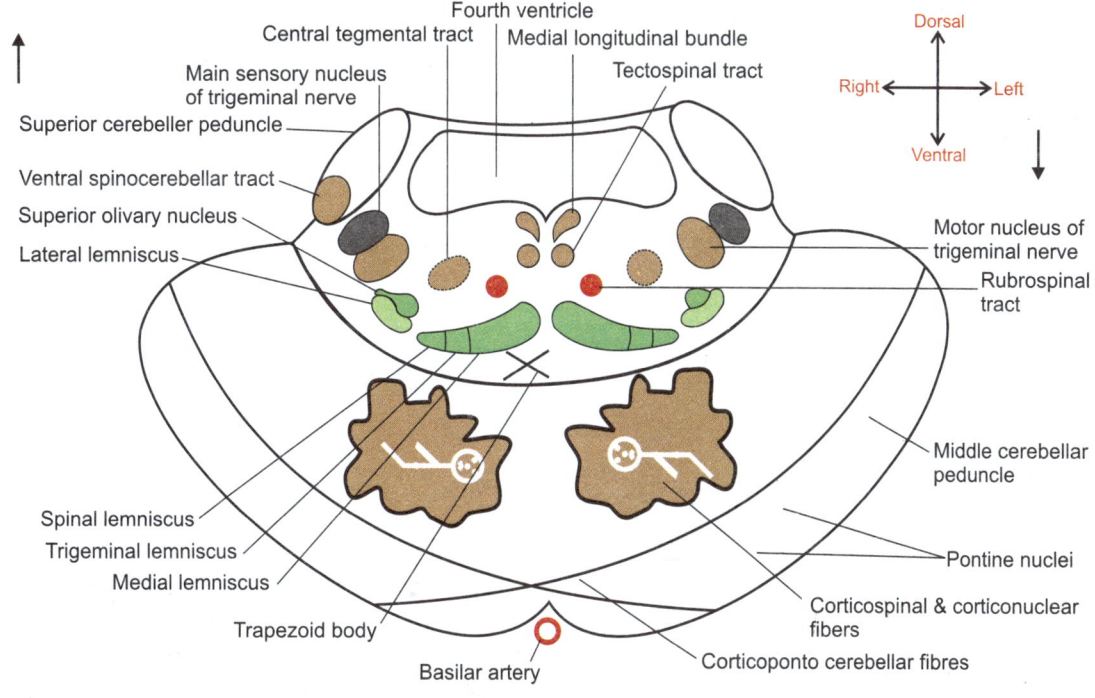

Fig. 4.13 : T. S. at upper level of pons.

LAQ-8 : Draw and label a transverse section of midbrain at the level of inferior colliculus.

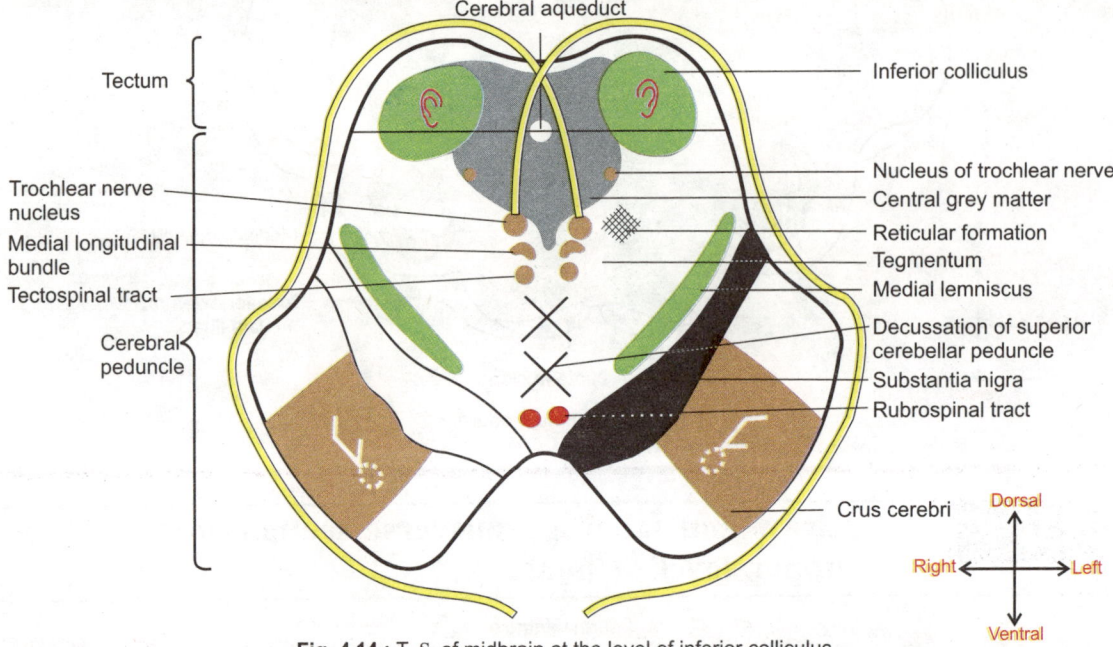

Fig. 4.14 : T. S. of midbrain at the level of inferior colliculus.

SAQ-2 : Trapezoid body

1. **Introduction :** It is a transverse band of fibers lying just behind the ventral part of pons.

2. **Formation :** It is formed by the fibers that arise in the cochlear nuclei of both the sides. Most of the axons arising in these nuclei cross to the opposite side (in the trapezoid body) and terminate in the superior olivary nucleus. Many fibers end in the nucleus of trapezoid body.

3. **Situation :** In mid line of the tegmental part of pons. Most of the fibers of the trapezoid body ascend upward as the lateral lemniscus.

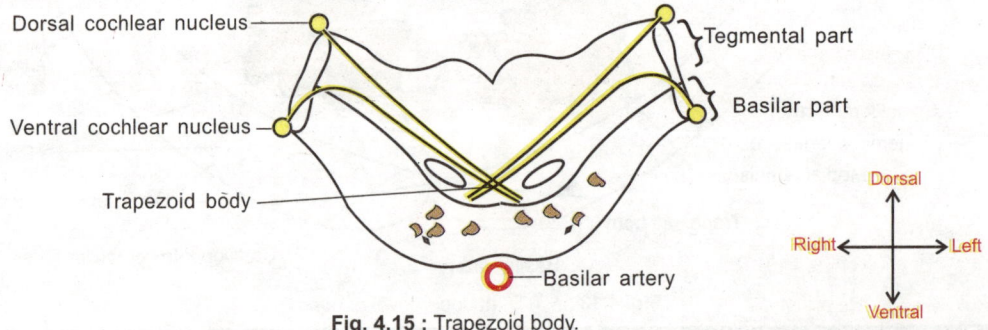

Fig. 4.15 : Trapezoid body.

SN-7   Crus cerebri (*crus* - leg, *cerebri* - cerebrum)

1. **Introduction :** It is a white matter present on ventral part of cerebral peduncle. It contains all descending tracts.

2. **Relations :**
   A. Medially it is related to interpeduncular fossa which contains
      a. Oculomotor nerve at the level of superior colliculus.
      b. Posterior cerebral artery (terminal branch of basilar artery).
   B. Laterally is trochlear nerve at the level of inferior colliculus.
   C. Posteriorly is substantia nigra.

3. **Divisions :** It is divided into three parts.
   A. Medial one sixth : It contains frontopontine fibers.

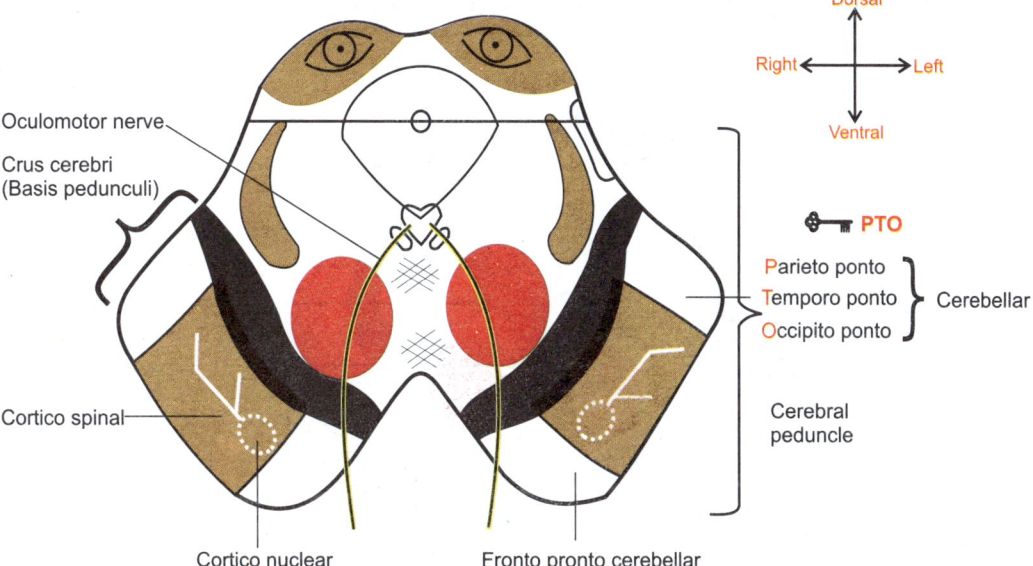

Fig. 4.16 : Crus cerebri.

   B. Middle two third : It contains
      a. Corticonuclear fibers going to different motor nuclei of cranial nerves.
      b. Corticospinal fibers : The fibers of the leg are placed laterally and   l for l
         the fibers of the upper limb are placed medially.
   C. Lateral one sixth : It contains
      a. Parietopontine.
      b. Temporopontine.
      c. Occipitopontine.

4. **Blood supply :** Short circumferential artery, a branch of posterior cerebral artery.

5. **Applied Anatomy :**
   Weber's syndrome : A lesion in the midbrain causes contralateral hemiplegia and ipsilateral paralysis of the muscles of the eyeball. This condition is known as Weber's syndrome. It includes
   A. Upper motor neuron lesion of cortico spinal tract.

B. Lower motor neuron lesion of third nerve and fourth nerve.

C. It results into : Contralateral hemiplegia with ipsilateral paralysis of muscles of eyeball.

D. Lesion of oculomotor nerve produces :
   a. Ptosis (pseudoptosis of eyelid).
   b. Strabismus : Squint due to unopposed action of lateral rectus.
   c. Loss of light & accommodation reflex due to involvement of ciliaris muscle & sphincter pupillae.
   d. Lesion of corticospinal tract produces increased deep reflex & loss of superficial reflex.

LAQ-9 **Draw and label a transverse section of midbrain at the level of superior colliculus.**

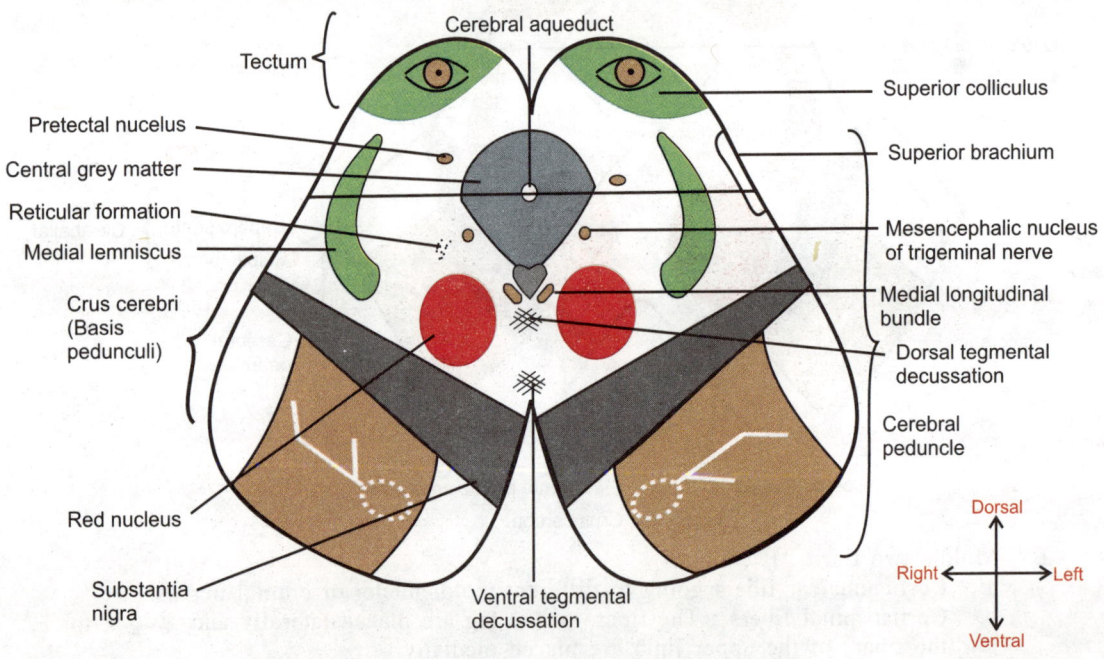

Fig. 4.17 : T. S. of midbrain at the level of superior colliculus.

SN-8 **Substantia nigra (*Substantia* substance + *nigra* black coloured)**

1. **Introduction :** It is a blackish area, present in the cerebral peduncle between tegmentum and crus cerebri.

2. **Shape :** It is broader on medial side.

3.   Parts : **Table 4.2 :** Table shows parts of substantia nigra.

Particular	Ventral part	Dorsal part
1. Synonym	Pars reticularis	Pars compacta
2. Neuron	Few, large and multipolar	More, smaller and multipolar
3. Type of fibres	Majority are GABA and some are dopaminergic	Medium sized dopaminergic and cholinergic neurons
4. Pigment	Iron and little melanin pigment	Deeply pigmented neuromelanin granules
5. Structure	Structurally it resembles globus pallidus of basal ganglion	----
6. Connections	Pallidonigral Corticonigral	Pallidonigral Nigrostriate

4.   Applied : Parkinsonism is a degenerative disease of substantia nigra.
It is characterised by
A.   Rigidity and tremor.
B.   Rigidity is due to increased muscle tone with normal deep reflexes.

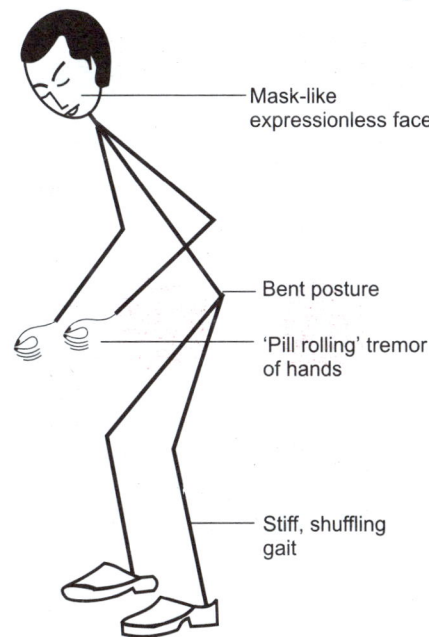

Mask-like
expressionless face

Bent posture

'Pill rolling' tremor
of hands

Stiff, shuffling
gait

Fig. 4.18 : Characteristic features of Parkinson's disease.

C. Rigidity of parkinsonism affects all muscles with poor movements. The patient possesses masked face (appearance with no emotional response), walks with short, quick steps and experiences difficulty in taking initial steps and terminating the movements.

D. Tremor occurs with regular frequency when the subject is at rest.

5. **Treatment :** Administration of L - dopa in low quantity diminishes rigidity and in high doses reduces tremor.

6. **Connections :**
    A. Afferent : Strionigral.
    B. Efferent : Nigrostriate fibres are dopaminergic.

SN-9   Tectum of midbrain / colliculi / corpora quadrigemina

1. **Introduction :** The tectum is the part of midbrain, posterior to the horizontal line passing through the cerebral aqueduct. It consists of the two pairs of rounded elevations called as corpora quadrigemina.

2. **Relations :**
    A. Rostral : Pineal gland,
    B. Caudal : Superior medullary velum,
    C. Behind : Splenium of corpus callosum and
    D. Overlapped on each side : Pulvinar of the thalamus.

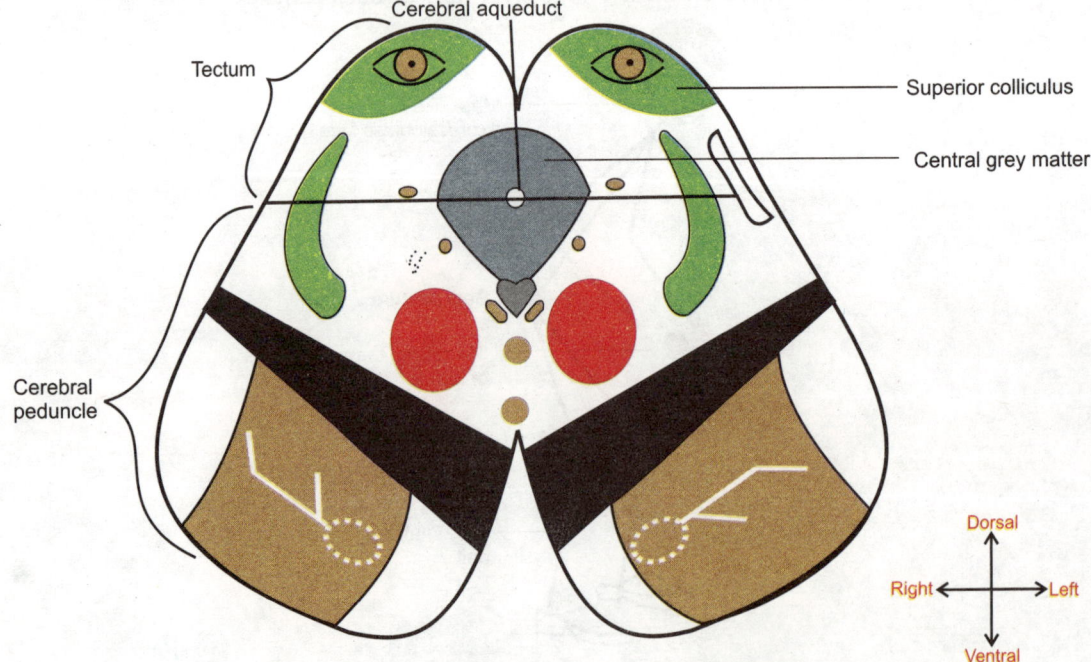

Fig. 4.19 : Tectum of midbrain / colliculi / corpora quadrigemina

3. **Divisions :** It consists of
   A. Superior colliculi,
   B. Inferior colliculi.

4. **Connection :**
   A. Superior colliculus.
      a. Afferents
         I. Retina via optic tract.
         II. Visual cortex via optic radiation and superior brachium.
         III. Spinal cord via spinotectal tract.
         IV. Inferior colliculus of the same side.
         V. Lateral geniculate body.
      b. Efferents
         I. Motor nuclei of IIIrd, IVth, VIth, VIIth and XIth cranial nerve nuclei via tectobulbar tract.
         II. Motor cells of spinal cord via tectospinal tract.
         III. Nuclei of the extra pyramidal system.
         IV. Superior colliculus of the opposite side.
         V. Lateral geniculate body.
   B. Inferior colliculus.
      a. Afferents : Lateral lemniscus.
      b. Efferents
         I. Medial geniculate body of the same side via inferior brachium.
         II. Superior colliculus of the same side.
         III. Cerebellum through tectocerebellar fibers.

5. **Functions :**
   A. Superior colliculus is the center for visual reflexes. Because of its connections with various nuclei it acts as an important integrating sensory center.
   B. Inferior colliculus is associated with
      a. Auditory pathway.
      b. Auditory reflexes.
      c. Audio visual reflexes.

SN-10   Pretectal nucleus

1. **Introduction :** It is small group of cells which lies deep to the upper and lateral part of the superior colliculus and extends slightly upwards beyond its limits.

2. **Connections :**
   A. Afferent fibers from
      a. Retina (via optic tract and superior brachium).
      b. Visual cortex (via optic radiation and superior brachium).
   B. Efferent fibers to
      a. Edinger Westphal nucleus (parasympathetic nucleus of the IIIrd cranial nerve) of the same and opposite side.
      b. Tectospinal and tectobulbar tracts.

3. **Function :** Pretectal nucleus from part of a reflex pathway for the pupillary response to light (light reflex).

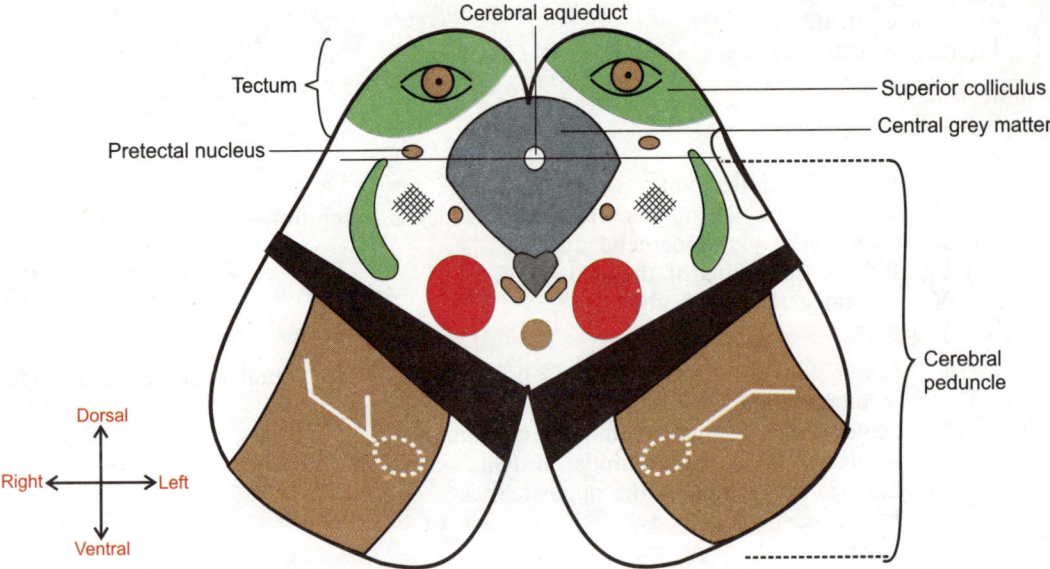

Fig. 4.20 : Pretectal nucleus

SN-11   Red nucleus

1. **Introduction :** It is a collection of pinkish cell bodies, present in the midbrain at the level of superior colliculus, which is one of the important relay station, for extra pyramidal system.

2. **Gross anatomy :**
   A. Number : One on each side.

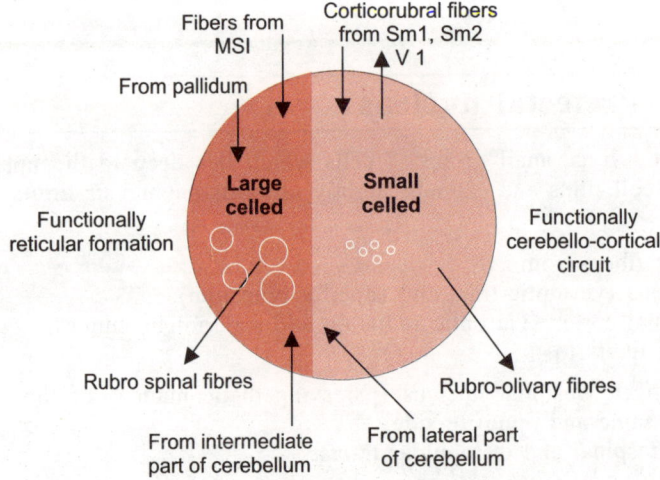

Fig. 4.21 : Divisions of red nucleus.

B. Capsule : Formed by white matter i.e. fibers of superior cerebellar peduncle.
C. Colour : Pinkish in fresh specimen because of iron content.
D. Dimension : 1 x 0.5 cm.
E. Extent : From subthalamic nucleus to lower part of superior colliculus.
F. Situation : Tegmentum of midbrain (dorsal part of cerebral peduncle).
G. Shape : Oval.

3. **Relations** :
   A. Dorsally : Peri aqueductal grey matter.
   B. Ventrally : Substantia nigra.

4. **Parts :**

Table 4.3 : The table shows divisions of red nucleus.

Particulars	Cranial	Caudal
Cell - Type	Parvocellular	Magnocellular
Neuron	Small	Large, multi polar
Origin	Recent	Old

5. **Connections :**
   A. Afferents.

Table 4.4 : The table shows afferent connections of the red nucleus.

Fibres	Origin	Destination
a. Cortico rubral	Motor area 4 & 6	Entire red nucleus.
b. Pallido - rubral	Globus pallidus Corpus striatum	Red nucleus.
c. Tectorubral	Tectal nucleus of superior colliculus	Red nucleus.
d. Cerebello rubral	Dentate nucleus Globose nucleus	Parvocellular.
	Emboliform nucleus	Magnocellular.

Table 4.5 : The table shows efferent connections of the red nucleus.

Fibers	Origin	Destination
a. Rubrothalamic	Red nucleus	Ventral nucleus of thalamus
b. Rubrobulbar	Caudal 3/4 of red nucleus	Motor nucleus of trigeminal (V), Facial (VII) nerve
c. Rubro-olivary	Caudal 3/4 of red nucleus	Inferior olivary nucleus
d. Rubrospinal	Caudal 3/4 of red nucleus	Dorsomedial thoracic nucleus Intermediate thoracic nucleus Ventrolateral lumbosacral nucleus

6. **Functions** :
   A. Monitors cerebellar functions.
   B. Influence lower motor neuron for facilitating flexor muscle of limbs. } Extra pyramidal function

7. **Applied** :
   A. Weber's syndrome :
      a. Upper motor neuron lesion of corticospinal tract leading to contralateral hemiplegia and
      b. Lower motor neuron lesion of oculomotor nerve leading to paralysis of muscles of eyeball of the same side.
   B. Benedikt's syndrome :
      Lesion of tegmental part of midbrain affects -

Table 4.6 : The table shows clinical manifestations of the midbrain at the level of red nucleus.

a. Oculomotor nerve	Ipsilateral oculomotor palsy.
b. Red nucleus	Tremor, chorea and athetosis.
c. Medial lemniscus	Contralateral loss of touch, vibration and proprioceptive sensation.
d. Fibres of superior cerebellar peduncle	Ataxia and vertigo.

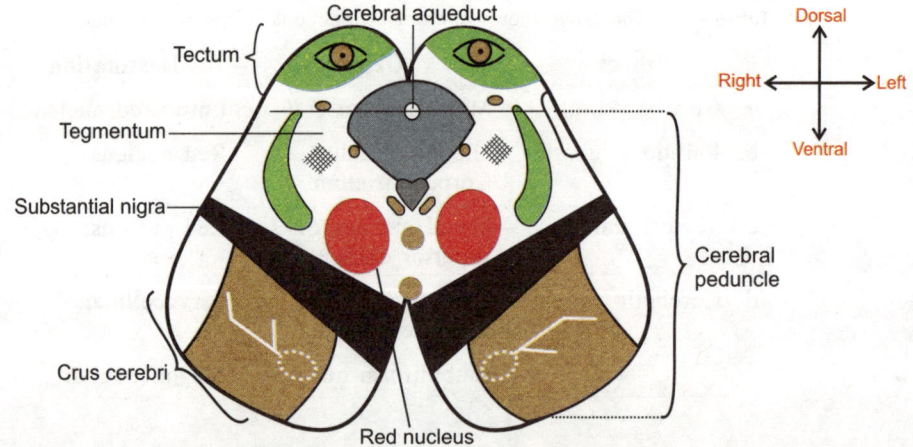

Fig. 4.22 : T. S. of midbrain at the level of red nucleus.

LAQ-10 | **Describe reticular formation under**
1. Gross anatomy   2. Connections   3. Functions
4. Applied anatomy

1. **Gross anatomy** :
   A. Definition : It is a network of small cells with fibres of ascending, descending, crossed, transverse and uncrossed mixed with numerous poorly defined nuclei.
   B. Evolution : Phylogenetically it is the oldest part.

C. Location : It is present mainly in the deep and dorsal part of brainstem. It can be traced cranially to the brain and caudally to the spinal cord.

2. **Connections :** It has afferent and efferent connections
   A. Afferent :
      a. Spinoreticular
      b. Cerebelloreticular
      c. Vestibuloreticular
      d. Thalamoreticular (from thalamus, subthalamus and hypothalamus.)
      e. Strioreticular
      f. Septoreticular
   A. Efferent : 🔑 **BMC**
      a. Brainstem
         I. Reticulo bulbar
         II. Reticulo spinal
      b. Midbrain
         Reticulo mesencephalic (to red nucleus and tectum of midbrain)
      c. Cerebral cortex
         I. Reticulocortical
         II. Reticulostriate
         III. Reticulothalamic

3. **Functions :**
   It is the ascending activating system responsible for alertness and awareness which boosters the activities. It can be summarized as
   🔑 Somatomotor
      Somatosensory
      Visceromotor
      Neuroendocrinal
      Alertness
      Awareness
      Consciousness
      Reward and
      Award

   A. Somatomotor : Certain areas of reticular formation inhibit voluntary and reflex activities of the body and some areas facilitate them.
   B. Somatosensory : It has connections with sensory tracts with number of collaterals.
   C. Visceromotor : It influences respiratory and vasomotor activities.
   D. Neuroendocrinal : It takes part in the neuroendocrinal reegulations and the development of conditioned and learned reflexes.
   E. Alertness : It is responsible for maintaining the state of alertness through its collaterals.
   F. Awareness : It maintains the state of wakefulness.
   G. Consciousness : It maintains mental consciousness, attention, sleep and waking.
   H. Reward.
   I. Award.

4. **Applied anatomy :**
   A. Reticular system is affected in brainstem injury and results in loss of consciousness or interference in arousal mechanism.

B. Disorders of reticular system manifests as
    a.   Narcolepsy : It is recurrent, uncontrollable, brief episodes of sleep.
    b.   Cataplexy : A condition in which there are abrupt attacks of muscular weakness and hypotonia triggered by an emotional stimulus such as anger, fear or surprise.

SN-12   Archicerebellum

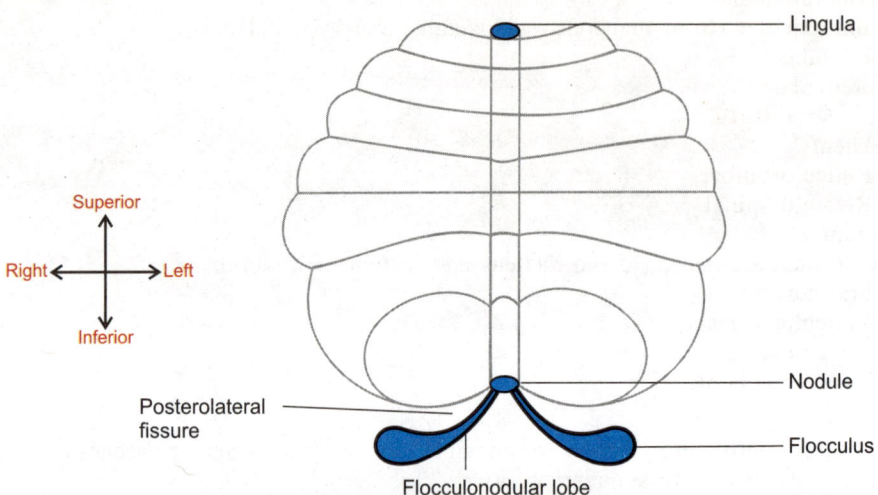

Fig. 4.23 : Parts of the archicerebellum

1. **Evolution :** It is the oldest part of cerebellum.

2. **Parts :**
    A. Parts of vermis
        a.   Lingula and
        b.   Nodule.
    B. Part of hemisphere : Flocculus, sometime paraflocculus.

3. **Nucleus :** Fastigii

4. **Connections :**
    A. Afferent : Vestibulo cerebellar.
    B. Efferent : Cerebellar vestibular.

5. **Functions :** It controls the axial musculature and the bilateral movements used for locomotion and maintenance of equilibrium.

6. **Applied anatomy :** Lesion of the archi cerebellum is called archi cerebellar syndrome.
It is affected by tumor, medullo blastoma, particularly in childhood.
It is characterized by
    A. Failure of maintenance of equilibrium.
    B. Failure to walk on a normal base.
    C. Unable to maintain the upright posture.

7. **Morphology :** Archi cerebellum is separated by rest of the cerebellum by posterolateral fissure. This is the first developed part of the cerebellum.

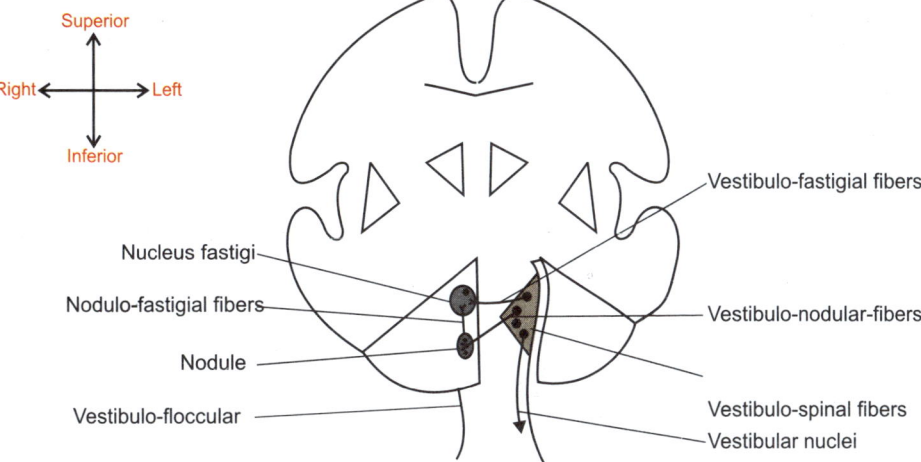

Fig. 4.24 : Afferent and efferent connections of archicerebellum.

| SN-13 | Paleocerebellum |

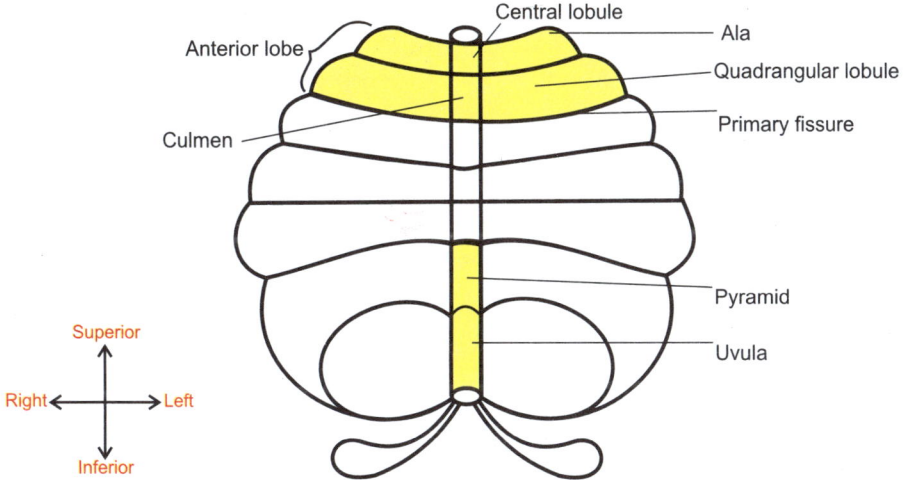

Fig. 4.25 : Parts of the paleocerebellum.

1. **Evolution :** It is the older part of cerebellum, evolved next to archicerebellum.

2. **Parts :** 🔑 **Anterior lobe + UP**

   A. Parts of vermis
      a. Central lobule.
      b. Culmen.
      c. Pyramid.
      d. Uvula.

B.   Parts of hemisphere :
    a.   Ala.
    b.   Quadrangular lobule.

3.   Nucleus interpositus which consists of
    A.   Globose nucleus.
    B.   Emboliform nucleus.

4.   **Connections :**
    A.   Afferents :
        a.   Anterior spino cerebellar.
        b.   Posterior spino cerebellar.
        c.   Cuneo cerebellar.
        d.   Par olivo cerebellar.
        e.   Reticulo cerebellar.
    B.   Efferents : Cerebello spinal.

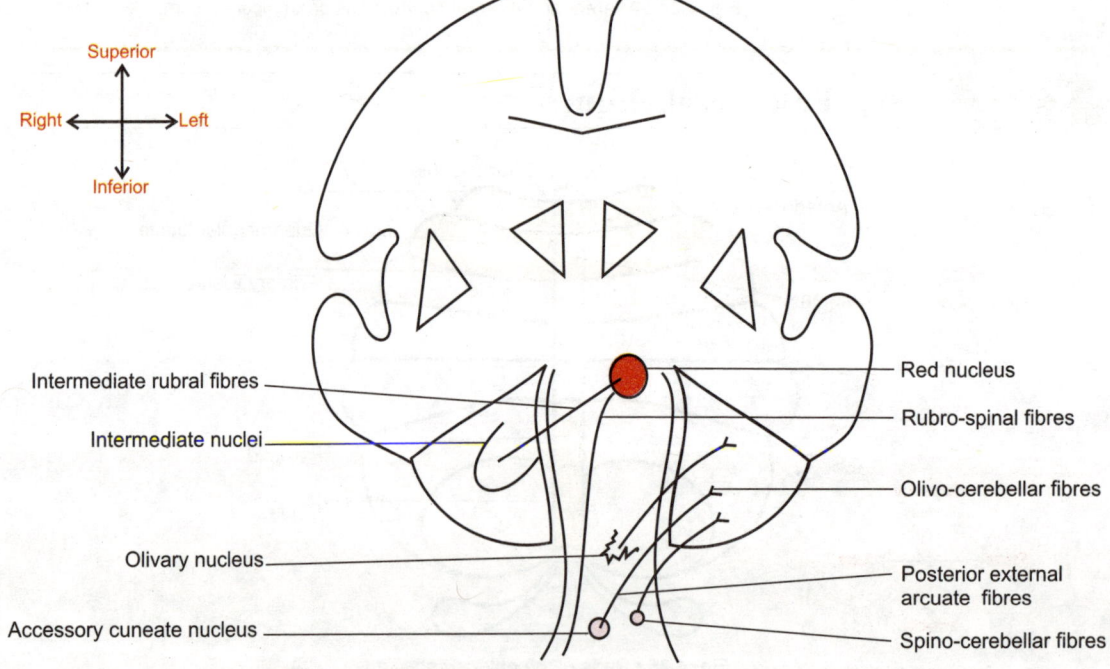

Fig. 4.26 : Afferent and efferent connections of paleocerebellum.

5.   **Functions :** It has a significant role in muscle tone and posture of the limbs.

6.   **Applied anatomy :**
Lesion of the paleocerebellum is due to excessive intake of alcohol or in malnutrition. It is characterized by
Alteration of gait. Individual movements of legs are much affected with increase in tone of extensor group of the muscle.

SN-14 Neocerebellum

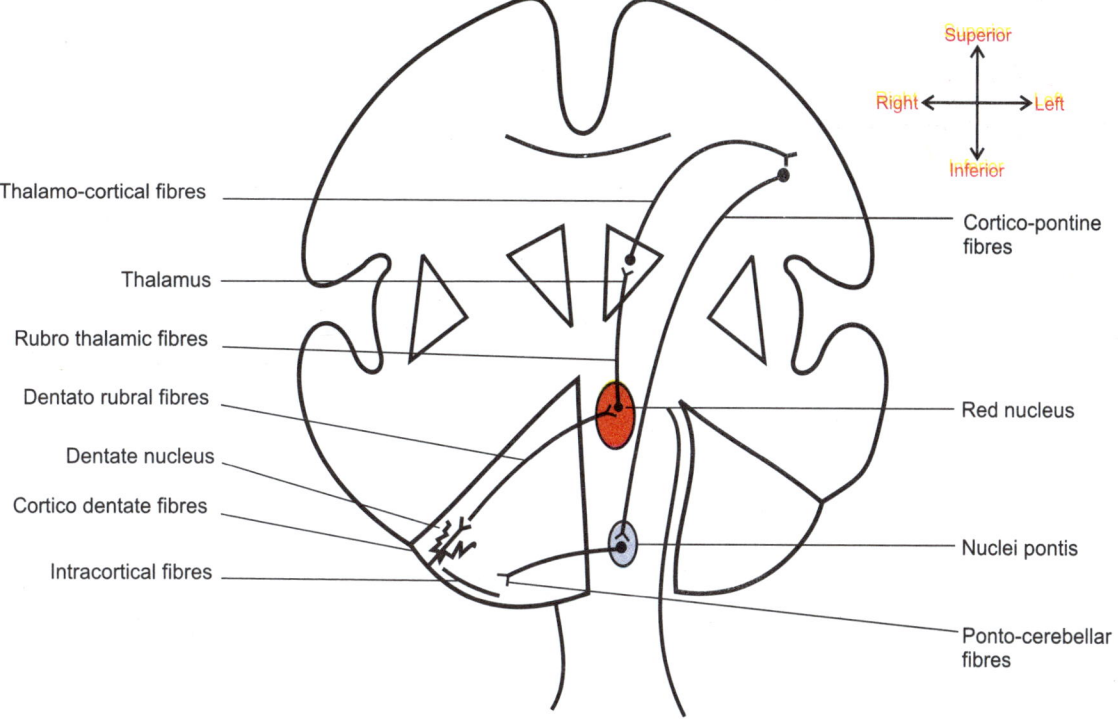

Thalamo-cortical fibres

Thalamus

Rubro thalamic fibres

Dentato rubral fibres

Dentate nucleus

Cortico dentate fibres

Intracortical fibres

Superior

Right ← → Left

Inferior

Cortico-pontine fibres

Red nucleus

Nuclei pontis

Ponto-cerebellar fibres

Fig. 4.27 : Afferent and efferent connections of neocerebellum.

1. **Evolution :** It is most recently developed during evolution.

2. **Parts :** 🔑 **Middle lobe - UP** (i.e. Uvula and pyramid)
   A. Parts of vermis
      a. Declive
      b. Folium
      c. Tuber
   B. Parts of hemisphere :
      a. Simple lobule.
      b. Superior semilunar lobule.
      c. Inferior semilunar lobule.
      d. Tonsil.

3. **Nucleus :** Dentate nucleus.

4. **Connections :**
   A. Afferent :
      a. Cortico ponto cerebellar.
      b. Anterior external arcuate fibers.
      c. Stria medullaris.
      d. Olivo cerebellar.

      e.   Trigemino cerebellar.

B. Efferent :

      a.   Dentato rubro thalamo cortical.

      b.   Dentato rubro spinal.

5.   Functions : It is primarily concerned with the regulation of fine movements of the body.

6.   Applied anatomy :

Lesion of the neo cerebellum is called neo cerebellar syndrome. It is characterized by

A. Hypotonia : Diminished muscle tone.

B. Asynergia : Loss of muscular coordination.

      a.   Ataxia : Loss of coordination of muscles of trunk, pectoral and pelvic girdle.

      b.   Dysmetria : Loss of ability to measure the distance for reaching an intended goal.

      c.   Decomposition of movements : Loss of coordination of series of movement.

      d.   Dysdiadochokinesis : Loss of ability to execute alternate movements in rapid succession, such as pronation and supination of forearm.

      e.   Dysarthria or scanning speech : Loss of coordination of muscles concerned with speech. The speech is slurred, prolonged and explosive.

      f.   Nystagmus : Involuntary, rhythmical and oscillatory movements of the eyeball.

C. Intensional tremor is evident during purposeful movements and is diminished or absent with rest.

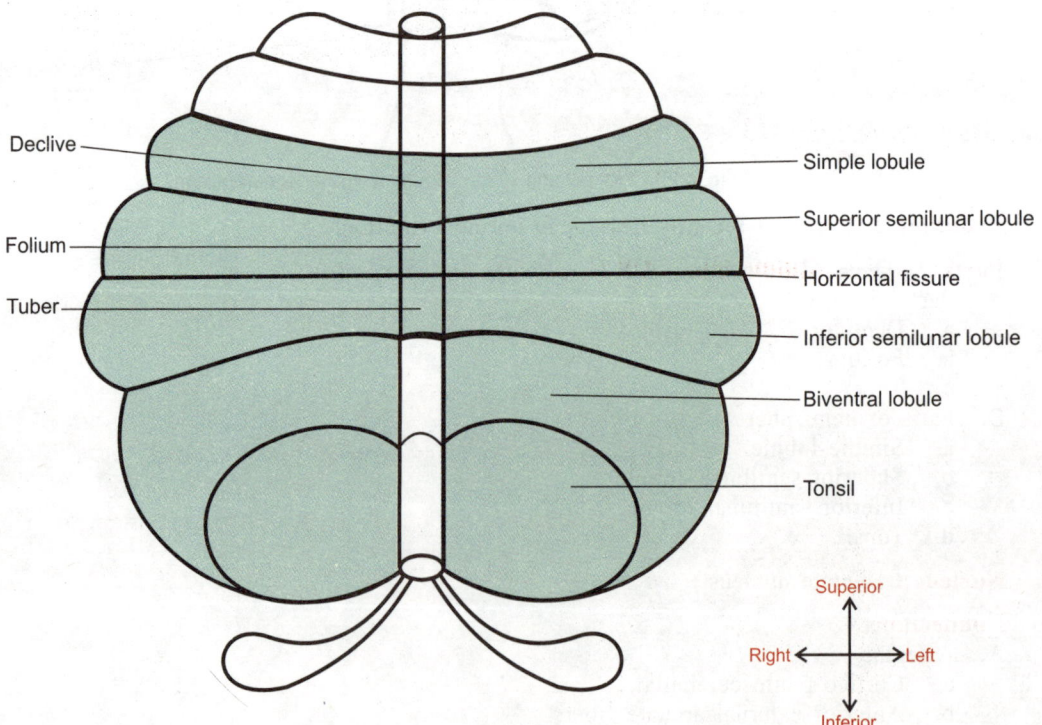

Fig. 4.28 : Parts of neocerebellum.

SN-15   Inferior cerebellar peduncle

1. **Introduction :** This is the largest collection of white fibers which connect the cerebellum to medulla.

2. **Fibers :**
   A. Afferent fibres

Table 4.7 : The table shows afferent connections passing through Inferior cerebellar peduncle

Fibres	Origin	Destination	Nucleus	Crossing	Function
a. Vestibulo cerebellar	Medial and inferior vestibular nuclei	Archice-rebellum	Fastigius	-----	Sensation from ampullary crest of semicircular ducts.
b. Posterior spino cerebellar	Thoracic nucleus of spinal cord (Clarkes column)	Paleocereb-ellum	Inter positus	-----	Position of individual muscle of lower limb.
c. Cuneocerebellar [posterior external arcuate fibres]	Accessory cuneate nucleus at lower medulla	Paleocer ebellum	Inter positus	-----	Position of individual muscle of upper limb.
d. Anterior external arcuate fibres	Arcuate nuclei of both sides	Neocere bellum	Dentate	-----	Information to cerebellum.
e. Striamedullaris	Arcuate nucleus	Neocere bellum	Dentate	Yes	Information to cerebellum.
f. Olivo-cerebellar	Inferior olivary nucleus of medulla	Neocere bellum	Dentate	Yes	-----------
g. Par-olivocerebellar	Medial and dorsal accessory olivary nuclei	Paleocer ebellum	Inter positus	Yes	-----------
h. Trigeminocerebellar	Spinal nucleus of trigeminal nucleus	Paleo	Dentate	-----	Unconscious proprio- ception of TM joint.
I. Reticulo cerebellar	Lateral reticular and paramedian nucleus of medulla	Paleocer ebellum	Inter positus	Yes	-----------

B.   Efferent fibers are

Table 4.8 : The table shows efferent connections passing through Inferior cerebellar peduncle.

Fibres	Origin	Destiny
a. Cerebello vestibular	Flocculo nodular lobe (same side) Fastigial nuclei of opposite side.	Vestibular nuclei.
b. Cerebello olivary	Middle lobe	Inferior olivary nucleus.
c. Cerebello reticular	Fastigial nucleus of both sides.	Medullary reticular fibers.

3. **Blood supply :**
   A. Superior cerebellar artery.
   B. Posterior inferior cerebellar artery (branch of vertebral artery).

4. **Applied :**
   A. A lesion causes loss of co-ordination and truncal ataxia.
   B. Lateral medullary syndrome.
   C. Medial medullary syndrome.

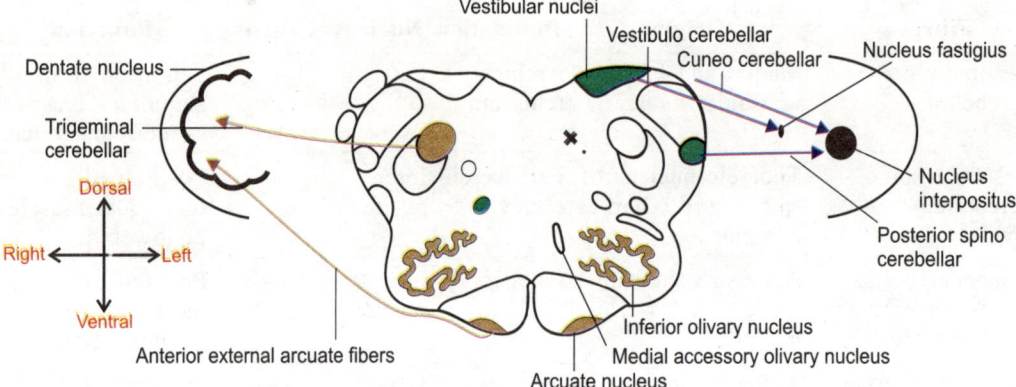

Fig. 4.29 : Afferent uncrossed fibers passing through inferior cerebellar peduncle

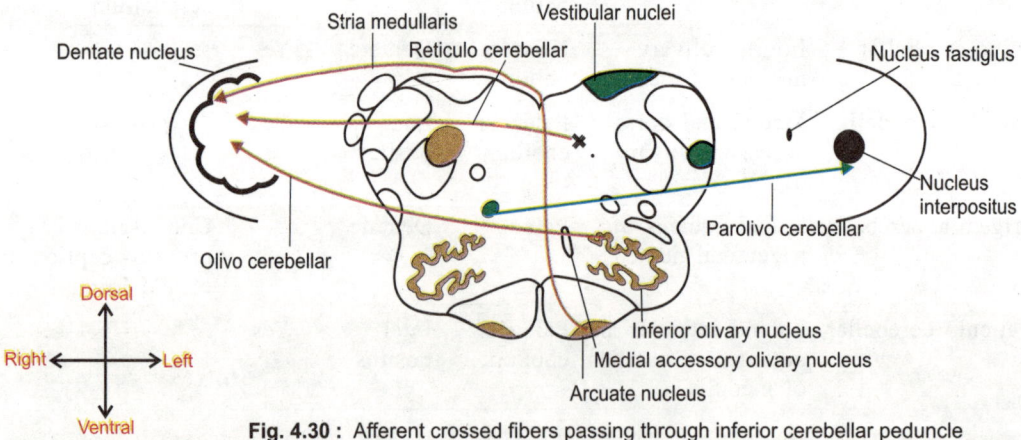

Fig. 4.30 : Afferent crossed fibers passing through inferior cerebellar peduncle

SN-16   Lateral medullary syndrome (Wallenberg's syndrome)

Lateral medullary syndrome : The lateral part of the medulla oblongata receives blood from posterior inferior cerebellar artery and occlusion of the vessel produces damage of the posterolateral part of the medulla.

     VC SC ST NT (*VC* verification committee for SC, ST and NT)

Table 4.9 : The table shows tracts and effects of the lesion.

Tracts	Effects
1. **V**estibulo **c**erebellar	Vertigo, vomiting and nystagmus on the side of lesion
2. **S**pino **c**erebellar	Ataxia of limbs (on the side of lesion).
3. **S**pino **t**halamic i.e. spinal lemniscus (lateral spinothalamic tract)	Contralateral loss of pain and temperature from upper and lower limbs.
4. **N**ucleus ambiguus	Paralysis of muscles of soft palate, pharynx, larynx on the side of lesion.
5. **T**rigemino thalamic tract (Spinal nucleus and its tract of trigeminal nerve)	Ipsilateral loss of pain and temperature from the face and forehead.

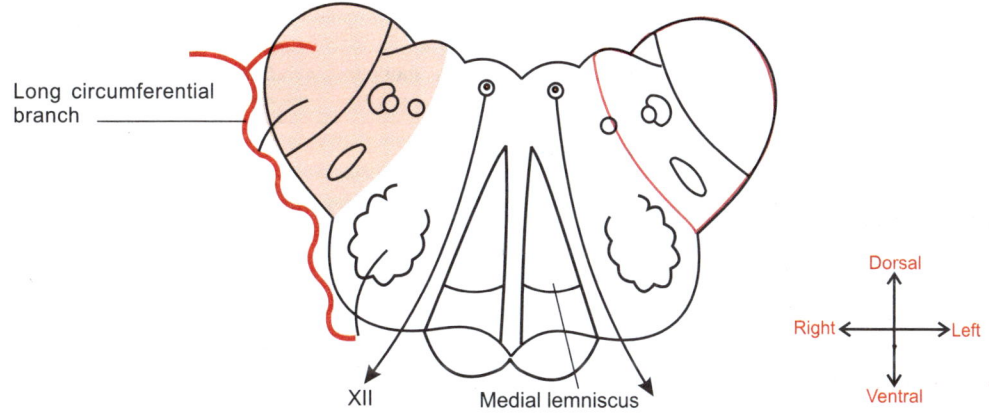

Fig. 4.31 : Lateral medullary syndrome.

SN-17	**Medial medullary syndrome**

Medial medullary syndrome : The medial part of the medulla oblongata receives blood from anterior spinal artery and its paramedian branches. The occlusion of the artery leads to medial medullary syndrome. ⚷ **HMC** (HM**C** Hindustan motor corporation)

Table 4.10 : The table shows tracts and effects of the lesion.

Tracts	Effects
a. Hypoglossal nerve nucleus	Wasting of the tongue muscles on the side of lesion
b. Medial lemniscus	Loss of sense of position of limbs on the opposite side of lesion
c. Cortico spinal tract	Hemiplegia on the contralateral side. The muscles of the face are unaffected.

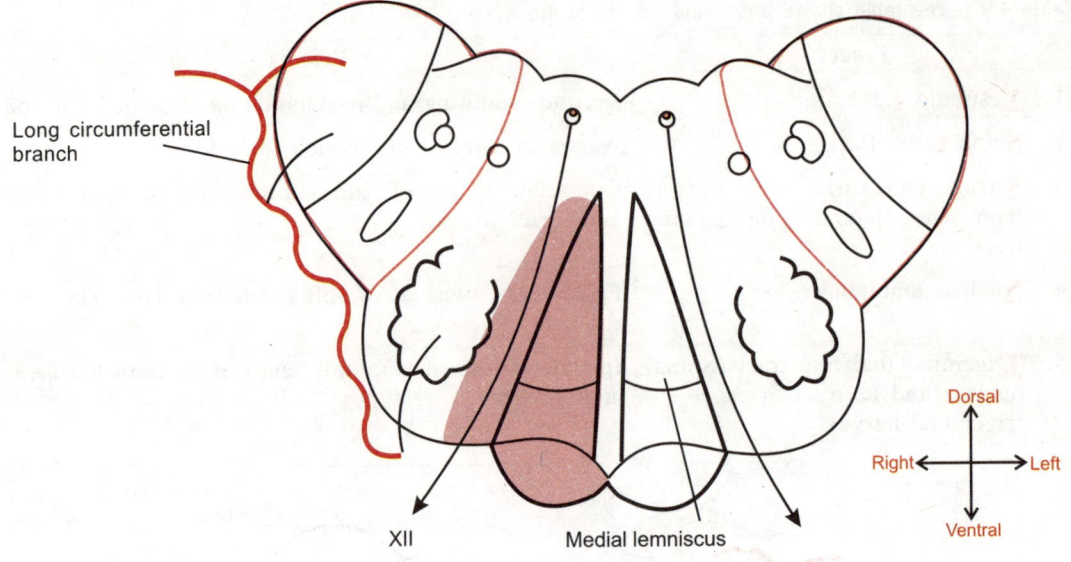

Fig. 4.32 : Medial medullary syndrome.

| SN-18 | **Dentate nucleus** |

1. **Introduction :**
   A. It is the chief and largest nucleus of cerebellum.
   B. It is situated in deep part of cerebellar hemisphere.
   C. It is present in white matter of cerebellum.
   D. It belongs to neocerebellum.

2. **Gross anatomy :**
   A. Location : It is located in the roof of fourth ventricle, just lateral to emboliform nucleus.
   B. Size : 3 - 4 cm.
   C. Shape : It gives appearance like a crumpled bag, the hilum directed medially. It resembles inferior olivary nucleus.

3. **Connections :**

Table 4.10 : The table shows afferent and efferent connections of dentate nucleus

Particular	Fibers	Origin	Destiny	Decussation
A. Afferent	a. Corticoponto cerebellar.	Cerebral cortex	Dentate nucleus	Yes
	b. Olivocerebellar.	Inferior olivary nucleus of medulla oblongata.		Yes
B. Efferent	a. Dentato rubro thalamo cortical tract.	Dentate nucleus	Cerebral cortex	Yes
	b. Dentato rubro spinal tract.	Dentate nucleus	Spinal cord	Yes

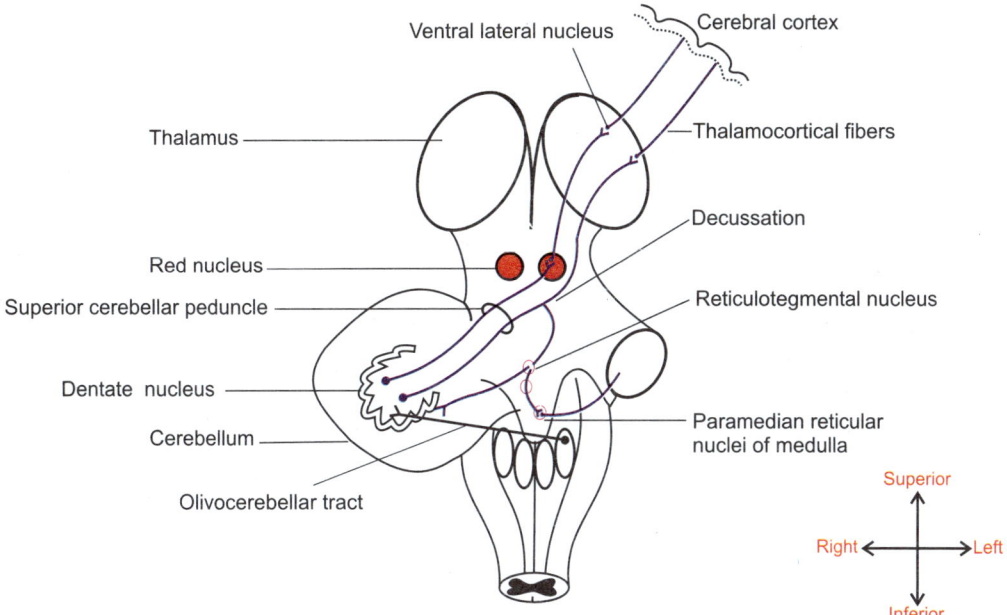

Fig. 4.33 : Afferent and efferent connections of dentate nucleus.

4. **Histology :**

A. It consists of large and multipolar neurons with branching dendrites.

B. The axons acquire myelin sheath within the nucleus.

5. **Applied anatomy :** The lesion of dentate nucleus produces.

A. Hypotonia : Diminished muscle tone, which produces pendular jerk.

B. Asynergia : Loss of muscular co-ordination.

C. Ataxia : In coordination of muscles of trunk.

LAQ-11 **Describe floor of IVth ventricle under**
1. Gross anatomy 2. Development
3. Communications & 4. Applied anatomy.

1. **Gross anatomy :**

A. Introduction : Fourth ventricle is a cavity of rhombencephalon, situated between pons, medulla infront and cerebellum behind.

B. Morphology :

  a. Shape : Rhomboid.

  b. Angles : It has four angles.

    I. One rostral,

    II. One caudal and

    III. Two lateral.

C. Formation : It is formed by

   a. Posterior surface of lower part of pons.

   b. Posterior surface of upper part of medulla.

D. Contents : Nuclei of VIth, VIIIth, IXth, Xth & XIIth cranial nerve.

E. Features :

   a. Median sulcus : It divides entire floor into two equal parts.

   b. Median eminence : It is a longitudinal elevation on either side of median sulcus.

   c. Sulcus limitans : It limits the median eminence laterally.

      It divides each half into medial and lateral area.

      Medial area contains **m**otor nuclei ⚷ m for m and lateral area contains sensory nuclei.

   d. Superior fovea : It is the depression present at intermediate widest part present on the sulcus limitans.

   e. Inferior fovea : It is the depression present on the caudal part of sulcus limitans.

F. Division : The floor is described into

   a. Upper triangular area

      I. It is formed by posterior surface of lower part of pons.

      II. In the upper part of superior fovea, it presents a bluish grey discoloured area called locus ceruleus (*Locus* point, *ceruleus* dark colour).

      III. Colour is due to melanin formed by substantia ferruginea (blue).

      IV. It belongs to reticular formation.

      V. It is rich in nor adrenaline.

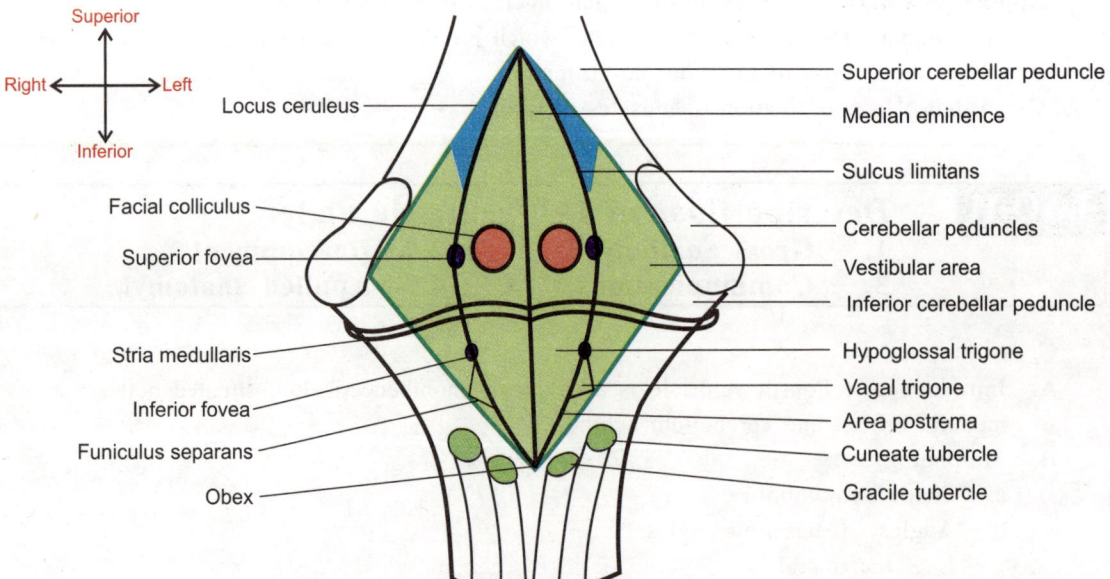

Fig. 4.34 : Floor of the fourth ventricle.

    b. Lower triangular area

        I. It is formed by posterior surface of upper part of medulla oblongata.

        II. It consists of a raised triangular area present on the median eminence called hypoglossal triangle.

        III. It shows following nuclei deep to the triangle.

            i. Hypoglossal nuclei situated medially.

            ii. Inter-calatus nuclei (perihypoglossal nuclear complex) situated laterally.

        IV. Vagal triangle : It is the area between hypoglossal triangle and vestibular area. It overlies dorsal nucleus of vagus.

        V. Funiculus separans : It is a narrow ependymal thickening and separates vagal triangle and area postrema.

        VI. Area postrema (*post* beyond, *trema* opening) :

            i. It is a small tongue shaped area, present inferolaterally.

            ii. It is composed of highly vascular neuroglial & neuronal tissue.

            iii. It is devoid of blood brain barrier.

            iv. It is closely related to vomiting and respiratory centres.

        VII. Calamus scriptorius (*Calamus* reed बोरू, *scriptorius* relating to script) : It is lowest part of floor which resembles the pointed nib of a writing pen called calamus scriptorius.

        VIII. Obex (*Obex* bolt) : It is meeting point of lower triangular area.

    c. Junction of upper and lower part :

        I. Facial colliculus : Present on the median eminence at the level of superior fovea. It is caused by -

            i. Axons of facial nerve (VIIth cranial nerve) and

            ii. Nucleus of abducent nerve (VIth cranial nerve).

        II. Vestibular area : Rounded elevation present lateral to sulcus limitans overlies vestibular nuclei.

        III. Striae medullaris (Auditory striae)

2. Development :

  A. Upper triangular : Isthmus rhombencephalon.

  B. Intermediate part : Metancephalon.

  C. Lower triangular : Myelencephalon.

4. Applied :

  A. Lesion of floor of IVth ventricle may result into loss of control of swallowing, respiration, movements of tongue.

  B. The tumor in the floor may produce symptoms and signs of cerebellar deficiency or may press vital nuclear centre and produce cardiac irregularities, tachycardia and irregular respiration.

Table 4.12 : The table shows the communication of the fourth ventricle at different angles.

Location	Through	To
A. Superior angle	Cerebral aqueduct	3rd ventricle.
B. Inferior angle	Central canal	Medulla oblongata.
C. Each side	Foramen of Luschka	Subarachnoid space.
D Roof	Foramen of Magendie	Subarachnoid space.

C. Hydrocephalus : The blockage of the foramina leads to accumulation of cerebro spinal fluid in the brain.

LAQ-12 Describe superolateral surface of cerebral hemisphere and show different sulci, gyri and functional areas.

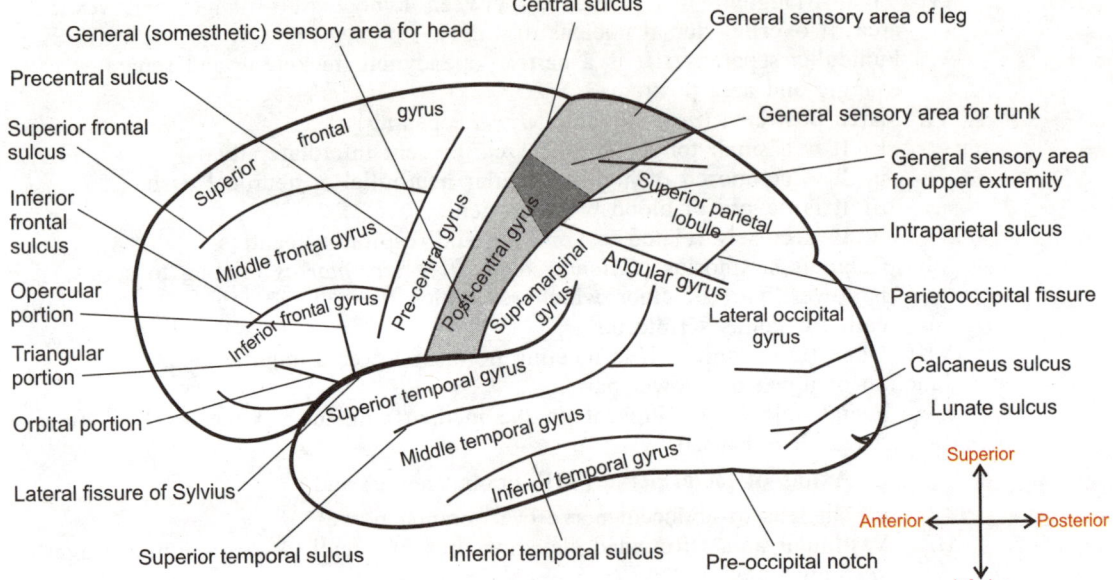

Fig. 4.35 : Superolateral surface of cerebral hemisphere showing sulci, gyri and functional areas.

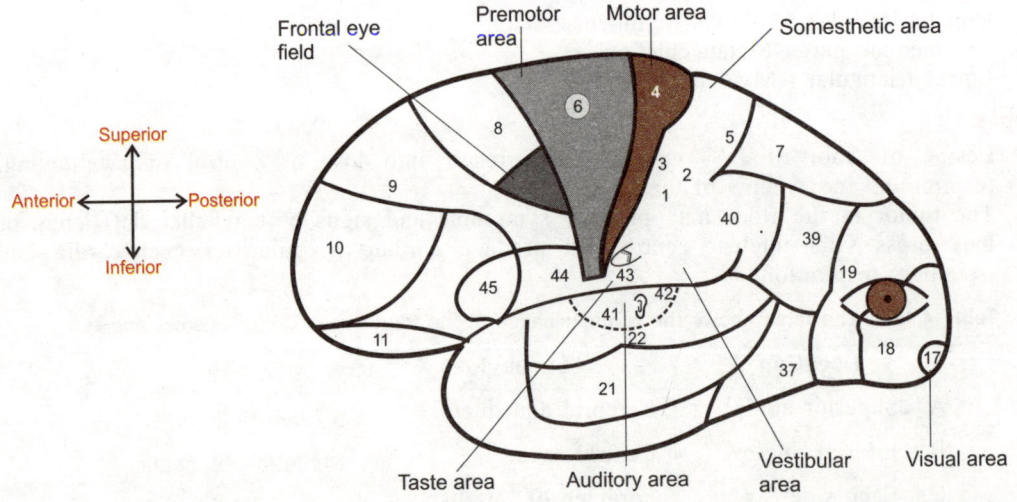

Fig. 4.36 : Superolateral surface of cerebral hemisphere showing functional areas.

SN-19   Primary motor area

1. **Location :**
   A. Precentral gyrus.
   B. Anterior wall of the central sulcus.
   C. Anterior part of the paracentral lobule.

2. **Arterial supply :**
   A. Branches of the anterior cerebral artery.
      They supply the paracentral lobule and upper parts of the motor area (about a finger's breadth area near the upper border of the hemisphere).
   B. Branches of the middle cerebral artery.
      They supply the rest of the motor area.

3. **Representation** of body in the motor area is in an inverted manner as follows :
   A. In paracentral lobule :
      a. Centres for micturition and defecation and
      b. Foot movements.

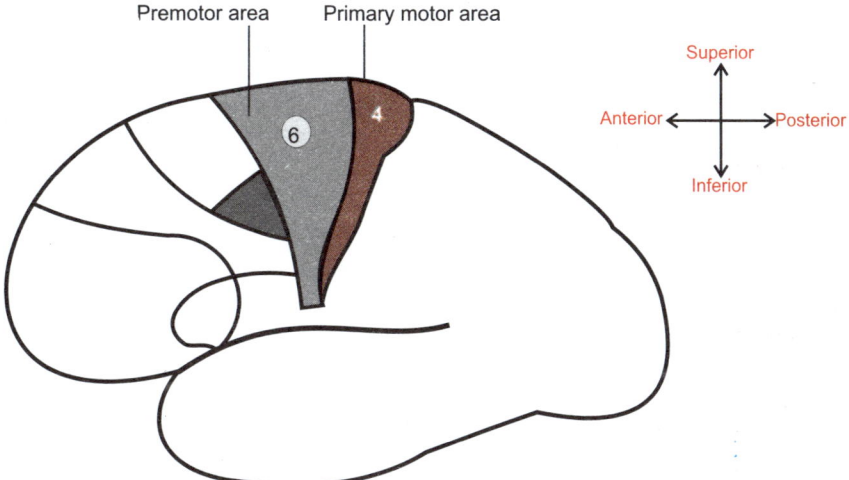

Fig. 4.37 : Superolateral surface of cerebral hemisphere showing primary motor area.

   B. In precentral gyrus : The sequence from above downwards is leg, thigh, trunk, upper limb, face, larynx, lips, jaws, tongue and pharynx.
      The area of cortex representing a part of the body is not proportional to the size of that part, but rather to intricacy of movements in that region. Thus movements in the hand or the lips are represented by relatively large area of the cortex.

4. **Functions :**
   A. The primary motor area controls voluntary movements of the opposite side of the body.
   B. It also controls micturition and defecation..

5. **Applied anatomy :** A lesion in this area gives rise to upper motor neuron type of paralysis on the opposite side of the body.

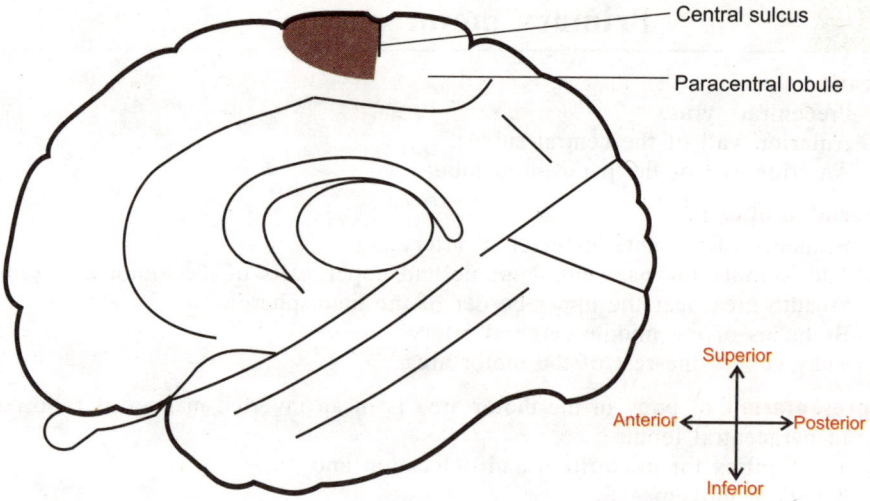

Fig. 4.38 : Medial surface of the cerebral hemisphere showing motor area.

SN-20   Premotor area

1. **Location :** The premotor area (Brodmann's area no. 6) is located in posterior part of the
   A. Superior,
   B. Middle and
   C. Inferior frontal gyri and extends on the superolateral surface of the cerebral hemisphere.

2. **Fibers :** It is the main site for the cortical origin of the extrapyramidal fibers. It helps to perform successful voluntary motor activities.

3. **Function :** These fibers are responsible to carry out complex, skilled or learned movements, especially related to manual dexterity.

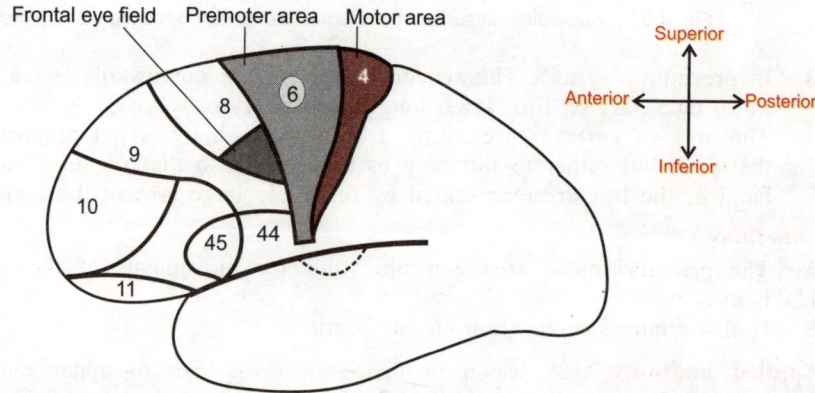

Fig. 4.39 : Superolateral surface of cerebral hemisphere showing premotor area.

4. **Applied anatomy :**
    Apraxia : A lesion in the premotor area results into impairment in the performance of learned movements. It is characterized by hesitancy in performing these movements.

SN-21   Sensory speech area of Wernicke

1. **Situation :**
    A. It is situated on the posterior part of the superior temporal gyrus of the dominant cerebral hemisphere.
    B. The parts of the inferior parietal lobule including the angular and supramarginal gyri. The latter gyri correspond to Brodmann areas 39 and 40 respectively.

2. **Functions :**
    A. Understanding the written and spoken languages, i.e. it is concerned with the interpretation of language through visual and auditory input.
    B. It is also essential for constant availability of learned word patterns.
    C. The angular and supra marginal gyri are essential for the process of learning such as reading, writing and computing.

3. **Applied anatomy :**
    A. Receptive or sensory aphasia : Affected individuals cannot understand spoken words although his hearing is normal,
    B. Alexia : Disabilities in reading,
    C. Agraphia : Disabilities in writing,
    D. Acalculia : Disabilities in computing and
    E. Anomia : Recognition of names of objects.

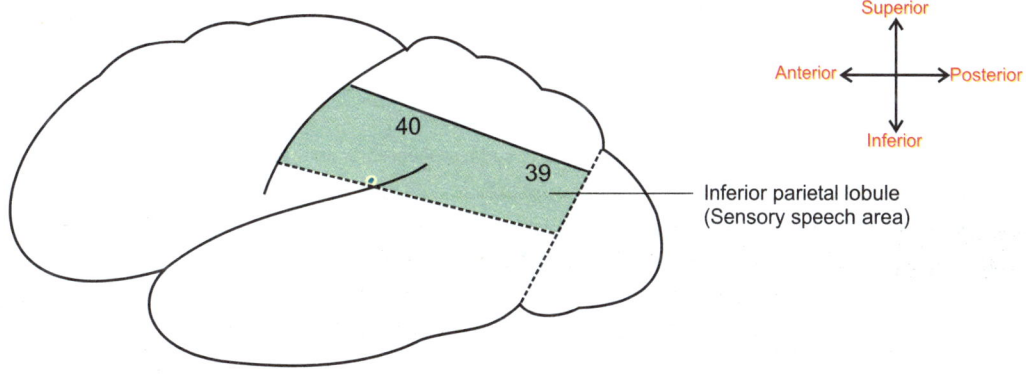

Fig. 4.40 : Sensory speech area of Wernicke.

SN-22   Motor speech area of Broca

1. **Location :** The motor speech area (Brodmann's area 44 & 45) is located in the
    A. Pars triangularis (area 45) and
    B. Pars posterior (area 44) in the inferior frontal gyrus of the dominant hemisphere (i.e. left in right handed persons).

2. **Functions :** The motor speech area is essential for production of speech, i.e. It controls the expressive speech.

3. **Blood supply :** Branches of middle cerebral artery.

4. **Applied anatomy :** If this area is damaged, the person will suffer form motor aphasia i.e. inability to articulate properly though there is no paralysis of muscles of lips, tongue, palate and vocal cords.

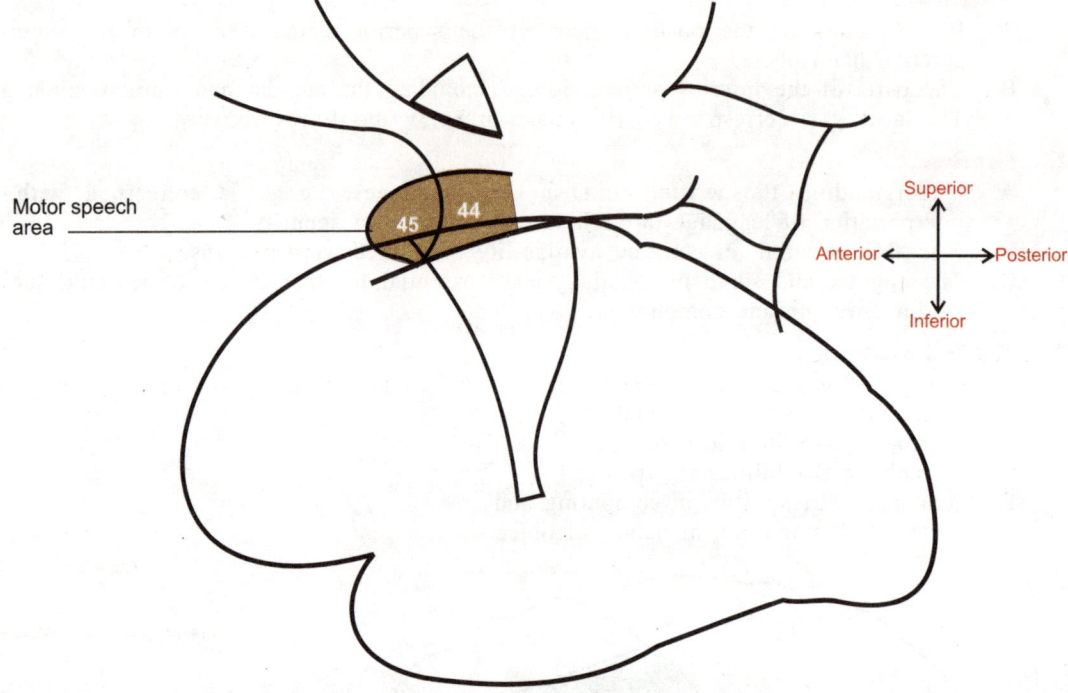

Fig. 4.41 : Superolateral surface of cerebral hemisphere.

| **LAQ-13** | **Describe limbic system under** |

Describe limbic system under
1. **Characteristics**   2. **Components**   3. **Connections**
4. **Functions and**   5. **Applied anatomy.**

1. **Characteristics :** Part of cerebrum situated at the   LIMBIC
   A. **L**imbus (junction) of diencephalon & telencephalon for
   B. **I**ntegration of olfactory, visceral & somatic information for
   C. **M**aking homeostatic response for short term & long term & includes
   D. **B**ehavioural &
   E. **I**motional response & consists of
   F. **C**ore of
      a. Archi cortex and
      b. Peleo cortex.

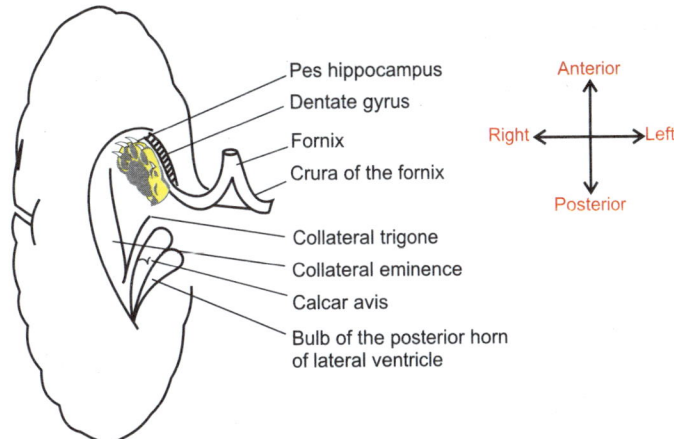

Fig. 4.42 : Inferior horn of the lateral ventricle showing parts of limbic system.

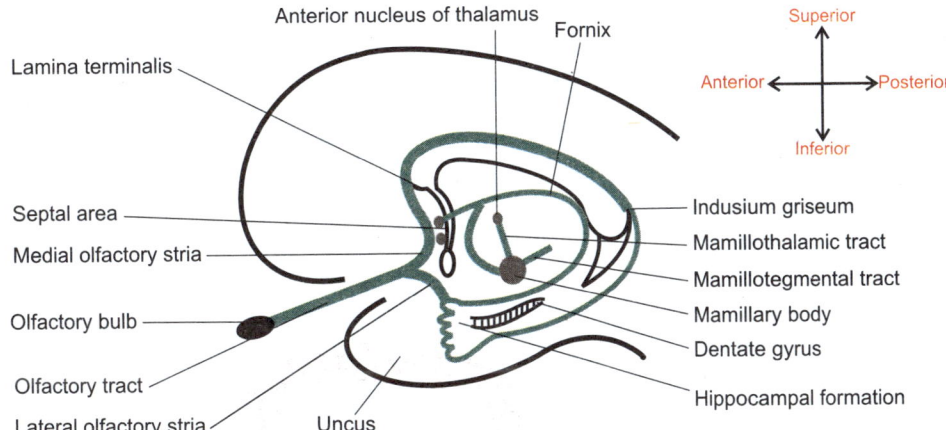

Fig. 4.43 : Parts of limbic system and fornix.

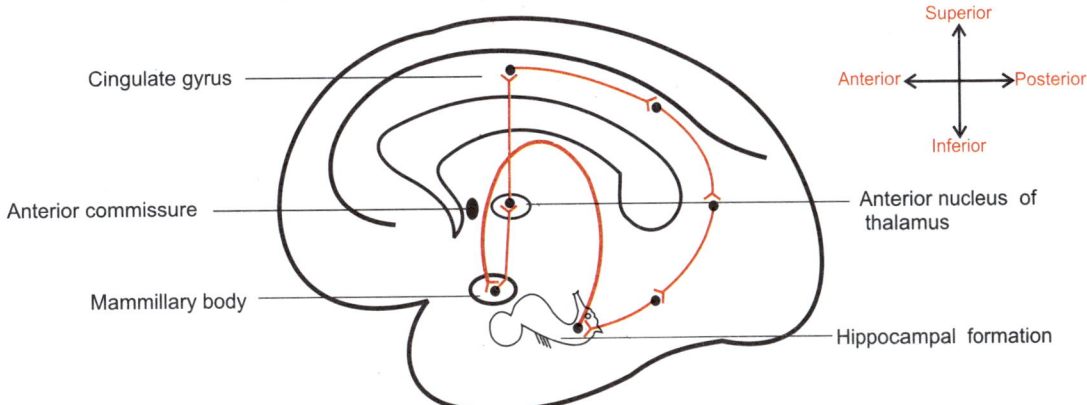

Fig. 4.44 : Papez circuit.

2. **Components :**

A. Archi cortex consists of hippocampal formation which includes -
   a. Hippocampus,
   b. Dentate gyrus,
   c. Splenial gyrus, indusium griseum and
   d. Longitudinal stria (White matter in the indusium griseum).

B. Paleo cortex
   a. Olfactory nerves & olfactory bulb.
   b. Olfactory tract.
   c. Olfactory striae.
   d. Pyriform cortex (olfactory cortex) septal area (medial olfactory area).
   e. Septal nuclei.

3. **Connections :**

A. Afferent :
   a. Pyriform area.
   b. Septal area.
   c. Hypothalamus.
   d. Tegmentum of midbrain.

B. Efferent :
   a. Hippocampus.
   b. Fornix.
   c. Hypothalamus.
   d. Cortical areas of frontal lobe.

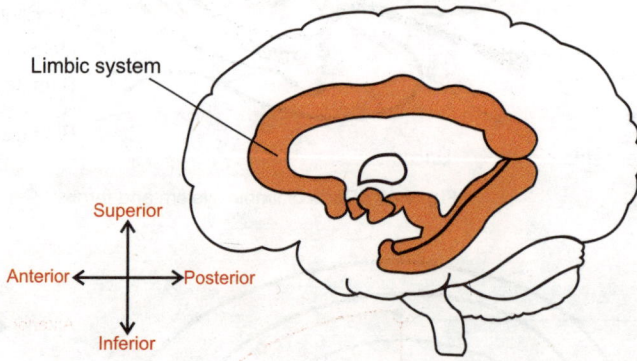

Fig. 4.45 : Limbic system.

4. **Functions :** The functions of the limbic system are not exactly known. However the following functions are attributed to the system.

A. It is responsible for emotional reactions with respect to preservation of individual and the species.

B. It integrates olfactory, visceral and somatic impulses reaching the brain.

C. It controls visceral functions associated with emotions.

D. It is suggested that a normally functioning hippocampus - fornix - mamillary body - thalamus - cingulate gyrus connections are necessary for retaining recent memory.

5. **Applied anatomy :** A lesion of limbic system results into,
    A. Psychomotor seizures, marked by occasional attacks of violent behavior, which are not remembered by the patient. In between the attacks, the patient is normal.
    B. Uncinate fits, consisting of attacks of olfactory hallucinations.
    C. Unreal fear : The patient gets attacks in which he is afraid of non existent conditions, and has a feeling of unreality, as if he is in a dream.
    D. De ja vu or seen it before phenomenon. The patient may get an unreal feeling of familiarity with an object, or an event and feels as if he has experienced it before.
    E. Automatism : Paroxysmal attacks in which the patient automatically performs complex activity, without being aware of what he is doing. Later, on recovery from the attacks he does not remember anything about it.

SN-23   Fornix

1. **Definition :** It is a bundle of white matter lying beneath the corpus callosum.

2. **Parts of fornix :**
    A. Alveus,
    B. Fimbria,
    C. Crus,
    D. Body and
    E. Column.

3. **Content :** It contains
    A. Association fibers arising from dentate gyrus.

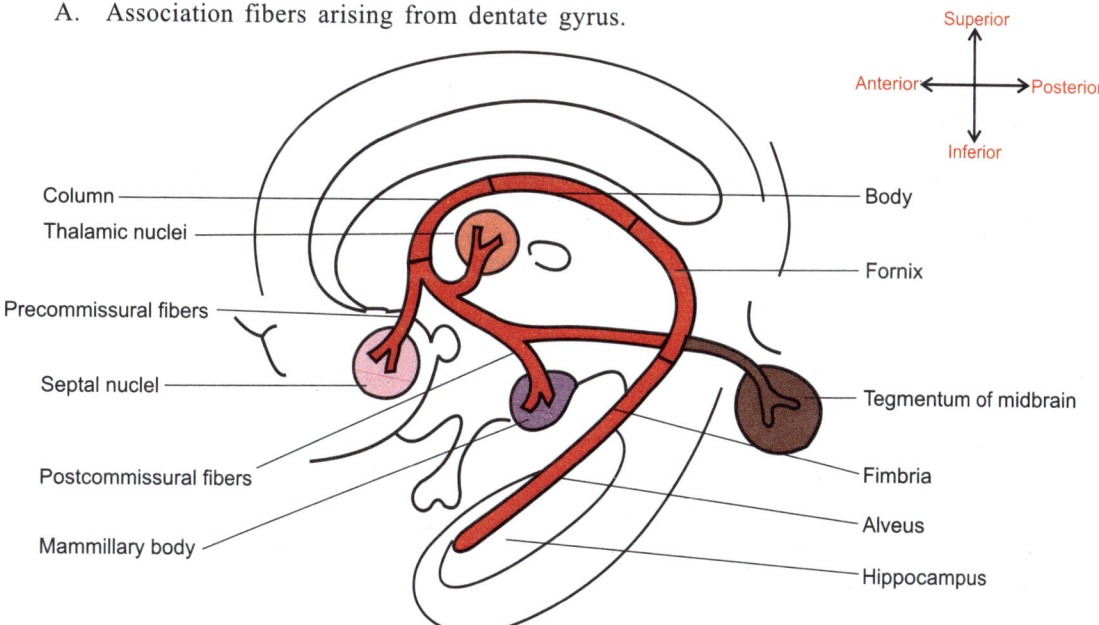

Fig. 4.46 : Fornix.

B. Commisural fibers which connect two hippocampus.
C. Projection fibers which project to tegmentum of midbrain. It consists of
    a. Mamillo-tegmental tract.
    b. Mamillo-reticular tract.
    c. Papez circuit : It is a neuronal circuit in the limbic system. It consists of
        I.   Hippocampus.
        II. Fornix.
        III. Mamillary body (mamillothalamic tract).
        IV. Anterior thalamic nuclei.
        V.   Cingulate gyrus.
        Through cingulum again to hippocampus.
        Function : It is involved with the experiencing of emotions and response to them.

SN-24   Thalamus

1. **Definition :** It is a large mass of grey matter, which integrates all the sensory information and acts as a great sensory relay station.

2. **Gross anatomy :**
    A. Length : 4 cm antero-posteriorly.
    B. Ends : Two.
        a. Anterior end
        b. Posterior end (pulvinar).
    C. Surfaces : Four.
        a. Superior,
        b. Inferior,
        c. Medial and
        d. Lateral.

3. **Structure :**
    A. White matter :
        a. Stratum zonale on the superior surface.
        b. External medullary lamina on the lateral surface.
        c. Internal medullary lamina (a vertical sheet of white matter which bifurcates antero-superiorly to divide the grey matter of thalamus into 3 large parts -
            I.   Anterior,
            II. Medial and
            III. Lateral.
    B. Grey matter : There are 7 main groups of thalamic nuclei :
        a. Anterior,
        b. Medial,
        c. Lateral,
        d. Ventral,
        e. Intralaminar,
        f. Midline and
        g. Reticular.

4. **Connections :**
    A. Afferent :

a. Sensory relay :
    I.   Medial lemniscus.   } Ends in 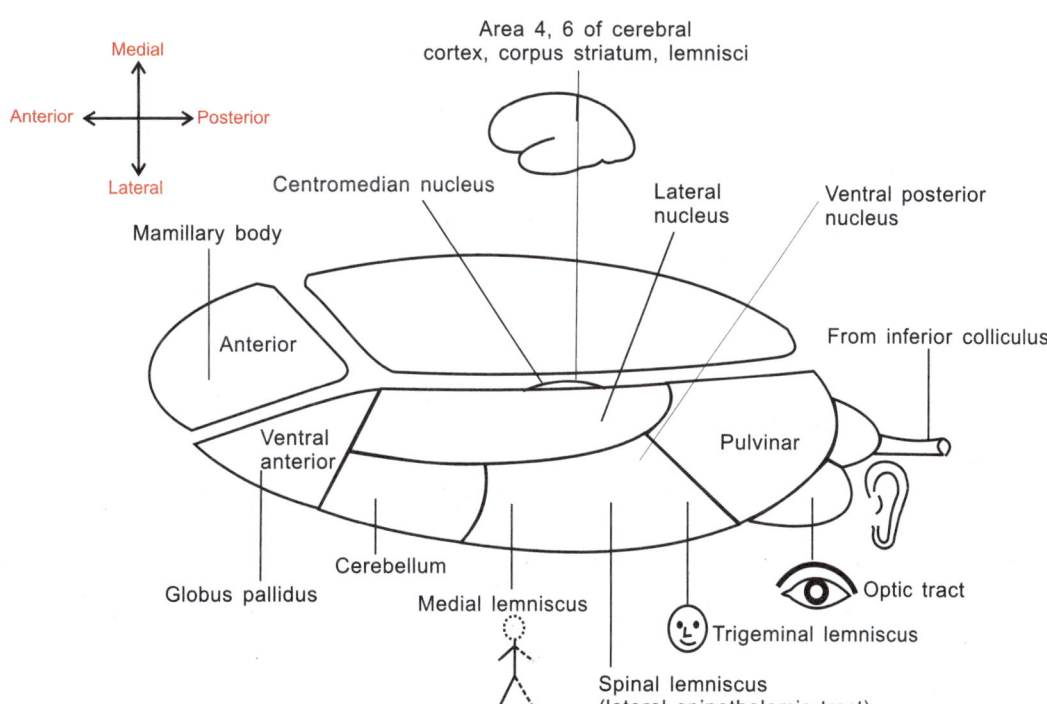 VPL (ventropostero lateral)
    II. Spinal lemniscus.   nucleus of thalamus
    III. Solitario thalamic.   } Ends in VPM (ventropostero medial)
    IV. Trigeminal lemniscus : } nucleus of thalamus
    V. Cochlear nuclei.
    VI. Retina.
    VII. Vestibular.
b. Motor :
    I.   Cerebellum.
    II. Parietal cortex.
c. Emotion :
    I.   Mamillary body : Anterior nucleus of thalamus.
    II. Hypothalamus.

B. Efferent :
a. Thalamic radiation.
    I.   Anterior,
    II. Superior,
    III. Posterior and
    IV. Ventral.
b. Corpus striatum.
c. Hypothalamus.
d. Reticular formation.

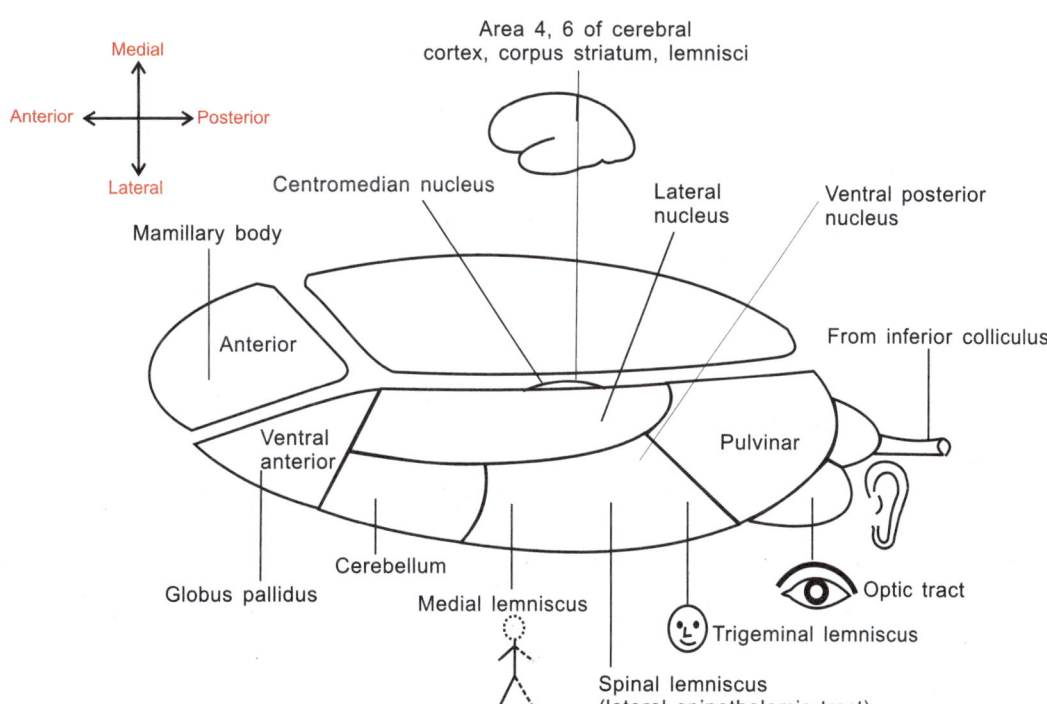

Fig. 4.47 : Thalamus and its afferent and efferent connections.

5. **Functions :**
    A. It serves as a great relay station for all sensory impulses (except olfactory)
    B. It acts as a correcting and integrating center.
    C. It influences motor activities from its sensory experience.
    D. It maintains a state of wakefulness and alertness through reticular activating system. (RAS)
    E. It plays an important role in the control of emotional behavior and recent memory mechanism.

6. **Applied anatomy :**
    A. Thalamic lesions produce impairment of all types of sensations.
    B. Thalamic syndrome : This is caused by a vascular lesion of thalamo-geniculate branch of posterior cerebral artery. It is characterized by -
        a. Disturbance of sensations : Hyperaesthesia and severe spontaneous pain on the opposite side of the body.
        b. Emotional instability : i.e. Spontaneous or forced laughing or crying.

SN-25   Medial geniculate body

Geniculate body (*genu* knee) : The lamellae are arranged like knee, hence geniculate body.

1. **Definition :** It is a small oval collection of cell bodies present in the metathalamus. It consists of lamellae, which are arranged in the form of bend, hence it is called geniculate body.

2. **Gross :**
    A. Location : It is situated below the pulvinar of the thalamus.
    B. Relations :
        a. Superior :
            I.   Pulvinar of thalamus and
            II. Pineal body.

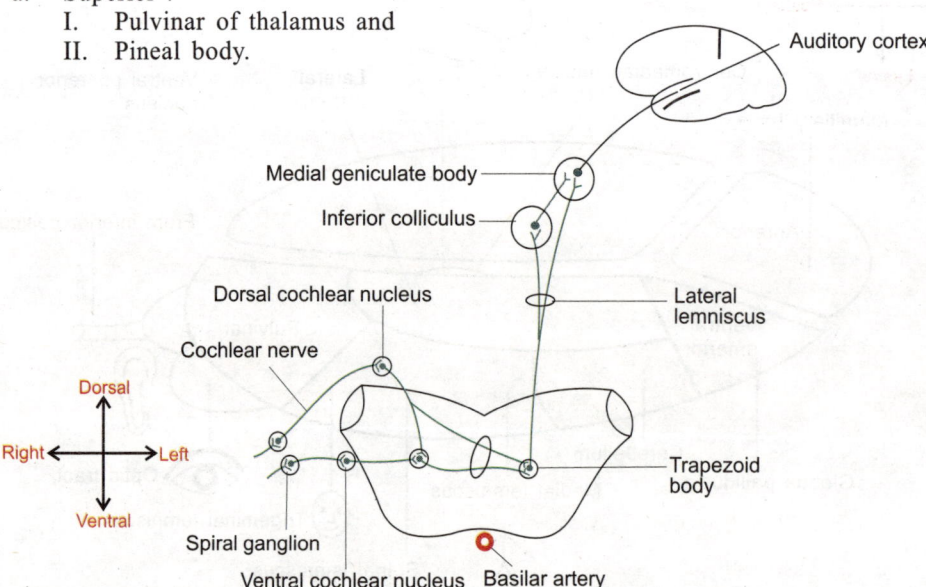

Fig. 4.48 : Afferent and efferent connections of medial geniculate body.

b. Lateral : Lateral geniculate body.

c. Medial : Midbrain (cerebral peduncle).

3. Connections :

a. Afferent : Inferior colliculus through lateral lemniscus.

b. Efferent : To the auditory area of the cortex through the auditory radiation.

4. Function : It is the final relay center in the pathway of hearing.

SN-26   Lateral geniculate body

Geniculate body (*genu* knee) : The lamellae are arranged like knee, hence geniculate body.

1. Definition : It is a small oval collection of cell bodies present in the metathalamus. It consists of lamellae which are arranged in the form of bend, hence it is called geniculate body.

2. Gross anatomy:

A. Location **:** It is situated below the pulvinar of the thalamus.

B. Relations :

a. Superiorly : Thalamus.

b. Medially : Medial geniculate body.

C. Structure :

a. It is composed of 6 layers of nerve cells.

b. They are numbered from its ventral aspect.

c. The layers are well defined only in the central region.

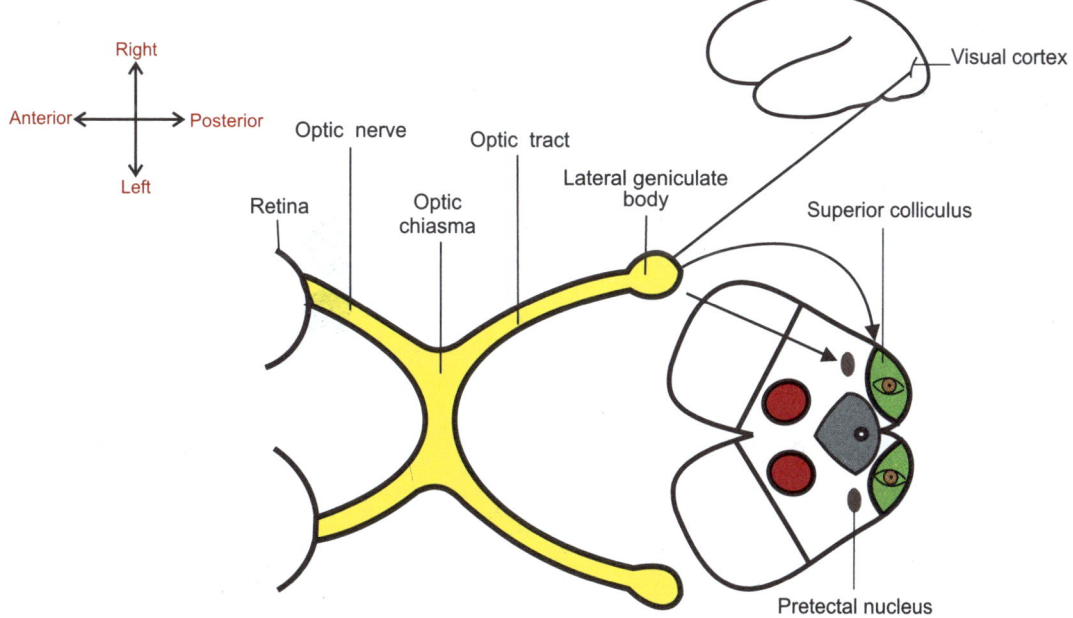

Fig. 4.49 : Afferent and efferent connections of lateral geniculate body.

3. **Connections :**
    A. Afferent :
        a. Optic tract : It consists of two types of fibers :
            I. The crossed fibers (nasal fibers of the opposite retina) terminate in layers 1, 4 and 6.
            II. The uncrossed fibers (temporal fibers) of the ipsilateral retina terminate in the layers 2, 3 and 5 of the LGB.
              There is a point to point projection of the retina in the LGB.
              i. Superior retinal quadrant project to the medial side of the nucleus.
              ii. Inferior retinal quadrant project to the lateral part.
              iii. The macular area projects to the central part of nucleus.
        b. Superior colliculus.
    B. Efferent :
        a. Optic radiation to visual area of the occipital lobe (areas 17, 18 & 19) through geniculo calcarine tract.
        b. Superior colliculus.

4. **Function :** It is a final relay center in the visual pathway.

5. **Applied anatomy :** Lesion of the LGB causes contralateral homonymous hemianopia.

SN-27   Pineal body

1. **Definition :** It is a small conical organ formed by collection of cell bodies, present between and above two superior colliculi.

2. **Gross anatomy :**
    A. It has
        a. Superior lamina, which consists of habenular commissure.
        b. Inferior lamina, which consists of posterior commissure.
    B. Morphological significance :
        a. Anterior part : It represents parietal eye, which has disappeared in evolution.

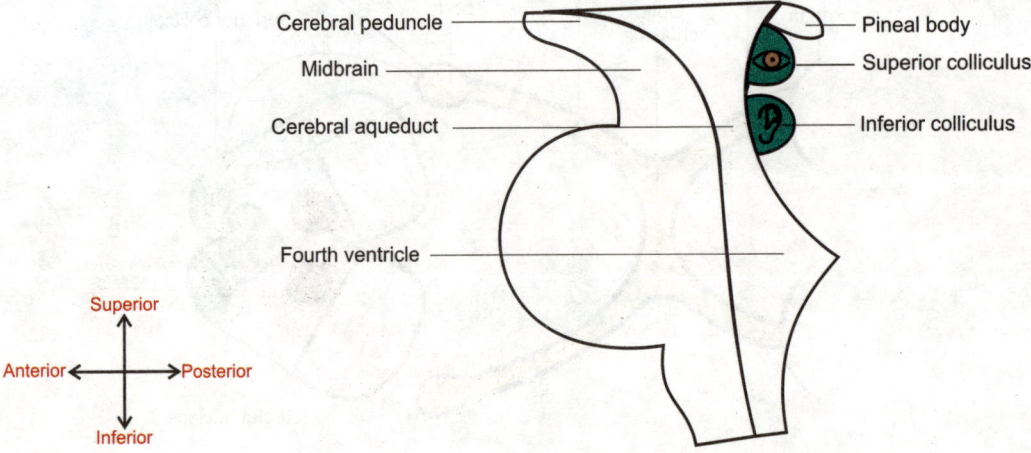

Fig. 4.50 : Position of pineal body.

      b.   Posterior part : It is now recognized as endocrine gland. It consists of 2 types of cells.
         i.   Pinealocyte and
         ii. Neuroglial cell.

3. **Development :** It develops from roof of diencephalon (ectodermal).

4. **Functions :**
    A. It contains melatonin & serotonin, which play role in the development of gonads.
    B. It also produces hormones that may have an important regulatory influence on many other endocrine organs (including adenohyposis, neurohypophysis)

5. **Applied :**
    A. Tumor of pineal body causes precocious puberty.
    B. Calcification in pineal is seen in X-ray.

LAQ-14	Describe hypothalamus under
	1. Boundaries **2. Parts**
	3. Connections **4. Functions**

1. **Boundaries :** It is bounded as follows :
    A. As seen on the base of the brain :
       a. Anteriorly : Optic chiasma.
       b. Posteriorly : Posterior perforated substance.
       c. On each side :
         I.   Optic tract.
         II. Crus cerebri.
    B. As seen in a sagittal section :
       a. Anteriorly : Lamina terminalis.
       b. Inferiorly : By the floor of third ventricle.

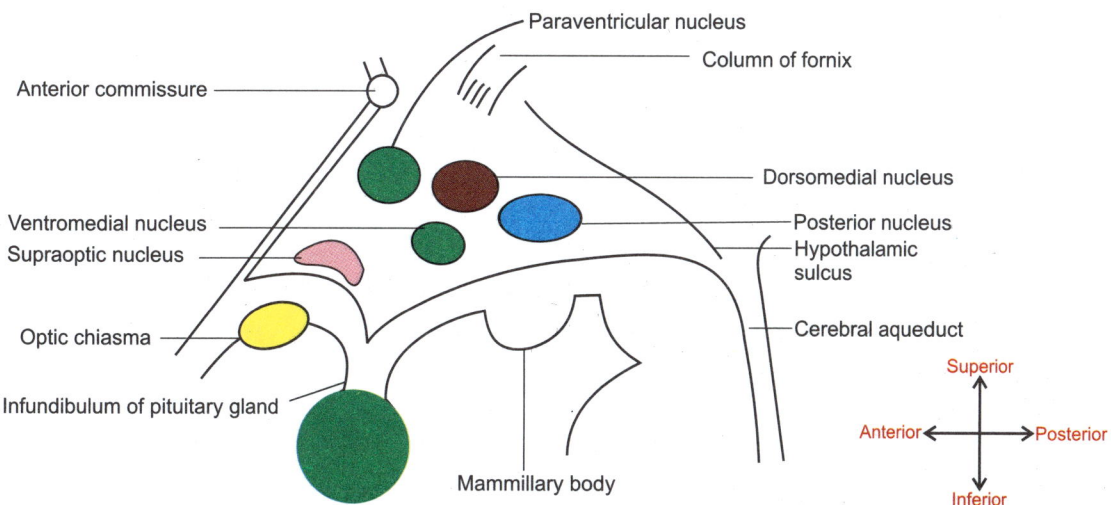

Fig. 4.51 : Nuclei of hypothalamus.

2. Parts and location :

Table 4.13 : The table shows nuclei of hypothalamus and their locations.

Nucleus	Location
A. Preoptic	Caudal to lamina terminalis.

B. Supraoptic
  a. Supraoptic nucleus
  b. Paraventricular
  c. Anterior nucleus
  d. Suprachiasmatic nucleus
	
	Above optic chiasma.
	Just above the supraoptic nucleus.
	Continuous with preoptic area.
	Above optic chiasma.

C. Tuberal region
  a. Ventromedial
  b. Dorsomedial
  c. Arcuate
  d. Posterior hypothalamic
  e. Lateral hypothalamic
	
	Ventomedially.
	Dorsomedially.
	Floor of third ventricle.
	Dorsal to tuberal and mamillary region.
	Lateral to the posterior nucleus.

D. Mamillary region
  a. Lateral nucleus
  b. Posterior nucleus
	
	Lateral to the posterior nucleus.
	Caudal to ventromedial and dorsomedial nuclei.

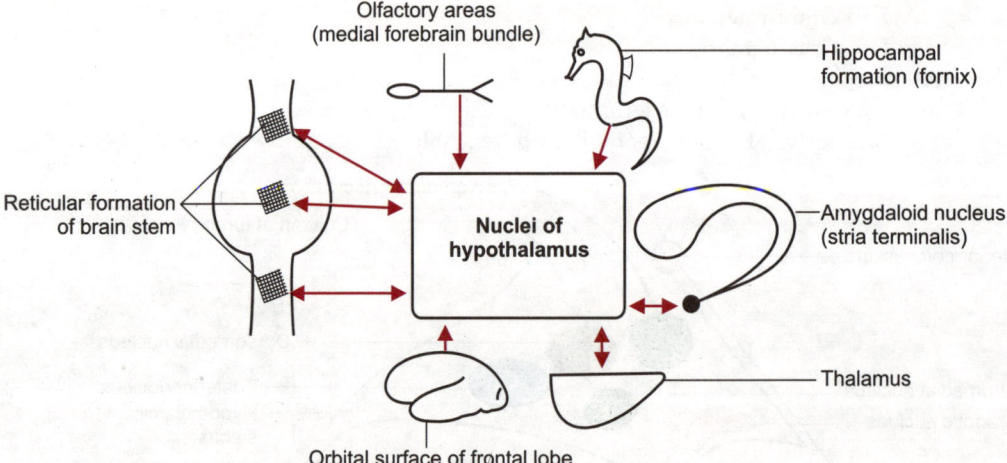

Fig. 4.52 : Important connections of hypothalamus.

3. Connections :

A. Afferent :

    a. Reticular formation : It receives visceral sensations from the reticular nuclei present in the spinal cord and brain stem.

    b. Olfactory pathways : It is also connected with the olfactory pathway which includes piriform cortex.

B. Efferent :
   a. Supraoptico-hypophyseal tract,
   b. Mamillothalamic tract and
   c. Mamillotegmental tract.

4. **Functions :** ⚷ A B C D E F G H
   A. **A**utonomic activity : Important subcortical centre for autonomous nervous system.
      ⚷ **VCR**
      a. **V**asomotor center,
      b. **C**ardio vascular center and
      c. **R**espiratory center.
   B. **B**iological clock. (Suprachiasmatic nucleus).
   C. **C**yclic variation (circadian rhythm).
   D. **D**rinking habit (lateral zone).
   E. **E**motional behavior (centromedian nucleus) (Fear, anger, pleasure)
      Endocrine activity.
      I. Supraoptic : It synthesize anti diuretic hormone.
      II. Paraventricular : It releases oxytocin.
   F. **F**ood intake (tuberal region)
      a. Ventromedian - satiety.
      b. Lateral nucleus - hunger centre.
   G. **G**amatogenesis (tuber cinereum).
   H. **H**omeothermic : Regulation of temp. (Pons)
      a. Preoptic nucleus is responsible for heat loss.
      b. Post hypothalamic nucleus is responsible for heat conservation.

LAQ-15 Describe basal nuclei under
1. Gross anatomy   2. Connections
3. Functions and   4. Applied anatomy.

---

1. **Gross anatomy :**
   A. **Inroduction :** It is a collection of grey matter, situated deeply at the base of brain. To begin with, they were situated at the base of the brain and as the development proceeds from all sides they were pushed inside but the name continues as the basal ganglia. They are better called as basal nuclei.
      They include subcortical masses of grey matter which are situated in white matter.
      a. Corpus striatum
         I. Caudate nucleus.
         II. Lentiform nucleus.
            The head of caudate nucleus and lentiform nucleus are connected by a band of white matter, situated deep to the anterior limb of internal capsule. They give the appearance of the striations as gray, white and gray. Hence, these nuclei forming the striations are called nuclei corpus striatum.
      b. Claustrum (*claustrum* barrier; barrier between external and extreme capsule) : It is a thin sheet of grey matter which intervenes between putamen and insular cortex. It is related medially to external capsule and laterally to extreme capsule. It is derived from detached part of
         I. Either insular cortex or

II.   Corpus striatum or

III. From both.

Function : Its significance is not known.

c. Amygdaloid body (*amygdaloid* almond) : It is apparently continuous with tail of caudate nucleus, but is entirely connected with limbic system. It is a part of archistriatum.

B. Evolution : Functionally corpus striatum is subdivided into

a. Neostriatum : It is an area, which is developed recently and consists of putamen and caudate nucleus.

b. Paleostriatum : It is an old part of corpus striatum and consists of globus pallidus (pallidum) ⚷ p for p

c. Archistriatum : It is an oldest part of corpus striatum and consists of amygdaloid nucleus.   ⚷ a for a

2. Connections : The connections of the basal ganglion are described as

A. Connections of the neostriatum

Table 4.14 : The table shows afferent connections of the neostriatum. ⚷ **NTC**

Fibers	Origin	Route	Features
I. Nigrostriate	Pars compacta of substantia nigra.	i. Caudate nucleus ii. Putamen and partly iii. Globus pallidus	Fibers are dopaminergic and exert inhibitory influence to the striate and pallidal fibers.
II. Thalamostriate	Fibres arise from i. Centromedian ii. Intralaminar iii. Mid line iv. Dorsomedial nucleus	Reach caudate nucleus and putamen.	Fibers are excitatory.
III. Corticostriate	All areas of cerebral cortex are predominant, except sensorimotor area.	i. External capsule ii. Internal capsule iii. Subcallosal	Connections are ipsilateral and are excitatory.

Table 4.15 : The table shows efferent connections of the neostriatum.   ⚷ **NTP**

Fibers	Origin	Route	Features
I. Strio nigral	Striate neuron	i. Pars reticularis & ii. Substantia nigra.	Convey neuro transmitter substance GABA (gamma amino butyric acid) which inhibits the dopaminergic neurons. (No back)
II. Striothalamic	Caudate nucleus and putamen	————	————
III. Striato pallidal	Outer part of putamen.	Outer part of globus pallidus.	The chief efferent connections are to globus pallidus

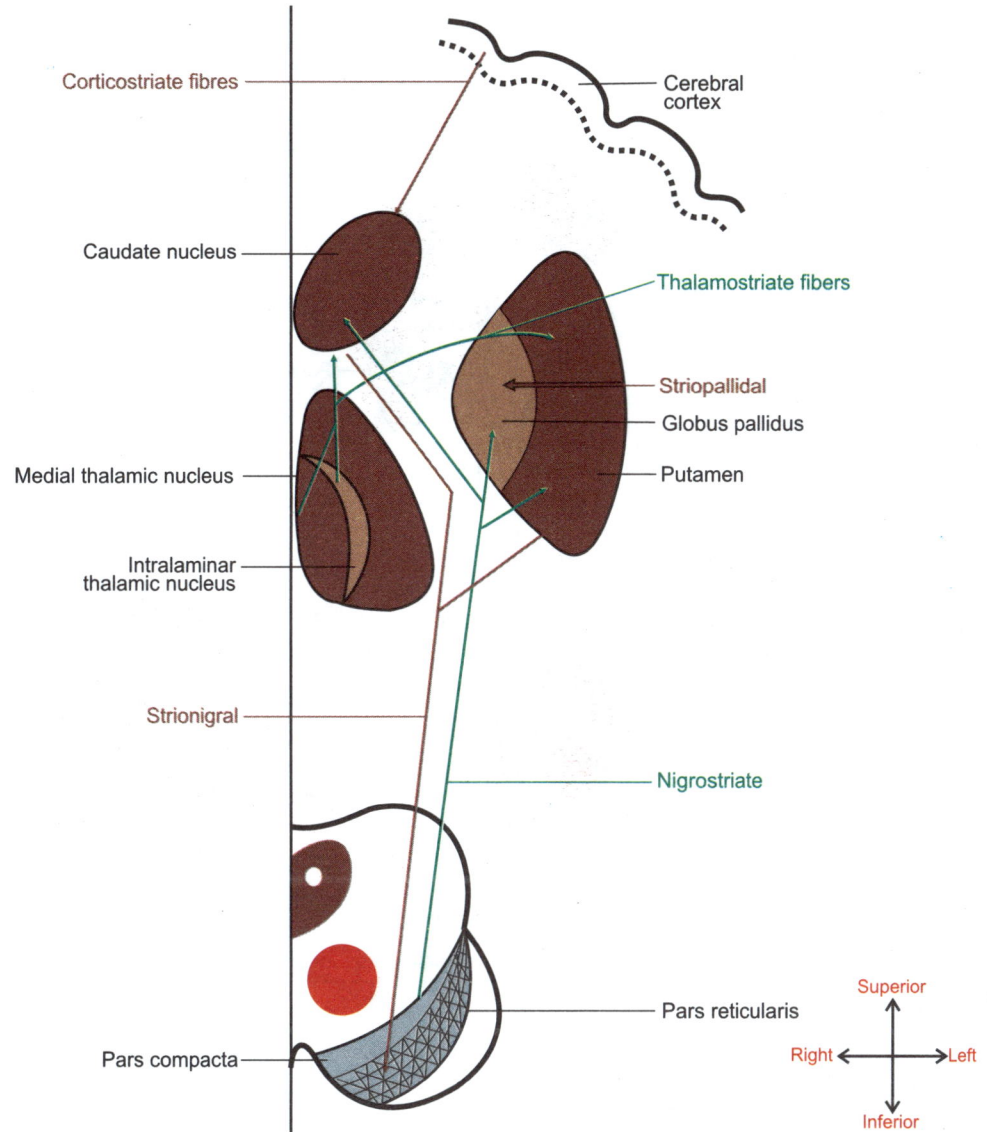

Fig. 4.53 : Connections of neostriatum.

B.   Connections of paleostriatum :

Table 4.16 : The table shows afferent connections of the paleostriatum

Fibers	Origin	Destiny
I. Striatum	Putamen.	Globus pallidus.
II. Pars compacta of substantia nigra.	Substantia nigra.	Globus pallidus.

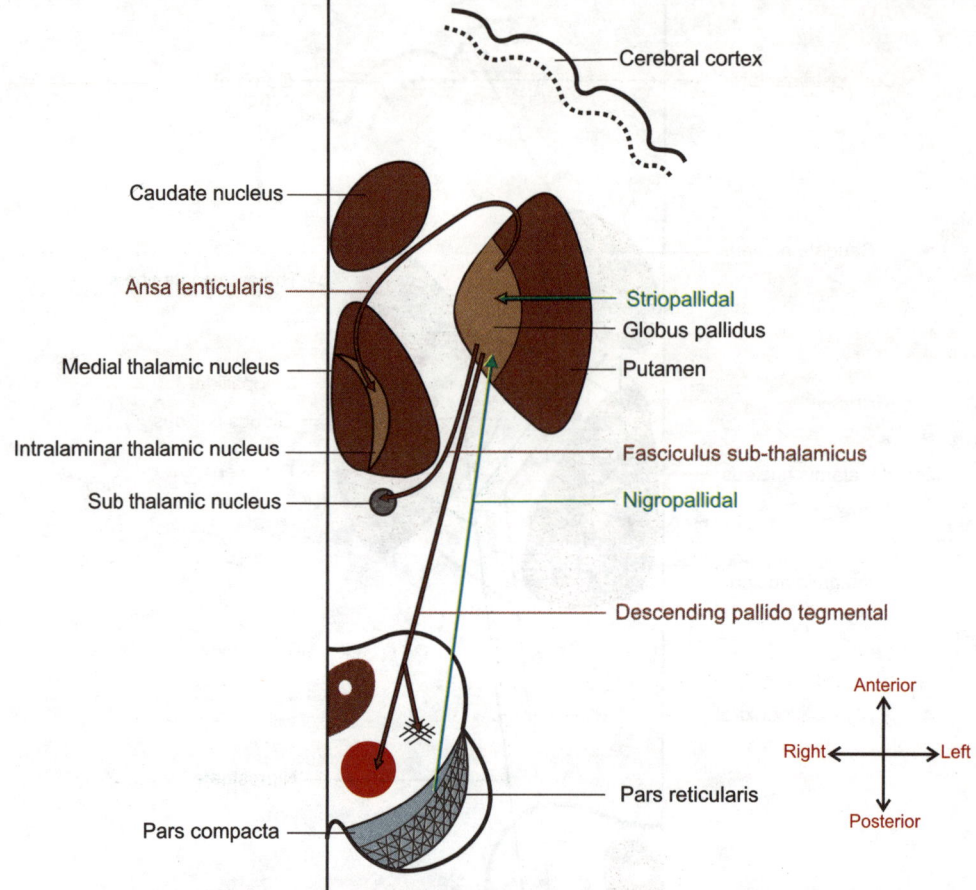

Fig. 4.54 : Connections of paleostriatum.

Table 4.17 : The table shows efferent connections of paleostriatum.

Fibers	Origin	Destiny
I. Fasciculus lenticularis.	Inner segment of globus pallidus.	
II. Ansa lenticularis	Both segments of globus pallidus join with dentato-rubro- thalamic fibres.	Thalamus i. Ventroanterior, ii. Ventrolateral and iii. Centromedian nuclei of thalamus.
III. Fasiculus subthalamic.	Globus pallidus.	Sub thalamic nuclei.
IV. Descending pallido tegmental.	Globus pallidus.	i. Red nucleus. ii. Reticular nuclei of midbrain. iii. Inferior olivary nucleus.

3. **Functions :** Basal nuclei are considered as important parts of the extrapyramidal system. They have the following functions :
    A. Control reflex and voluntary muscular activity.
    B. Control skilled and manipulative movements of the body e.g. threading a needle.
    C. Control automatic associated movements as co-ordinated movements of legs or swinging of arms during walking.
    D. Control abnormal involuntary movements.
    E. Control movements of emotional expression.

4. **Applied anatomy :** In lesions of basal ganglia, abnormal manifestations are observed. They are of two types.
    A. Hyper tonic and hypo kinetic : Increased muscle tone without alterations of deep reflexes e.g.
        Parkinson's disease (Paralysis agitans). It is characterised by
        a. Rigidity and tremors. Rigidity is due to increased muscle tone.
        b. It affects all muscles with poor movements. It results into cogwheel rigidity.
        c. Patient has masked face appearance with no emotional response.
        d. He walks with short and shuffling gait (quick steps).
        e. He experiences difficulty in taking initial steps and in terminating movements.
            Tremors occur with regular frequencies when subject is at rest. Tremors disappear during movements. They increase in emotions.
    B. Abnormal involuntary movements or dyskinesis are in the form of -
        a. Athetosis : Slow, worm like writhing movements of extremities, affecting chiefly fingers and the wrist. It is seen due to damage of putamen.
        b. Ballism : It is a rare disease manifested by wild, flail like movements of one arm and is caused by degeneration of subthalamic nucleus of opposite side.
        c. Chorea : It is characterized by brisk, jerky, purposeless and graceful movements of the distal parts of the extremities and associated with twitching of face. They are cardinal signs of two diseases.
            I. Sydenham's chorea : It is one of the complications of rheumatic fever.
            II. Huntigton's chorea : It is a dominant hereditary disorder. It first appears in middle age and become worse in advanced age. It results into mental deterioration. It is due to degeneration of striatum and due to reduced GABA.

SN-28   Caudate nucleus (*Caudate* tail)

Caudate tail
1. **Definition :** It is a large mass of grey matter situated deeply within the cerebral hemisphere. It forms part of the basal nuclei and belongs to neostriatum.

2. **Parts** of caudate nucleus
    A. Head : It is a large, globular part, forms floor of anterior horn of lateral ventricle.
        a. Situation :
            I.   It lies on medial side of anterior limb of internal capsule.
            II. It is separated from lentiform nucleus by anterior limb of internal capsule.
            III. In the upper part, it is continuous with putamen of lentiform nucleus and in the lower part it gives stripped appearance in horizontal section.

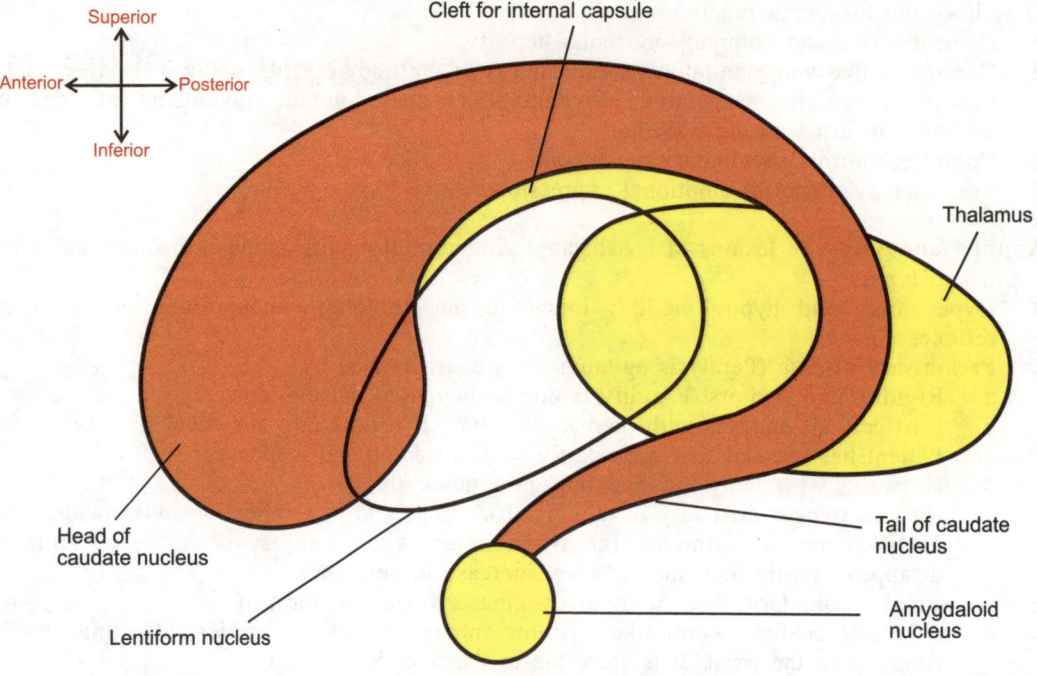

Fig. 4.55 : Caudate nucleus.

B.   Body :
Relations :
I.   Medially : Thalamostriate groove containing
i.   Thalamostriate vein.
ii. Stria terminalis : It is a white matter and connects amygdaloid nucleus
to septal nuclei.
II. Laterally : Fronto occipital bundle above and corona radiata below.
III. Posteriorly : Continuous with the tail.
C.   Tail : It forms roof of inferior horn of lateral ventricle and ends in amygdaloid body
Relations :
I.   Medially : Stria terminalis.
II. Laterally : Tapetum (*Tapetum* carpet).
III. Superiorly :
i.   Sublentiform part of internal capsule and
ii. Globus pallidus.

3.   **Structure :**
Putamen (*Putamen* shell) : It contains mostly small stellate cells and only few large cells,
whose fibers pass on to the globus pallidus.

4.   **Connections :** Please refer connections of neostriatum.

5.   **Applied anatomy :** In Huntington's chorea, the small cells of caudate nucleus and
putamen are affected due to the disease process and there is marked decrease of GABA

(Gama aminobutyric acid) in the striatonigral neurons. Chorea is intermittent, brisk, jerky, purposeless involuntary movements of the distal parts of the extremities.

SN-29   Amygdaloid body

1. **Introduction :** It is an almond shaped nucleus present at the end of tail of caudate nucleus.

2. **Location :** Temporal lobe, lying anterosuperior to the inferior horn of the lateral ventricle.

3. **Topographically :** It is continuous with the tail of the caudate nucleus, but functionally it is related in the stria terminalis. It is a part of the limbic system. It is continuous with the cortex of the uncus of the temporal lobe, the limen insulae and the anterior perforated substance.

4. **Evolution :** It is the part of archi striatum.

5. **Connections :**
   A. Afferent : From the olfactory tract.
   B. Efferent : It gives rise to the stria terminalis which ends in the anterior commissure, the anterior perforated substance and in hypothalamic nuclei.

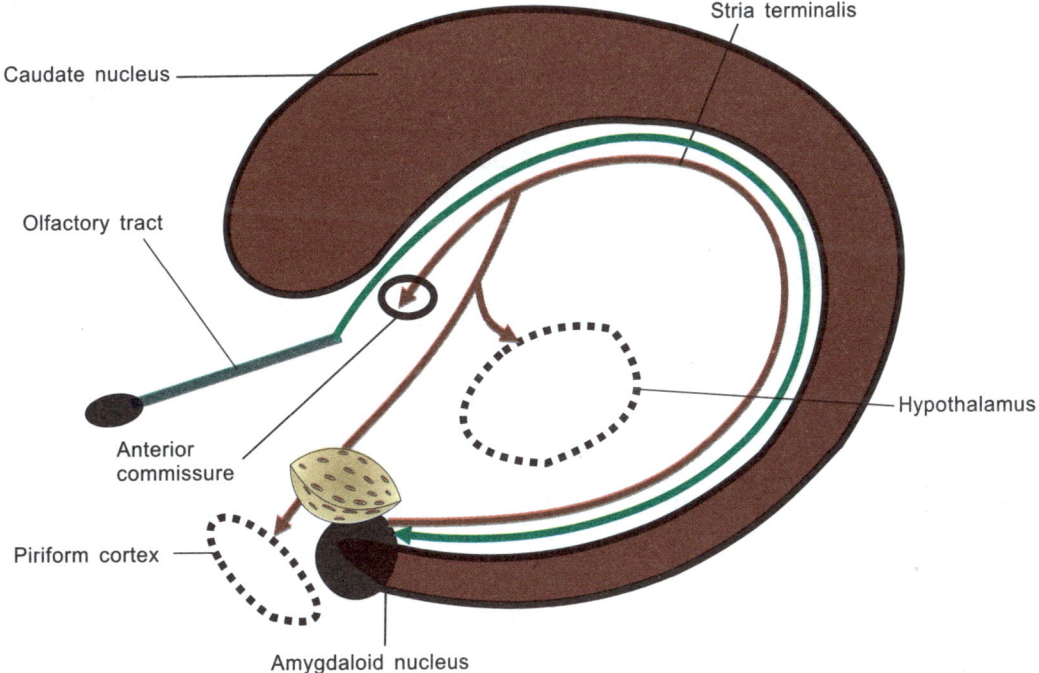

Fig. 4.56 : Main connections of the amygdaloid body

SN-30   Trigeminal nucleus

Table 4.18 : The table shows parts of trigeminal nucleus and their location and functions.

Particulars	Spinal	Sensory	Motor	Mesencephalic
1. Location	Pons to the second or third segment of spinal cord.	Pons.	Pons.	Midbrain.
2. Cell body	Trigeminal ganglion.	Trigeminal ganglion.	Motor nucleus.	Mesencephalic nucleus. *It lies within CNS which is exception for its location.*
3. Development	Myelencephalon.	Metancephalon.	Metancephalon.	Mesencephalon.
4. Functions	Pain and temperature from the skin of face and neck.	Touch and pressure from the skin of face and neck.	Movements of the muscles of mastication.	Proprioception from A. Muscles of mastication. B. Facial expression. C. Muscles of eye ball and D. Temporomandibular joint.
5. Lesion	Loss of pain and temperature from the skin of the face on the side of lesion.	Loss of touch and pressure from the skin of the face on the side of lesion.	Paralysis of muscle of mastications on the side of lesion.	Loss of proprioception.
6. Homologus tract in the limbs	Lateral spinothalamic tract.	Anterior spinothalamic tract.	Corticospinal.	Posterior column.

LAQ-16   Define and classify white matter of cerebrum?

1. **Definition** : These are myelinated fibers, which connect various parts of the cortex on the same side, opposite side and also other parts of the central nervous system.

2. **Classification** : It is classified as,
    Association fibers : They connect gyrus of the same side of the cerebral hemisphere. They are
    a.   Short association fibers : They connect the different areas of the same gyrus or adjacent gyri, e.g. superior frontal gyrus to inferior frontal gyrus.

b. Long association fibers :

Table 4.19 : The table shows examples of long association fibers.

Particulars	Connects	To
I. Superior longitudinal fasciculus.	Frontal lobe.	Occipital and temporal lobe.
II. Inferior longitudinal fasciculus.	Occipital lobe (area 18 & 19).	Temporal lobe.
III. Uncinate fasciculus.	Broca's area and gyri on the orbital surface of frontal lobe.	Temporal lobe.
IV. Cingulum fasciculus.	Gyrus cingulum.	Parahippocampal gyrus.

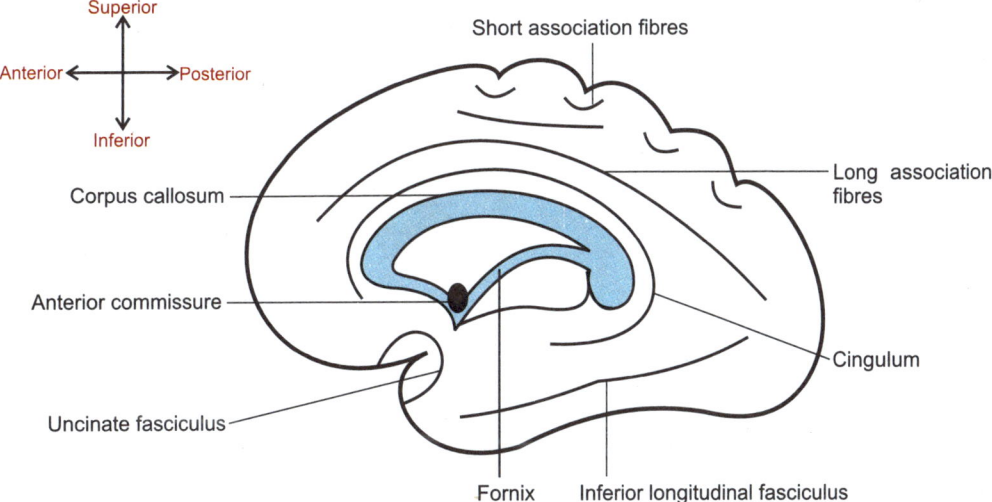

Fig. 4.57 : Medial surface of cerebral hemisphere showing whitematter.

3. **Commissural (transverse) fibres :** They connect two identical areas of one cerebral hemisphere to the other cerebral hemisphere.
   A. Corpus callosum : It is the biggest bundle of commissural fibers and connects frontal, temporal and occipital lobes.
   B. Anterior commissure : Round bundle of white matter formed by
      a. Archipallial (archi cortex) belongs to rhinencephalon and connects olfactory bulb & piriform area of both sides. It is pearshaped paleocortex present on the anterior part of parahippocampal gyrus.
      b. Neopallial : It is a larger bundle and connects two temporal lobes.
   C. Posterior commissure : It connects superior colliculi of both the sides and transmits
      a. Corticotectal fibres,
      b. Pretectal fibres.
   D. Hippocampal commissure : It is present at the junction of the posterior columns of fornix. It connects hippocampus of both sides.
   E. Habenular commissure : It connects habenular nuclei present in the Habenular triangle. It is responsible for visceral response to basic emotional drives and olfactory impulse.

4. **Projection fibres** : These are afferent and efferent fibres of cerebrum. They are
   A. Afferent :
      a. Thalamocortical :
      b. Auditory radiation
      c. Visual radiation
   B. Efferent :
      a. Corticobulbar or corticonucleur
      b. Corticospinal
      c. Corticoponto cerebellar

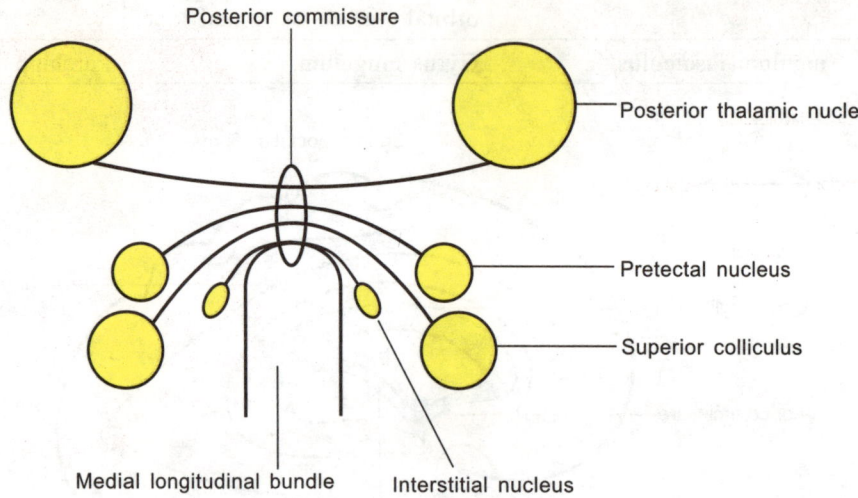

Fig. 4.58 : Commissural fibres.

LAQ-17 Describe corpus callosum under
1. Definition   2. Gross anatomy   3. Parts
4. Blood supply 5. Functions & 6. Applied anatomy.

1. **Definition** : It is the largest bundle of transverse commissural fibres which connects the two identical areas of neocortex, except the following area.
   A. *Lower and anterior parts of the temporal lobe which are connected by the anterior commissure.*
   B. *Primary visual cortex (area 17).*
   C. *Some parts of primary acoustic (area 41).*
   D. *Parts of primary somatosensory area (area 2, 1) especially those for the hand and foot.*
   E. *Part of the motor cortex (area 4) serving distal parts of the upper and lower limbs (excluding the shoulder and hip region).*

2. **Gross anatomy :**
   A. Situation : It is situated at the bottom of the median longitudinal fissure and lies nearer to frontal pole than to the occipital pole. Anterior end is about 4 cm. from frontal pole where as posterior end lies about 6 cm from occipital pole.

B.   Length : 10 cm.
C.   Type : Neopallial commissural fibres

3.   **Parts :** It has four parts.
A.   Rostrum : It extends from genu to lamina terminalis.
    a.   Fibers : It connects the orbital surfaces of frontal lobe.
    b.   Relations :
       I.   Upper surface :
          i.   In the median plane attachment of septum pellucidum and
          ii.   On each side forms floor of anterior horn of lateral ventricle.
       II.   Inferior surface :
          i.   Indusium griseum,
          ii.   Medial and lateral longitudinal striae.

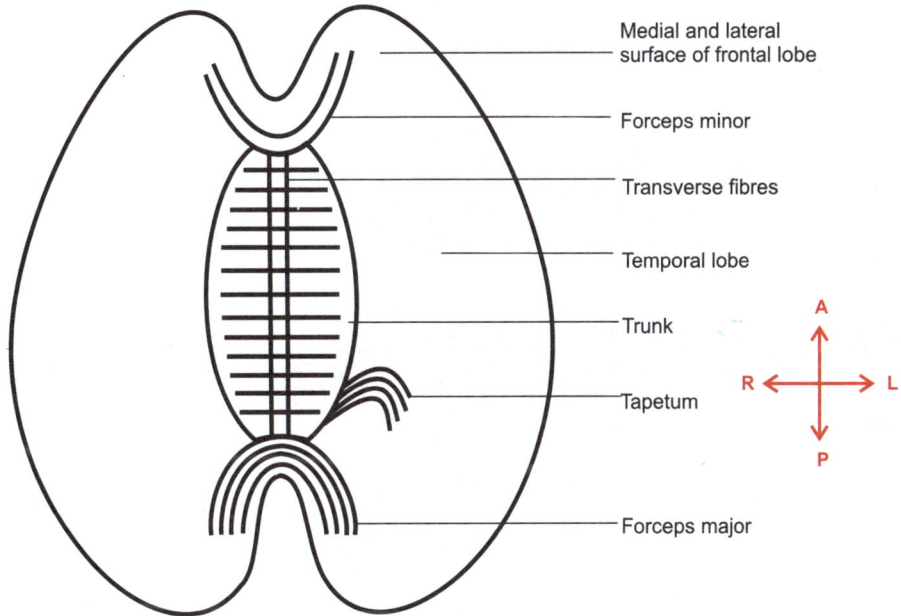

Fig. 4.59 : Fibres of corpus callosum.

B.   Genu : It is bend and thick part of corpus callosum. It is situated anteriorly and continues above and behind as trunk and below it continues as rostrum.
Fibers : It connects medial and lateral surface of frontal lobe. These fibers are called forceps minor.
C.   Trunk or body : It is major part of corpus callosum present between genu and splenium. It is one inch wide.
    a.   Fibers :
       I.   It connects the two temporal lobe.
       II.   Tapetum (*Tapetum* carpet) :
          i.   It is formed by posterior fibers of trunk and anterior fibers of splenium of corpus callosum.

    ii. These fibers run horizontally and do not intersect to the vertical running fibers of corona radiata.

    iii. They form
- Roof and lateral wall of posterior horn of lateral ventricle and the
- Lateral wall of inferior horn of the lateral ventricle.

  b. Surfaces : It has two surfaces

    I. Superior :
      i. It forms the floor of median longitudinal fissure.
      ii. It is related to anterior cerebral vessels and lower border of falx cerebri and inferior sagittal sinus.
      iii. It is covered by indusium griseum and medial and lateral longitudinal striae.
      iv. It is overlapped by cingulate gyrus but separated by callosal sulcus.

    II. Inferior : It forms roof of the body of lateral ventricle. It gives attachment to the following structures.
      i. Anteriorly and inferiorly, it gives attachment to septum pellucidum.
      ii. Posteriorly, it gives attachment to fornix and hippocampal commissure.

D. Splenium : It is posterior and thickest end of corpus callosum.

  a. Fibers : It connects the right and left occipital lobe. These fibers are called forceps major.

  b. Relations :

    I. Superiorly :
      i. It is covered by indusium griseum.
      ii. It is related to inferior border of falx cerebri which contains inferior sagittal sinus.
      iii. It is covered by cingulate gyrus on each side.

    II. Inferiorly : Formation of straight sinus.

4. Blood supply :

A. Arterial supply :

  a. Rostrum is supplied by central branches of anterior cerebral artery.

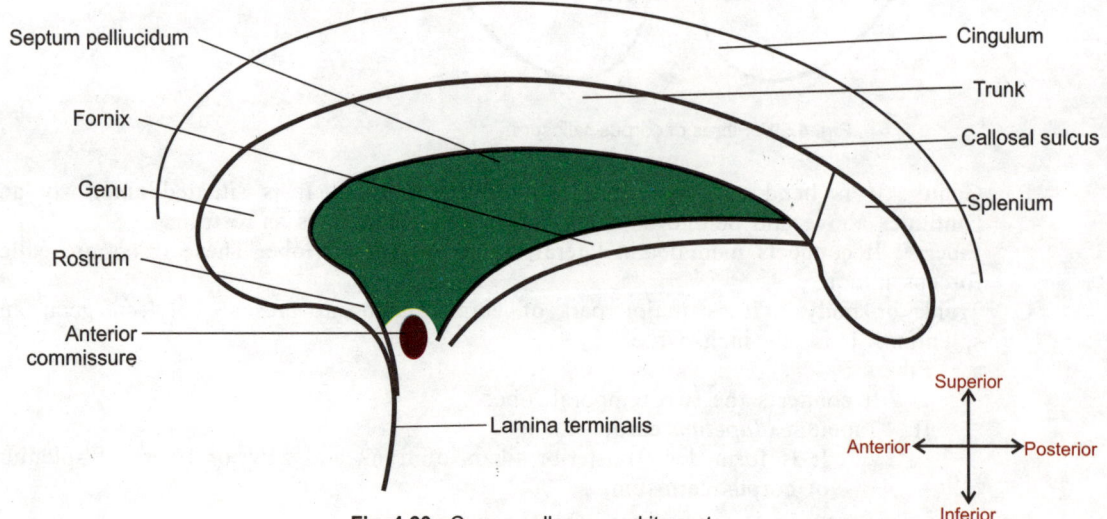

Fig. 4.60 : Corpus callosum and its parts.

b. Genu and trunk are supplied by frontal branches of anterior cerebral artery.

c. Splenium is supplied by posterior cerebral artery.

B. Venous drainage : It is drained by

a. Anterior cerebral vein and

b. Choroid vein.

5. **Functions :**

A. Transfer of learning process : The secondary sensory areas receive input, interprets and sends copy to the opposite cerebral cortex for processing and for storage in the form of memory through corpus callosum.

B. Transfer of speech function.

C. It possibly helps in coordination of activities of two cerebral hemisphere, but congenital absence of corpus callosum do not cause any functional disturbance.

6. **Applied anatomy :**

A. A lesion of the splenium of the corpus callosum affects the transfer of information from the right visual association cortex to the left side.

B. Patients with a lesion of the corpus callosum responds as if he or she has two separate brains called 'split brain'.

C. The section of the corpus callosum has been attempted surgically to prevent the spread of seizures from one hemisphere to the other.

LAQ-18 **Describe internal capsule under**
1. Definition **2. Gross anatomy** **3. Fibers**
4. Blood supply **5. Applied anatomy.**

1. **Definition :** It is a narrow gate, consists of compact bundle of ascending and descending fibers which connects the cerebral cortex to the brain stem and spinal cord.

2. **Gross anatomy :**

A. Communication :

a. It continues above as corona radiata.

b. It continues below as cerebral peduncle.

B. Shape : In horizontal section it appears 'V' shaped mass.

C. Parts and boundaries :

a. Anterior limb : Lies between head of caudate nucleus and lentiform nucleus.

b. Posterior limb : It is related medially to thalamus and laterally to lentiform nucleus.

c. Genu (Bend part of internal capsule) : It is present between anterior and posterior limb.

d. Retro lentiform part : It is present behind lentiform nucleus.

e. Sublentiform part : It lies deep to lentiform nucleus.

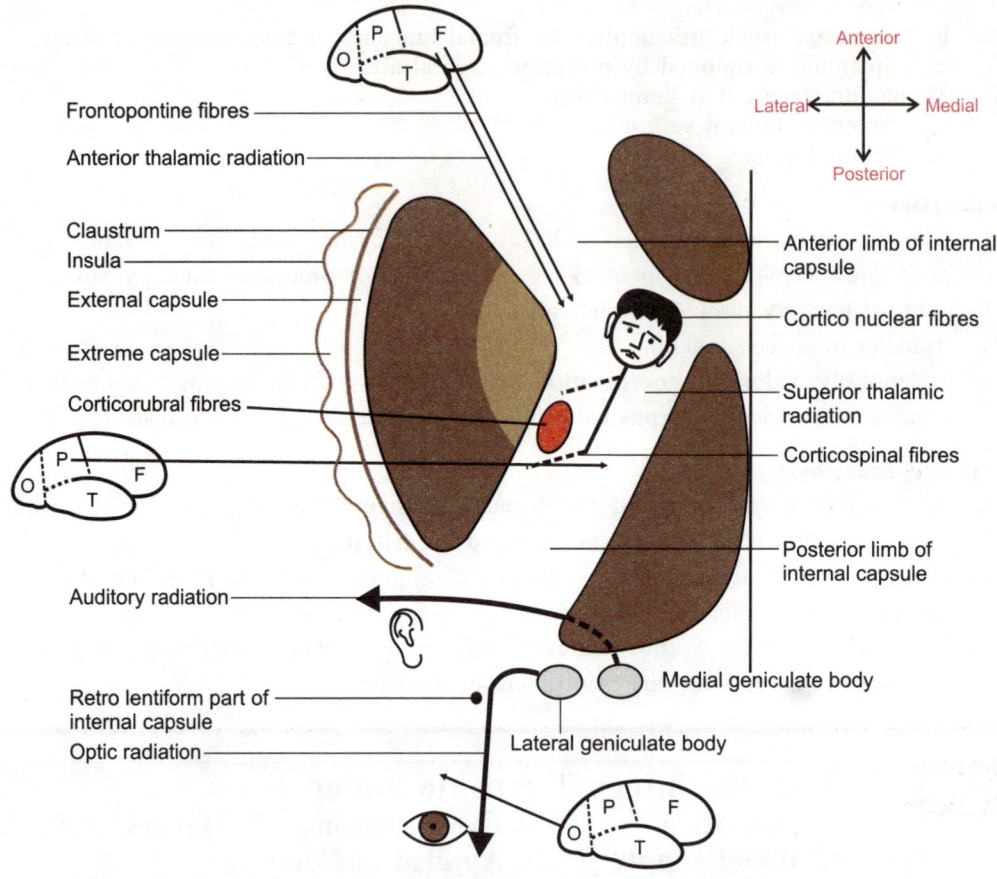

Fig. 4.61 : Internal capsule and its parts.

3. **Fibers :**

Table 4.20 : The table shows parts of internal capsule and fibers present in it.

Parts	Descending tract	Ascending tract
A. Anterior limb	Frontopontine fibres	Anterior thalamic radiation (from anterior & medial nucleus of thalamus).
B. Genu	a. Corticonuclear fibres and b. Corticoreticular	Anterior part of superior thalamic radiation (from posterior ventral nucleus of thalamus).
C. Posterior limb a. Anterior 2/3rd	a. Corticospinal tract b. Parieto pontine	Superior thalamic radiation.
b. Posterior 1/3rd	Corticorubral.	Thalamocortical fibres from ventroposterolateral nucleus to post central gyrus.

Table 4.21 : The table shows retrolentiform and sublentiform of the internal capsule and the tracts present in it.

Parts	Descending tract ↓	Ascending tract ↑
D. Retro lentiform part.	a. Occipitopontine fibres. b. Fibres from occipital cortex to superior colliculus & pretectal region.	Posterior thalamic radiation made up of a. Optic radiation b. Visual pathway : Connections between parieto occipital lobes to posterior part of thalamus.
E. Sublentiform part.	Temporopontine fibres : Inter connections between temporal lobe & thalamus.	Auditory radiation : Inferior thalamic radiation

4. Blood supply :

Table 4.22 : The table shows arterial supply to different parts of internal capsule.

Particulars	Upper	Lower
Anterior limb	Middle cerebral artery (Internal carotid artery)	Anterior cerebral artery (Internal carotid artery)
Genu	Middle cerebral artery (Internal carotid artery)	Recurrent branch of anterior cerebral (Heubner artery)
Posterior limb	*Artery of cerebral haemorrhage* (Middle cerebral artery)	Anterior choroidal artery (internal carotid artery)
Retro-lentiform	Posterior cerebral artery (Basilar artery)	
Sublentiform	Anterior choroidal artery (Internal carotid artery)	

5. Applied anatomy :

A. A small lesion in internal capsule results in widespread manifestation. The common lesion is due to cerebral haemorrhage or cerebral thrombosis. It results in complete hemiplegia on the opposite side. If the posterior part is involved, there will be hemianaesthesia.

B. There is homonymous hemianopia if the fibers of optic radiation are involved.

C. There is aphasia, if lesion is in dominant hemisphere.

D. *The artery commonly ruptured is medial striate artery, branch of middle cerebral artery.*
It is also called as artery of cerebral haemorrhage (Charcots artery). Following are the reasons for rupture of middle cerebral artery.
  a. It is a long artery,
  b. It is a thin artery,
  c. It is not supported by connective tissue and
  d. It is constantly exposed for the fluctuations of blood pressure.

E. Capsular lesions usually are vascular due to involvement of middle cerebral artery, giving rise to hemiplegia on opposite half of body. The condition is called upper motor neuron lesion.

SN-31   Choroid plexus

1. **Introduction :** It is tuft of capillaries covered by piamater and ependymal cells which are simple, ciliated columnar epithelium lining the ventricles of brain.

2. **Gross anatomy :**
    A.   Site : Present at the site where piamater and ependyma come close together.
         Examples :
         a.   Central part and inferior horn of lateral ventricle.
         b.   Roof of third ventricle.
         c.   Roof of fourth ventricle.
    B.   Structure : Consists of minute tuft of capillaries covered by piamater and ependyma.
    C.   Age changes : Calcification of choroid plexus occurs in late age.
         It is present at the junction of body and inferior horn of lateral ventricle.

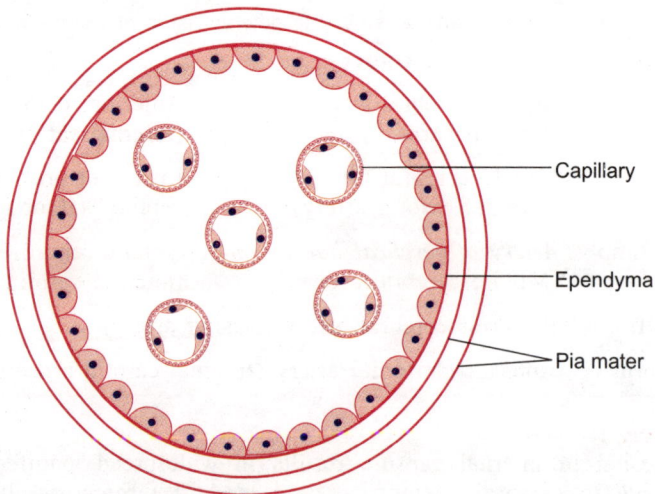

Fig. 4.62 : Choroid plexus.

3. **Blood supply :**
    A.   Arterial supply :
         a.   Anterior choroidal artery, branch of internal carotid artery.
         b.   Posterior choroidal artery, branch of posterior cerebral artery.
         c.   Posterior inferior cerebellar artery, (largest branch of vertebral artery).
    B.   Venous drainage by choroid vein, combines with thalamostriate vein - to form internal cerebral vein - great cerebral vein - straight sinus - transverse sinus - sigmoid sinus.

4. **Functions :** Formation of cerebrospinal fluid by ultrafiltration.

5. **Applied :**
    A.   Hydrocephalus : The blockage of cerebrospinal fluid is due to the choroid plexus tumour.
    B.   Calcification of choroid plexus can be visualised by radiography, which is important in differentiating tumor of pineal gland.

SN-32 Inter peduncular fossa

1. **Introduction** : It is a lozenge shaped space present between the cerebral peduncles of the midbrain.

2. **Gross anatomy :**
   A. Shape : Rhomboid.
   B. Boundaries :
      a. Anteromedially : Optic chiasma.
      b. Anterolaterally : Optic tract.
      c. Posteriorly : Upper border of pons.
      d. Postero laterally : Crus cerebri.
   C. Forms : Floor of IIIrd ventricle.
   D. Contents from before backward :
      a. Tuber cinerium : Slightly raised area of grey matter between mamillary body and optic chiasma.

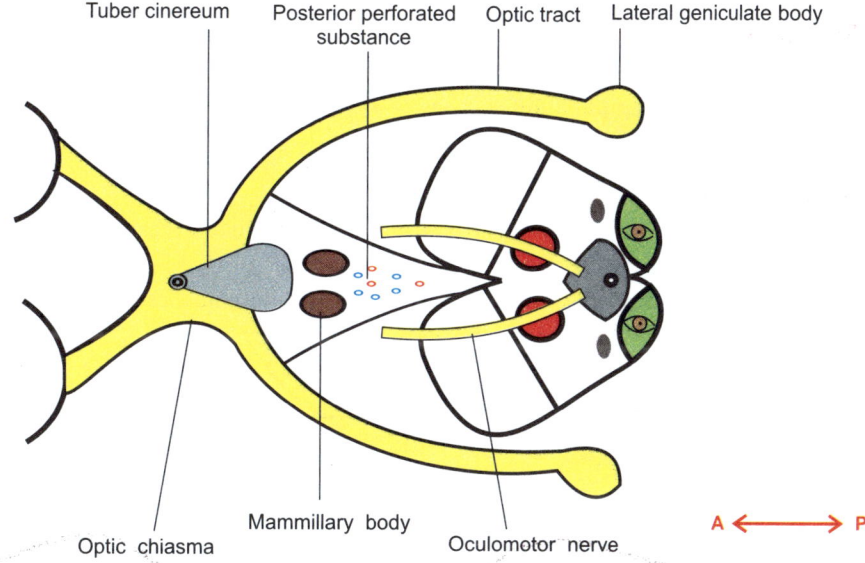

Fig. 4.63 : Inter peduncular fossa.

   b. Infundibulum : It suspends hypophysis cerebri.
   c. Posterior perforated substance : It is grey matter perforated by posterior cerebral arteries & inferior cerebellar arteries.
   E. Relations :
      a. Anterolateral : Anterior cerebral artery.
      b. Posterior : Posterior cerebral artery.
      c. Posterolateral : Posterior communicating artery.

3. **Applied :**
   A. Aneurysm of circle of Willis compresses optic chiasma and results into hemianopia.
   B. The pressure on hypophysis cerebri produces bitemporal hemianopia due to interruption of crossed nasal fibres.

SN-33   Arachnoid granulations (Pacchionian bodies)

1. **Introduction :** These are finger like projections, which project into dural venous sinuses. These are due to collection of arachnoid villi, which are the sites for the absorption of cerebro spinal fluid.

2. **Situation :** They are situated along the sides of superior sagittal sinus, present on the medial border of parietal bone.

3. **Structures :**
   A. These are small, granular bodies.
   B. Each arachnoid villus is a diverticulum in the subarachnoid space.
   C. It is covered by a thin cell layer which in turn is covered by endothelium of venous sinus.
   D. Age change : It erodes the inner table of skull as the age advances.

4. **Functions :**
   A. It is a main site for absorption of cerebrospinal fluid.
   B. It allows cerebrospinal fluid to pass to the venous spaces.
   C. It prevents reflux of blood.

5. **Applied Anatomy :**
   A. Clotting of blood in the superior sagittal sinus blocks these safety valves and causes rapid increase in cerebrospinal fluid.
   B. The granulations increase with the advance of age and therefore the age of person can be roughly determined by presence of granulations.
   C. Congenital absence of the arachnoid granulations is observed in hydrocephalus.

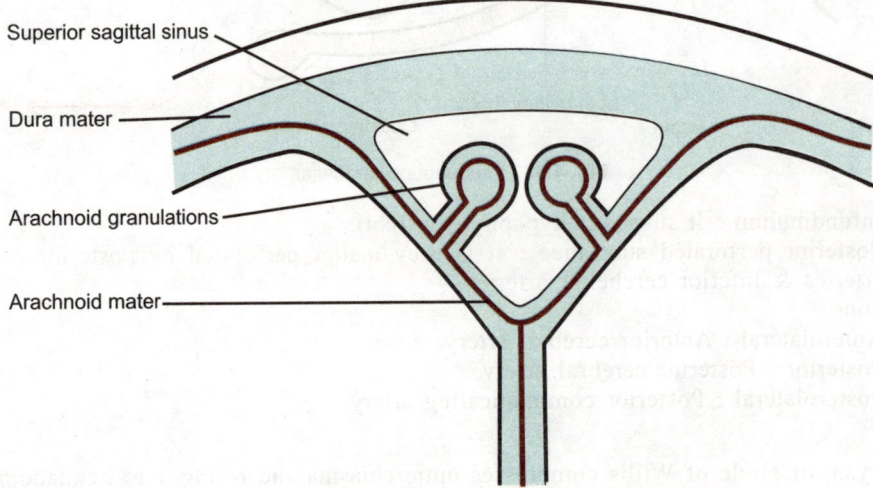

Fig. 4.64 : Arachnoid granulations.

SN-34   Cisterna magna (cisterna medullaris)

Cisterna Cavity, closed sac.

1. **Introduction :** It is an enlarged subarachnoid space between the anteroinferior surface of cerebellum and posterior surface of medulla oblongata.

2. **Shape :** It is triangular in sagittal section.

3. **Relations :**
   A. Anteriorly : Posterior surface of medulla oblongata.
   B. Posteriorly : Anterior and inferior surface of cerebellum.

4. **Communications :**
   A. It receives cerebrospinal fluid from -
      a. Roof of fourth ventricle (through foramen of Magendi).
      b. Lateral recess of fourth ventricle (through foramina of Lushka).
   B. It communicates
      a. Inferiorly : With spinal subarachnoid space.
      b. Anteriorly : With pontine cistern.

5. **Applied anatomy :**
   A. Cisternal puncture : Cerebrospinal fluid can be tapped through the posterior atlanto - occipital membrane.
   B. Tumour in the space obstructs the circulation of CSF and results into hydrocephalus.

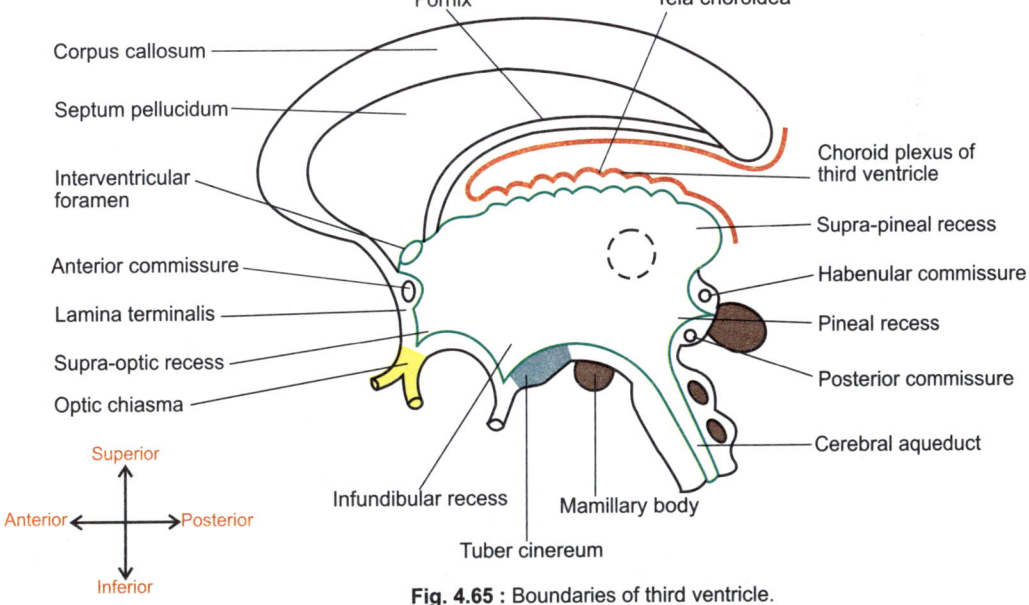

Fig. 4.65 : Boundaries of third ventricle.

LAQ-19 — Describe third ventricle under
1. **Gross anatomy**
2. **Boundaries**
3. **Recesses &**
4. **Applied anatomy.**

1. Gross anatomy :

A. **Introduction :** It is a narrow, midline cavity present between two diencephalon of cerebral hemisphere.

B. **Extent :** It extends from lamina terminalis to upper end of cerebral aqueduct.

C. **Communications :**

   a. Cranially it communicates with both lateral ventricles through interventricular foramen.

   b. Caudally it communicates, with fourth ventricle through cerebral aqueduct.

2. Boundaries :

A. **Roof is formed by**

   a. **Ependyma :** It is thin membrane lined by cuboidal or columnar epithelium. It lines the ventricle and stretches across the thalamus.

   b. **Tela choroidea :** It is a fold of piamater projecting into ventricle.

   c. **Body of fornix :** It is a prominent bundle of fibres present on the medial aspect of cerebral hemisphere. It arises from hippocampus and is suspended from corpus callosum by septum pellucidum.

B. **Floor is formed by following structures from anterior to posterior.** 🔑 **OT IMP**

   a. **O**ptic chiasma : Crossing of the optic nerves.

   b. **T**uber cinereum (*tuber* tubercle; *cinerieum* ash colour) : It is ash colored elevation formed by grey matter present between mamillary body and optic chiasma.

   c. **I**nfundibulum : It is a funnel shaped structure of the stalk of pituitary gland.

   d. **M**ammillary body : It is an important part of limbic system.

   e. **P**osterior perforated substance : It is a triangular interval between mamillary bodies and the midbrain which is pierced by numerous blood vessels.

   f. Tegmentum of midbrain : It is a part of cerebral peduncle of midbrain.

C. **Anterior wall : From above downwards**

   a. **Anterior column of fornix :** The body of fornix anteriorly divides into anterior column of fornix. It contains important connections of limbic system. It correlates olfactory and visceral activities.

   b. **Anterior commissure :** It is a round bundle of white matter formed by

   I. **Archipallial (archi cortex) :** It belongs to rhinencephalon and connects olfactory bulb and piriform area of both the sides (pearshape paleocortex present on the anterior part of parahippocampal gyrus).

   II. **Neopallial :** It is a larger commissure which connects two temporal lobes.

   III. **Lamina terminals :** *Thin plate derived from telencephalon (cranial end of neural tube)* extending from rostrum of corpus callosum to dorsum of optic chiasma. It is encroached by anterior commissure in the upper part.

D. Posterior wall :
  a. Pineal body : It is a small conical organ present between and above two superior colliculi.
  b. Posterior commissure : It connects two superior colliculi and also contains
     I. Corticotectal fibres and
     II. Pretectal fibres.
  c. Cerebral aqueduct.
E. Lateral wall :
  a. Anteriorly : Anterior column of fornix.
  b. In upper part :
     I. Anterior $2/3^{rd}$ of thalamus &
     II. Interthalamic connexus.
  c. Lower part :
     I. Lower part of thalamus.
     II. Hypothalamic sulcus : Separates thalamus & hypothalamus & represents sulcus limitans of diencephalon.

3. **Recesses :** These are prolongations of the 3rd ventricular cavity. These are described as :
   A. Anteriorly :
     a. Anterior recess : It is present between anterior column of fornix and anterior commissure.
     b. Optic recess : It is present at the junction of anterior boundary and floor immediately above optic chiasma.
   B. In the floor : Infundibular recess : It is present in the stalk of infundibulum.
   C. Posteriorly :
     a. Pineal recess : In stalk of pineal body.
     b. Suprapineal recess : It is present above the pineal body.

4. **Applied anatomy :**
   A. Ventriculography : It is a visualization of ventricles for determining obstruction or dilatation of third ventricle.
   B. Obstruction of third ventricle leads to raised intracranial pressure in adults and hydrocephalus in infants.

SN-35   Parts of lateral ventricle

1. **Introduction :** It is a cavity of telencephalon, situated one in each cerebral hemisphere.

2. **Communication :** It communicates with the third ventricle through interventricular foramen or foramen of Monro.

3. **Situation :** It is situated lateral to septum pellucidum and below corpus callosum.

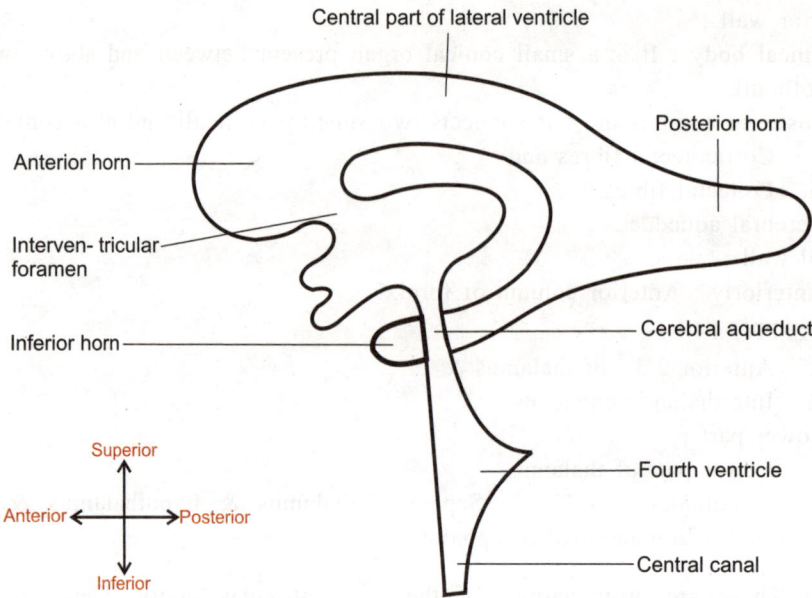

Fig. 4.66 : Parts of lateral ventricle.

4. **Content** : It contains
   A. Cerebrospinal fluid.
   B. Chlorid plexus in the central part and inferior horn of lateral ventricle.

5. **Lining** : It is lined by ependyma, a thin membrane.

6. **Parts** : It has
   A. Anterior horn.
   B. Central part.
   C. Posterior horn.
   D. Inferior horn.

7. **Development** : It is developed from cavity of telencephalon of neural tube.

8. **Applied anatomy** : The blockage of interventricular foramina results into
   A. Hydrocephalus : Excessive accumulation of cerebro spinal fluid into lateral ventricle.
   B. Increased intracranial pressure.

| SN-36 | **Inferior horn of lateral ventricle** | Imp. |

1. **Introduction** : It is the largest and longest of the three horns of lateral ventricle. It is direct continuation of the main ventricular cavity.

2. **Gross anatomy** :
   A. Situation : It is present in the temporal lobe.

B. Direction : It first extends backwards and laterally around the pulvinar (*pulvinar cushion*) the end of thalamus. It lies deep to the superior temporal sulcus and extends about an inch behind the temporal lobe.

3. **Boundaries :** It consists of roof and floor.

A. Roof : It is sloping and continues as lateral wall of inferior horn of lateral ventricle. It is formed by

    a. Lateral part of the tapetum of the corpus callosum. .

        I. The fibers of the tapetum are formed by posterior fibers of trunk and anterior fibers of splenium.

        II. These fibers do not intersect corona radiata fibers.

    b. The tail of caudate nucleus :

        It is a one of the important nucleus of basal nuclei. It is a part of neostriatum.

    c. Amygdaloid body : It is a part of limbic system and belongs to archistriatum.

    d. Stria terminalis : These are projection fibers of the amygdaloid nucleus. It connects amygdaloid nucleus to -

        I. Septal nuclei,

        II. Hypothalamic nuclei and

        III. Thalamic nuclei.

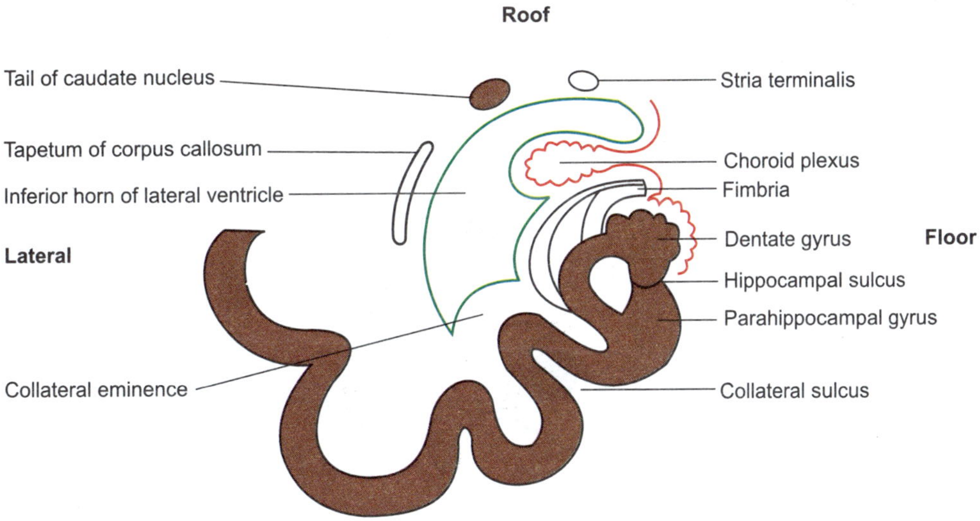

Fig. 4.67 : Inferior horn of lateral ventricle.

B. Floor : Floor of the inferior horn presents following feature from medial to lateral.

    a. Choroid plexus : It is present most medially, it extends into the inferior horn through a choroid fissure between the fimbria (fringe) and the stria terminalis.

    b. Fimbria (fringe) : The white matter of hippocampus is alveus. The fibers of the alveus (*alveus* trough द्रोण, पाट) converge backwards and medially to form fimbria. It is continuous with the crus of fornix below the splenium.

c. Hippocampus : It is an elevation belonging to limbic system. It resembles seahorse (पाणघोडा) hence called hippocampus. It lies medial to collateral eminence. It presents an enlarged anterior end with oblique grooves, which resembles paws of an animal. The fibers derived from the hippocampus form a thin sheath called alveus. It covers the ventricular surface of hippocampus.

d. Collateral eminence : It is an elevation formed by projection of collateral sulcus. It forms a triangular area called collateral trigon. It is present at the junction of the floor of the posterior and inferior horn of lateral ventricle.

4. **Surgical approach of the inferior horn** : A needle is introduced in the inferior horn through a hole at a point, 3 cm behind and above the center of external acoustic meatus. The needle is passed in the direction of apex of the opposite auricle. It is about 5 cm from the surface.

SN-37   Posterior horn of lateral ventricle

1. **Introduction** : It is a part of lateral ventricle which lies behind the splenium of corpus callosum.

2. **Gross anatomy :**
    A. Situation : It is present in the occipital lobe.
    B. Variation : It may be absent and may be of variable size.
    C. Direction : Backwards and medially.

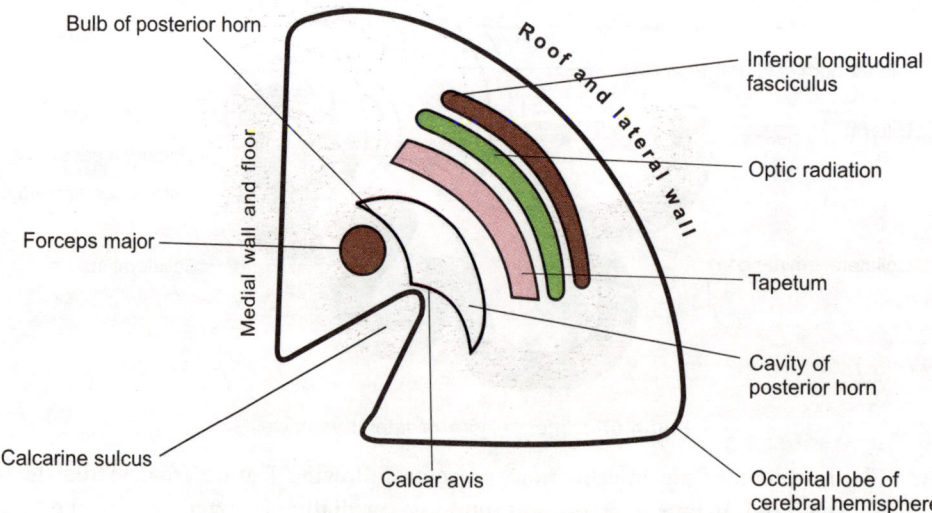

Fig. 4.68 : Posterior horn of lateral ventricle.

3. **Boundaries :**
    A. Medial wall and floor : It is formed by
        a. Bulb of the posterior horn :   ⚷━ **BPH**   It is a raised area formed by forceps major. These are commissural fibers connecting two occipital lobes.

b. Calcar avis (*calcar* spur काटा , *avis* bird) : It is a raised area formed by anterior part of calcarine sulcus.

B. Roof and lateral wall : It is formed by
   a. Inferior longitudinal fasciculus. (It is an example of association fibers).
   b. Optic radiation : The fibers of the optic radiation arises from lateral geniculate body and terminate in the visual area of the occipital lobe (areas 17, 18 and 19). (It is an example of projection fibers).
   c. Tapetum of the corpus callosum. (It is an example of commissural fibers).

SN-38   Central part of lateral ventricle

1. **Extent :** It extends from interventricular foramen (foramen of Monro) to splenium of corpus callosum.

2. **Roof :** It is formed by inferior surface of body of corpus callosum.

3. **Floor :** It is formed by
   A. Body of caudate nucleus. It is separated from corona radiata by the frontooccipital fasciculus.
   B. Thalamostriate groove which contains
      a. Striata terminalis : These are projection fibers of the amygdaloid body. It connects amygdaloid nucleus to
         I. Septal,
         II. Hypothalamic and
         III. Thalamic nuclei.
      b. Thalamostriate vein.

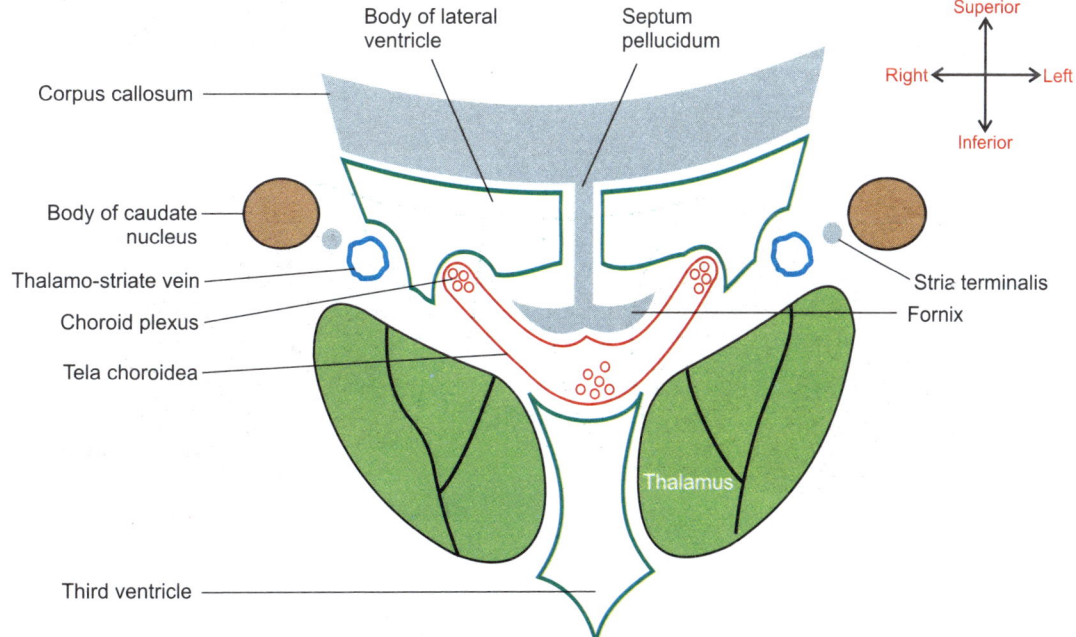

Fig. 4.69 : Central part of lateral ventricle.

C. Lateral part of upper surface of thalamus.
D. Fornix : It is a bundle of fibers connecting right and left hippocampus.
E. Choroid fissure : It is a slit like interval between the edge of the fornix and the upper surface of thalamus through which the choroid plexus enters the ventricles by invaginating the ependyma.

4. **Medial wall :** It is formed by
A. Posterior part of septum pellucidum is present antero-superiorly.
B. Body of fornix is present postero-inferiorly.

SN-39   Anterior horn of lateral ventricle

1. **Situation :** It is situated anterior to interventricular foramen.

2. **Extent :** It extends forwards, laterally and downward in the frontal lobe of the brain.
It is continuous with the central part posteriorly at the interventricular foramen.
It presents a triangular outline in coronal section and possesses a roof, a floor, medial wall, lateral wall and anterior wall.

3. **Roof :** It is formed by
A. Anterior part of body of corpus callosum and
B. Posterior part of genu of corpus callosum.

4. **Floor :** It is formed by
A. Medially : Rostrum of corpus callosum.
B. Laterally : Head of caudate nucleus.

5. **Medial wall :** Anterior part of septum pellucidum.

6. **Anterior wall :** Genu and rostrum of corpus callosum.

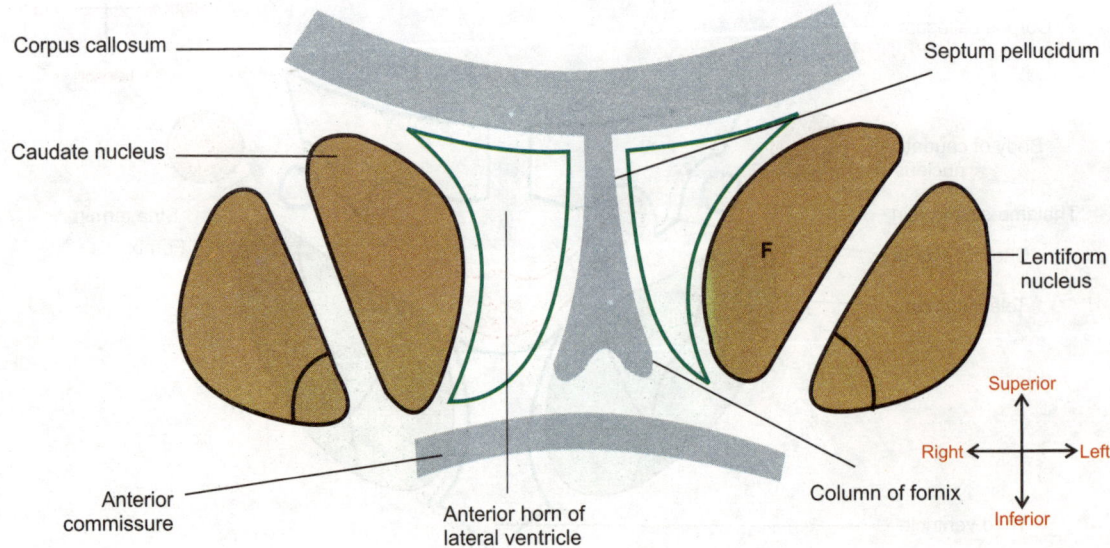

Fig. 4.70 : Anterior horn of lateral ventricle.

LAQ-20   Describe cortico spinal tract or pyramidal tract and the effects of the lesion.

1. **Functions :** The pyramidal tract is concerned with skilled, voluntary movements of non-postural type.

2. **Features :**
   A. Origin : The axons of the pyramidal tract arises from pyramidal cells of cerebral cortex.
   B. Source of the fibers :
      a. $1/3^{rd}$ fibers arise from upper $2/3^{rd}$ of pre-central gyrus. (area No. 4).
      b. $1/3^{rd}$ fibers arise from premotor cortex (area No. 6).
      c. $1/3^{rd}$ fibers arise from post central gyrus (somatosensory cortex area 3, 1, 2).
      d. Remaining fibers arise from adjacent parietal cortex (area No. 5).
   C. Types of fibers : Myelinated and relatively low conducting small fibers.
   D. Termination of fibers :
      a. 55% of the cortico spinal fibers are concerned with the muscles of the upper limb.
      b. 20% fibers are concerned with the muscles of the trunk.
      c. 25% fibers are concerned with the muscles of the lower limb.

3. **Course :**
   A. After arising from different areas of cerebral cortex, they pass through -
      a. Corona radiata, of cerebral cortex.
      b. Anterior $2/3^{rd}$ of posterior limb of internal capsule.
      c. Middle $2/3^{rd}$ of crus cerebri of cerebral peduncle of mid brain.
      d. Basilar part of pons through pontine nuclei.
      e. Anterior part of medulla oblongata and fibers start decussating.
      f. 90% fibres decussate and travel through lateral column of spinal cord and hence called lateral corticospinal tract.
      Almost 98% fibers end by synapsing with interneurons, which in turn project to alpha and gama motor neurons of the anterior horn.
      The 2% fibers that synapse directly with motor neurons are those which originate from the giant Betz cells.
   B. Termination : Most of the fibers terminate in the lamina of IVth to VIIth of spinal grey and through the interneurons. These fibers are connected to the alpha and gama motor neurons of the lamina IX.
   C. Somatotopic representation : It is represented as follows
      a. In cerebral cortex
         I. Paracentral lobule   - leg.
         II. Superomedial border   - knee joint
            i. Upper limb, $\Bigg\}$ On the precentral gyrus.
            ii. Hand,

      Representation depends upon the skilled activities of the muscles, not in proportion to the bulk of the muscle.

      Note : The muscles of the hand have more representation and thumb has maximum representation. The muscles of face have more representation and in face, upper and lower lip has maximum representation.

b. In internal capsule, it occupies anterior 2/3rd of posterior limb.
   I. Upper limb : Near genu,
   II. Lower limb : Posteriorly.
c. In midbrain, it occupies middle 2/3rd of crus cerebri
   I. Upper limb : Medially,
   II. Lower limb : Laterally.
d. In pons, through the pontine nuclei of basilar part.
e. The decussation of the fibres starts at the upper part and completes at lower part of medulla oblongata.
   I. Eighty five to ninety percent fibres cross and occupy lateral column - as lateral corticospinal tract.
   II. Fifteen percent of fibres do not cross and occupy anterior column and are called as anterior corticospinal tract.
f. In spinal cord, the arrangement in lateral corticospinal tract is as follows :
   I. Leg : Laterally,   L for L
   II. Upper limb : Medially.

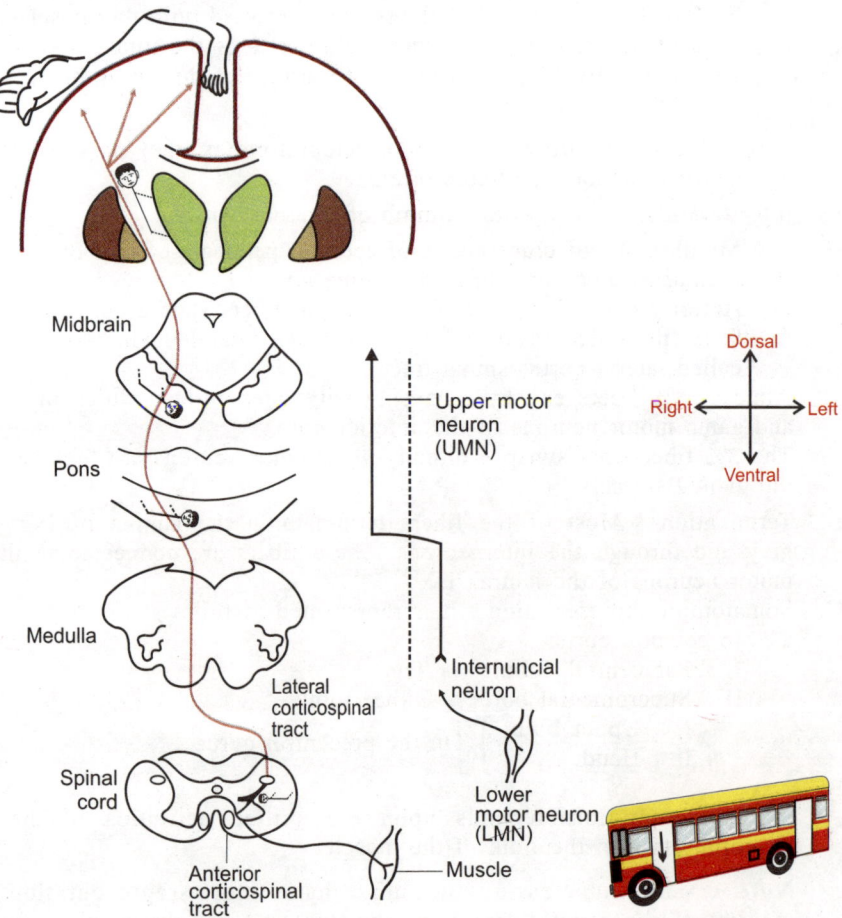

Fig. 4.71 : Cortico spinal tract.

4. **Applied** : Effects of lesion of corticospinal tract are
   A. The lesion anywhere above the synapse with the motor nuclei of lamina IX is called upper motor neuron lesion and the lesion anywhere after the synapse is lower motor neuron lesion.
   B. The most common cause for the upper motor neuron, is lesion in the internal capsule. The most common cause for the lower motor neuron is polio myelitis.
   C. The lesion above the level of decussation results into paralysis of the muscles of the upper and lower limbs on the opposite side.
   D. The lesions below the decussation results in the paralysis of the muscles of the limbs on the same side of the body.
   E. Characteristic features of upper motor neuron lesions are
      a. The muscles are not paralyzed but are weak and control on them is lost. Since upper motor neurons do not innervate muscles directly, there is no loss of muscle tone and no wasting of the affected muscles.
      b. The lower motor neurons are released from cortical control. As a result they become hyperactive leading to :
         I. Spasticity of muscles (spastic paralysis),
         II. Muscle twitching and
         III. Exaggerated tendon reflexes.
      c. Babinski sign is positive in lesion of corticospinal tract. It is clinical sign, in which great toe becomes dorsiflexed and other toes fan out in response to scratching of the skin along the lateral aspect of the sole of the foot. (The normal response is plantar flexion of all the toes).

LAQ-21 : Describe posterior column/tract of Goll and Burdach/fasciculus gracilis and cuneatus/tract of conscious proprioceptive impulses

1. **Introduction :** It is an ascending tract present in the posterior column of spinal cord and carries sensations from upper limb, lower limb and trunk.

2. **Functions :** It carries following sensations.

Table 4.23 : The table shows receptors of different sensations and their locations.

Sensations	Receptors	Situation
A. Pressure, B. Vibration.	Pacinian corpuscle.	Subcutaneous.
C. Movement, D. Position of body.	Muscles spindle, Golgi tendon organ.	Muscle.
E. Touch - a. Tactile localisation, b. Tactile discrimination, c. Stereognosis.	Meissner's corpuscle.	Dermis.
F. Sense of distension of bladder and rectum.	------	-----

3. **Origin** : The fibers of the posterior column arise from respective receptors present in the skin.

 A. Ist order neuron :
   a.   The peripheral process (of posterior column) begins from respective receptors and goes to cell body situated in dorsal root ganglion.
   b.   The central process enters the spinal cord and terminate in the nucleus gracilis and cuneatus located in medulla oblongata.

 B. IInd order neuron : It begins from nucleus gracilis and fibres deccussate in the medulla oblongata and form medial lemniscus, this is called sensory decussation.

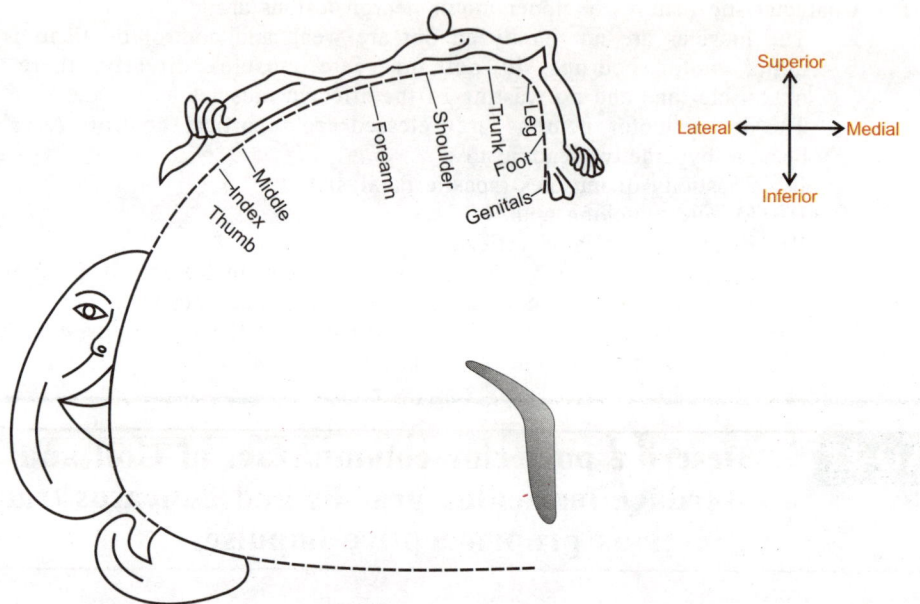

Fig. 4.72 : Sensory homunculus illustrating somatotopic organisation of the primary somatosensory cortex.

   a.   Pons : The fibres of the medial lemniscus ascend through tegmental part of pons and lies medial to the trigeminal lemniscus and lateral to trapezoid body.
   b.   Midbrain :
     I.   At the level of inferior colliculus : The medial lemniscus occupies tegmental part of midbrain and lies lateral to tegmental decussation and medial to trigeminal lemniscus.
     II. At the level of superior colliculus : The red nucleus appears and it pushes medial lemniscus laterally. And a band of lemniscus is placed antero-posteriorly.
   c.   Thalamus : ⚷ **VPL** The fibers reach to <u>v</u>entral <u>p</u>osterior <u>l</u>ateral nucleus of thalamus.

 C. IIIrd order neuron : The fibers start from ventro postero lateral nucleus of thalamus and passes through posterior 1/3rd of posterior limb of internal capsule and reach to post central gyrus of cerebral cortex (area 3, 1 and 2).

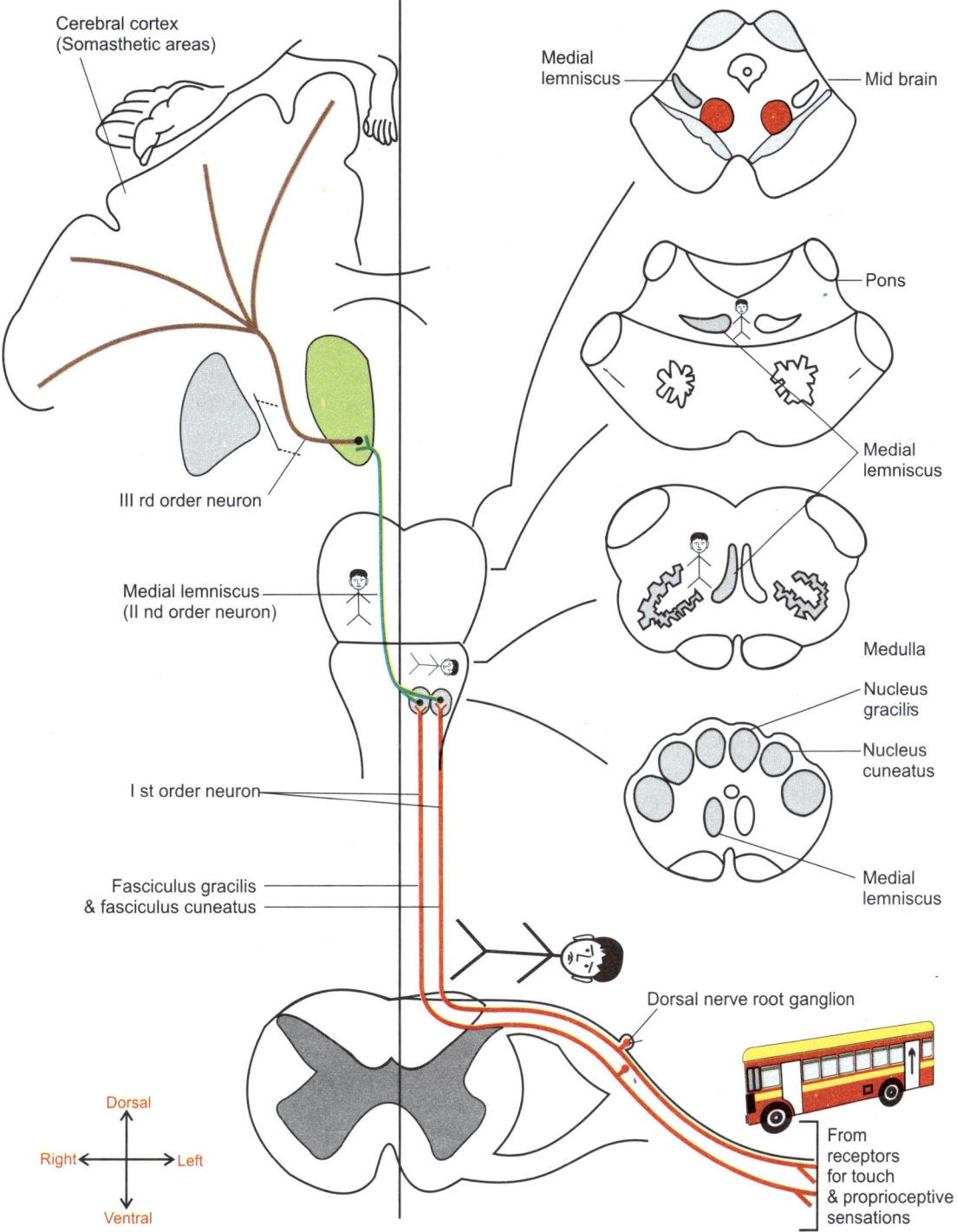

Fig. 4.73 : Posterior column.

4. **Somatotopic representation :**
   A. Spinal cord :
      a. The fasciculus gracilis carries fibres from lower limb, perineum and lower trunk. The fasciculus cuneatus carries fibers from upper limb and upper trunk.
      b. The fasciculus gracilis lies medially and fasciculus cuneatus lies laterally.
   B. Medulla oblongata and pons : In medial lemniscus, fibers of lower limb are placed anteriorly and the fibers of upper limb are placed posteriorly.
   C. Cerebral cortex : The fibers of the upper limb and lower limb, head, face and neck are arranged in upside down manner in the following sequence on post central gyrus.
      a. Lower limb : Paracentral lobule.
      b. Trunk : Superomedial border.
      c. Upper limb : On upper part of post central gyrus.
      d. Hand, thumb, face, larynx, pharynx : In the lower part of post central gyrus.
      Here representation is according to density of receptors.

5. **Modality representation :** In spinal cord, the fibers of the different modalities are arranged from posterior to anterior as follows :   🗝 **Pressure ViMP**
   A. Pressure,
   B. Vibration,
   C. Movement,
   D. Position and
   E. Touch.
      a. Tactile localisation.
      b. Tactile discrimination.
      c. Sterognosis.

6. **Applied anatomy :**
   A. Certain degenerative disorders selectively destroy the gracile and cuneate funiculi. These include
      a. Syphilis (tabes dorsalis),
      b. Vitamin B deficiency (subacute combined degeneration) etc.
      Characteristic features :
         I. There is impairment of proprioceptive sensibility. The patient loses the sense of tactile discrimination, vibration, passive movement and appreciation of posture.
         II. There is also an inability to maintain balance when the eyes are closed (Romberg's sign).
         III. Light and crude touch is not affected as this modality is also served by the spinothalamic tract.
         IV. There will be difficulty with walking in the dark or keeping the balance when washing the face with the eyes shut.
   B. Tabes dorsalis : It occurs in syphilis. The organisms responsible for syphilis cause selective destruction of dorsal nerve root fibers at the point of their entrance into the spinal cord, especially in the lower thoracic and lumbosacral regions.
      a. Stabbing pain in the lower limbs.
      b. Paraesthesia with numbness in the lower limbs.
      c. Hypersensitivity of skin to touch, heat and cold.
      d. Loss of cutaneous sensation in parts of trunk and lower limbs.
      e. Loss of awareness that the urinary bladder is full.
      f. Loss of appreciation of posture or passive movements of the limbs, especially the legs.

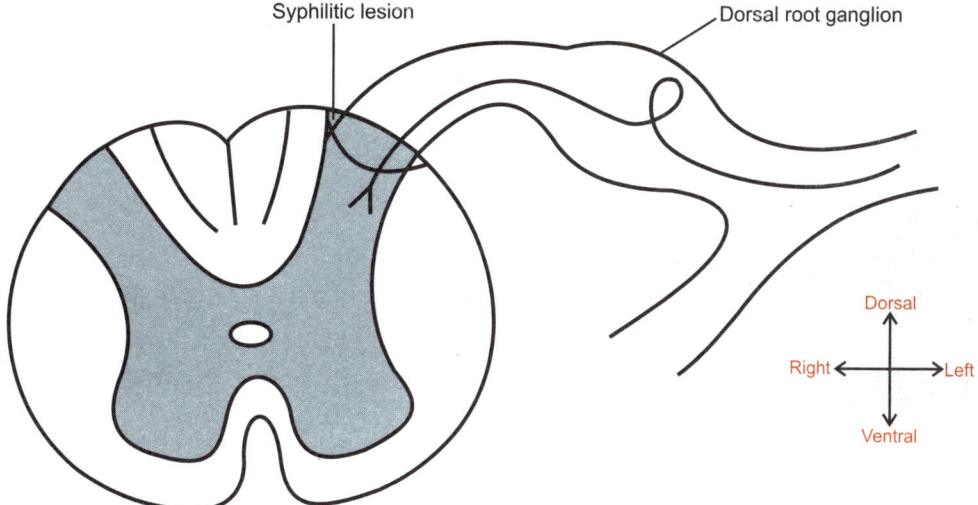

Fig.4.74 : Lesion of posterior column.

g. Impaired joint position sense. It results in stumbling and difficulty in walking, especially in the dark, when the visual compensation is imperfect.

h. Loss of sensations of deep and superficial pain.

i. Hypotonia and ataxia.

j. Loss of knee and ankle jerk.

LAQ-22 Describe lateral spinothalamic tract / describe the pathway of pain and temperature

1. **Introduction :** It is an ascending tract, carries sensations of pain and temperature from upper limb, lower limb and trunk.

2. **Receptors :**
    A. Pain : The receptors for pain are free nerve endings.
    B. Temperature :
        a. The receptors for cold are end bulbs of Krause.
        b. The receptors for hot are organs of Ruffini.

3. **Origin :** The fibers arise from the respective receptors.

4. **Course :**
    A. First order neuron : It is located in the dorsal root ganglion. The peripheral processes of the neurons, the cell bodies of which are situated in the dorsal ganglion form the sensory nerves. The central process of the neurons pass through the dorsal nerve roots and enter the spinal cord and synapse with the second order neuron.
    B. Second order neuron : It is located in the lamina I to VI of the grey matter of the spinal cord. The axons cross and go to the opposite side. It forms the lateral spinothalamic tract. It ascends through the lateral white column of the spinal cord and enters the brainstem. In the medulla oblongata, it forms a bigger bundle and is

called spinal lemniscus. The tract ends in the ventro posterolateral nucleus of thalamus.

C. Third order neuron : It lies in the ventro posterolateral nucleus of thalamus. The fibers arising from the nucleus pass through the posterior $1/3^{rd}$ of posterior limb of internal capsule. The fibers ascend through corona radiata and reach post central gyrus of the cerebral cortex (area 3).

5. **Somatotopic representation :**

Cerebral cortex : The fibers of the upper limb and lower limb are arranged in an upside down manner in the following sequence on post central gyrus.

A. Lower limb : Paracentral lobule.

B. Trunk : Superomedial border.

C. Upper limb : On upper part of post central gyrus.

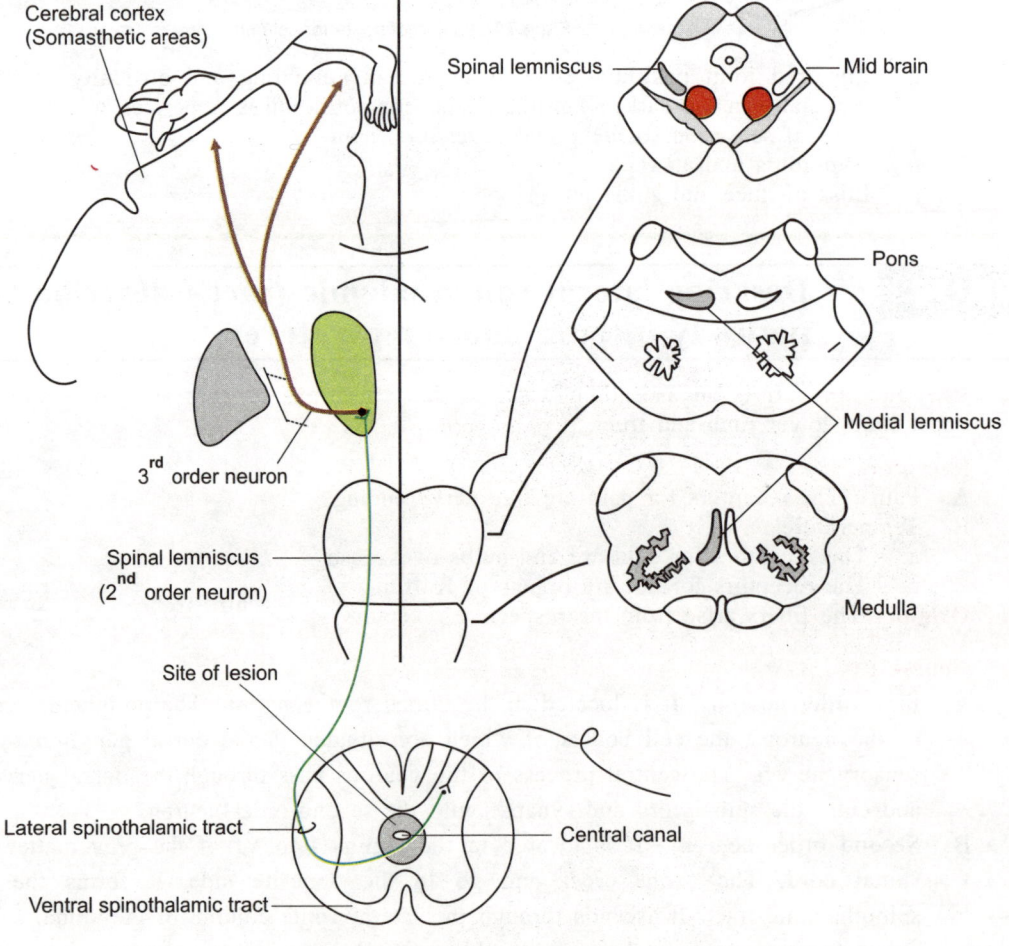

Fig. 4.75 : lateral spinothalamic tract.

The area of representation is according to density of receptors.

6. **Applied anatomy :**

Syringomyelia : This condition is characterized by the presence of elongated cavities involving the central canal of the spinal cord resulting in its dilatation. As the central canal dilates, it destroys the decussating spinothalamic fibers in the anterior white commissure.

   a. Although other sensations viz. touch and proprioceptive etc. are preserved, pain and temperature sensations are bilaterally affected, resulting in what is called 'dissociated sensory loss'.

   b. This lesion commonly involves the lower cervical and upper thoracic spinal segments. Therefore analgesia and thermo anaesthesia is usually seen in both upper limbs.

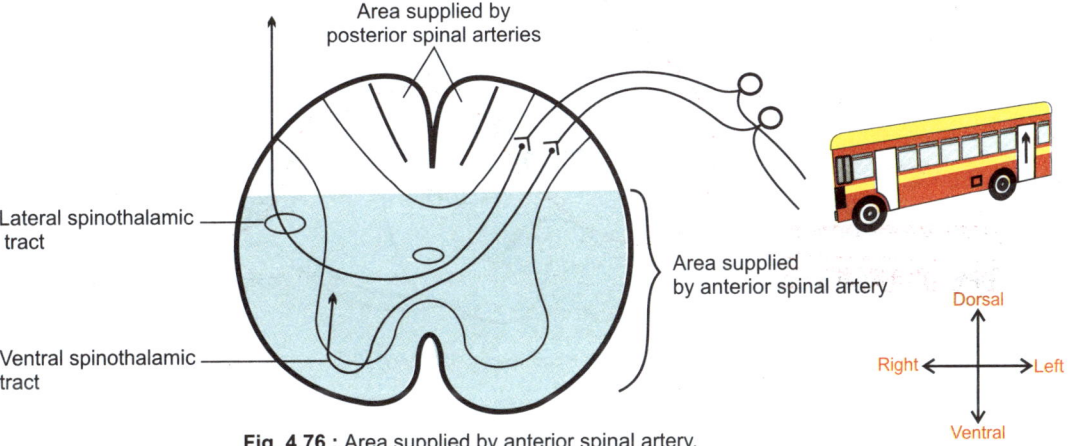

Fig. 4.76 : Area supplied by anterior spinal artery.

LAQ-23   **Describe pathway of unconscious proprioceptive impulses**

The unconscious proprioceptive impulses are carried by dorsal and ventral spinocerebellar tract and they are described as follows :

1. **Dorsal spinocerebellar tract :**

   A. Origin : This tract begins in the dorsal nucleus (Clarke's column cells) in the spinal segments C_8 to L_3.

   B. Function : It is responsible for the unconscious proprioceptive impulses from the lower limb and caudal part of the body.
      The tract is described as

   C. The fibers arise from the respective receptors. The peripheral process starts from the receptors and go to the cell bodies, which are situated in the dorsal root ganglion. The central process synapses in the cells present in the lamina I to VI of grey matter of the spinal cord.

D. Crossing of the fibers : *It is an uncrossed tract and lies at the periphery of the posterior half of the lateral funiculus.*

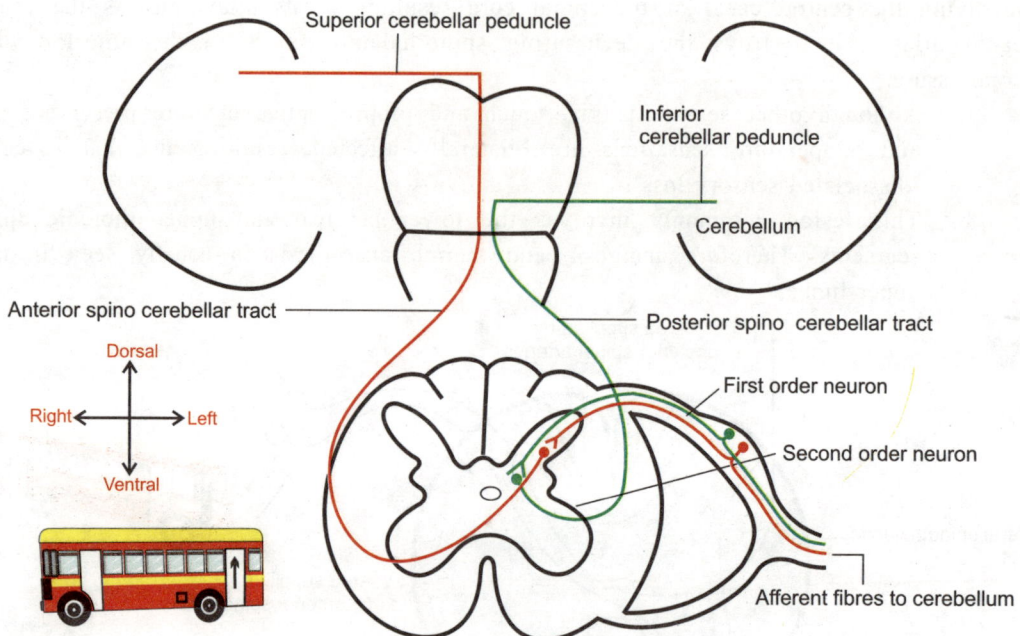

Fig. 4.77 : Spino cerebellar tract.

E. Course :

    a. It ascends through the lateral column of the spinal cord, dorsal to the ventral, spinocerebellar tract.

    b. The fibers ascend up to medulla oblongata and passes through the inferior cerebellar peduncle.

F. Termination : The fibers terminate in the nucleus interpositus of the cerebellum.

2. **Ventral spinocerebellar tract :** *This tract is predominantly crossed* and lies at the periphery of the anterior half of the lateral funiculus. The tract continues through the medulla and pons to the midbrain where it enters the cerebellum via the superior cerebellar peduncle.

It terminates in the nucleus interpositus of the cerebellum.

Both the dorsal and ventral spinocerebellar tracts carry proprioceptive impulses mainly from the lower limb; while the dorsal tract is concerned with movements of individual limb muscle and fine coordination of muscles controlling posture. The ventral tract is concerned with movement or posture of the whole limb.

3. **Cuneocerebellar tract (Posterior external arcuate fibers) :** It arises in the medulla from the accessory cuneate nucleus and conveys proprioceptive impulses from the upper limb

and neck to the cerebellum. It reaches the cerebellum as a component of inferior cerebellar peduncle.

Since Clarke's column cells are not present above C_8 level, cervical spinal fibers carrying proprioceptive impulses for cerebellum from the level above C_8 travel with the fasciculus cuneatus and relay in the accessory cuneate nucleus in the medulla.

Cuneocerebellar tract is regarded as the tract of upper limb equivalent of the dorsal spinocerebellar tract of the lower limb. In the cat a rostral spinocerebellar tract has been described as the fore limb equivalent of the ventral spinocerebellar tract.

LAQ-24 — Describe visual (optic) pathway and the effects of lesion of different parts of visual pathways

The visual pathway includes structures which are concerned with the reception, transmission and perception of visual impulses.

1. **Structures in visual pathway :**
   A. Retina : It is a thin, delicate inner layer of eyeball. It contains rods and cones which are receptors for the visual pathway. It contains bipolar cells and ganglion cells. The axons of the ganglion cells form optic nerve.
   B. Peculiarities of optic nerve :
      a. *It is thickest cranial nerve, hence whatever we see, we hardly forget.*
      b. *In a strict sense, the optic nerve is not a cranial nerve, but a prolongation of the white matter of the brain, because it is developed from the stalk of optic vesicle.*
      c. *It is the only cranial nerve covered by three meninges of the brain, hence the nerve undergoes atrophy in prolonged increase of cerebro-spinal fluid pressure.*
      d. *The myelination of the optic nerve is derived from the oligodenbroglia, but not from the schwann cells. Hence, it does not have endoneuriun and if damaged cannot regenerate.*
      e. *It has rich blood supply.*
      f. *It is a tract and not a nerve (The nerve is usually first order neuron).*
   C. Optic chiasma :
      In the chiasma, the nasal fibers of each optic nerve decussate and pass into the optic tract of the opposite side; The temporal fibers from each retina pass on to their own side.
   D. Optic tract :
      Each optic tract winds round the cerebral peduncle of the midbrain. It divides near the lateral geniculate body into
      a. Lateral root : It is thick and terminates in the lateral geniculate body. A few of its fibers pass to the superior colliculus, the pretectal nucleus and the hypothalamus.
      b. Medial roots : It is believed to contain the fibers of Gudden's commissure. (The fiber bundles situated dorsal to the optic chiasma.)
         Each optic tract contains temporal fibers of the same side and nasal fibers of the opposite side.

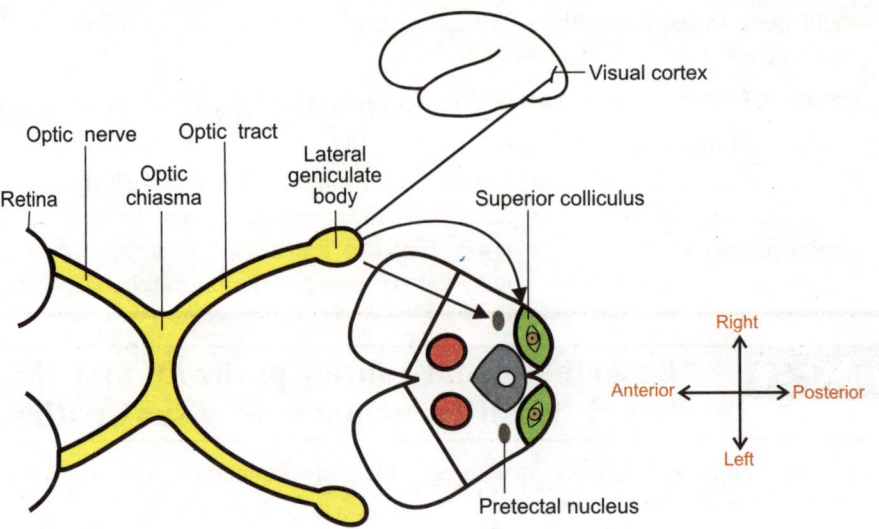

Fig. 4.78 : Visual pathway.

E. **Lateral geniculate body :** The larger fibers of the optic tract synapse in the lateral geniculate body. These are visual fibers.

F. **Optic radiation (Geniculo-calcarine tract) :** It begins from the lateral geniculate body, passes through the retro lentiform part of the internal capsule and ends in the visual cortex.

G. **Visual cortex :** The optic radiation ends in the striate area (area 17) where the colour, size, shape, motion, illumination and transparency are appreciated separately. Objects are identified by integration of these perceptions with past experience stored in the parastriate and peristriate areas (Areas 18, 19). The area of the visual cortex that receives impulses from the macula is relatively much larger than the part related to the rest of the retina.

Table 4.24 : The table shows site of lesion of optic nerve and their effects of lesion.

Site of lesion	Effects
A. Retina.	Scotoma. (*scotoma* small area of blindness).
B. Optic nerve.	Blindness on the same side; consensual reflex retained.

C. Optic chiasma.
   a. Central lesion.
 	
   b. Bilateral peripheral lesion.
	
	 Bitemporal hemianopia. (*Hemi* half, *a* not, *opia* vision) Blindness of the half of visual field of one or both eyes.
	 Binasal hemianopia.

D. Optic tract, lateral geniculate body and optic radiation.	Homonymous hemianopia on opposite side without macular sparing. Lesions of the optic radiation usually produce quadrantic visual defects.
E. Visual cortex.	Homonymous hemianopia with macular sparing.

SN-40   Pathway of light reflex

Light reflexes is mediated through the
- A.   Retina,
- B.   Optic nerve,
- C.   Optic chiasma,
- D.   Optic tract,
- E.   Lateral geniculate body,
- F.   Pretectal nucleus,
- G.   Edinger-Westphal nucleus of the third nerve,
- h.   Third cranial nerve,
- I.   Ciliary ganglion,
- J.   Short ciliary nerves and
- K.   Constrictor pupillae.

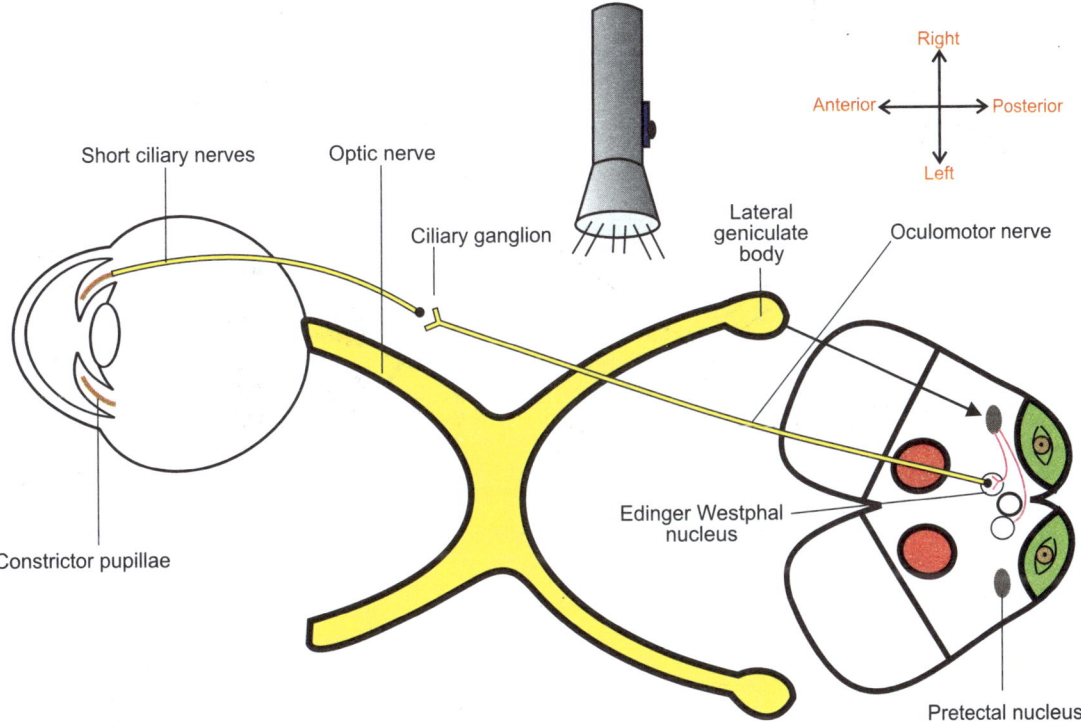

Fig. 4.79 : Light reflex.

Throwing light on one eye produces constriction of the pupil in both eyes (consensual reflex). This is due to bilateral connections of the pretectal nucleus with the Edinger-Westphal nuclei.

SN-41   Pathway of accommodation reflex

Constriction of the pupil also takes place when looking at near object. This is mediated through the
- A.   Retina,
- B.   Optic nerve,
- C.   Optic chiasma and tract,
- D.   Lateral geniculate body,
- E.   Optic radiation,

F.   Visual area of the cortex,
G.   Superior longitudinal bundle,
H.   Frontal eye field,
I.   Third nerve nucleus,   } Corticonuclear fibres
J.   Third cranial nerve,

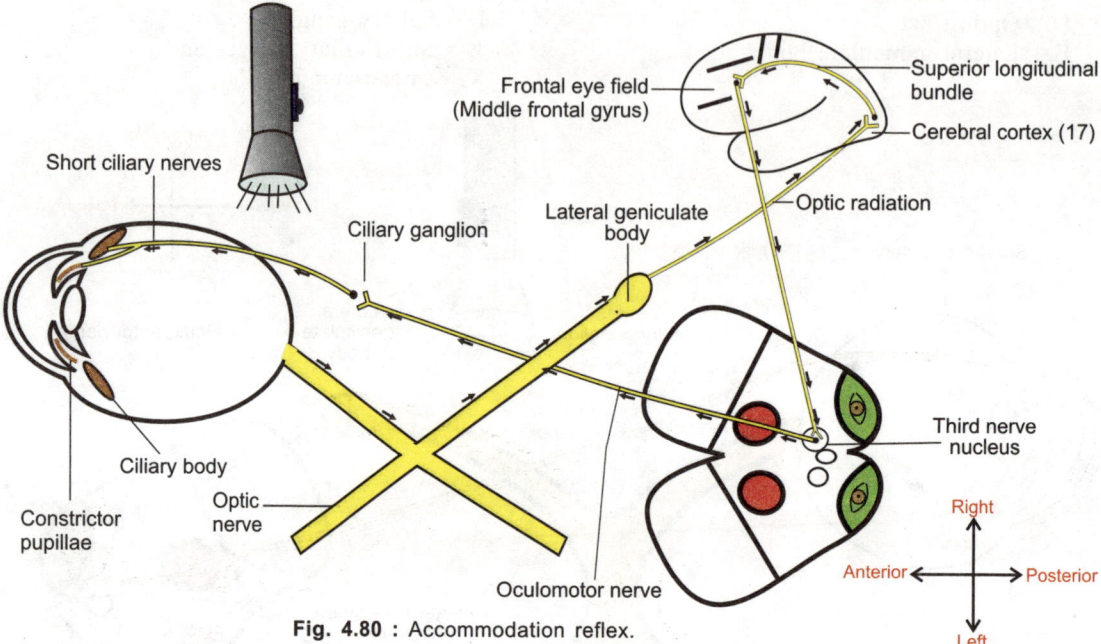

Fig. 4.80 : Accommodation reflex.

K.   Ciliary ganglion and
L.   Ciliaris and sphincter pupillae muscles.

Note that the pretectal nucleus is not involved in the accommodation reflex.

Applied anatomy : In lesions of the pretectal nucleus the light reflex is lost, but the pupil contracts on accommodation. This is called the **A**rgyll-**R**obertson **p**upil. (**A**ccommodation **r**eflex **p**resent) 🔑 **ARP**

SN-42   Pathway of hearing (Auditory pathway)

1.   The first order neurons of the pathway are located in the spiral ganglion. They are bipolar cells. The peripheral processes innervate the organ of Corti, while the central processes terminate in the dorsal and ventral cochlear nuclei.

2.   The second order neurons lie in the dorsal and ventral cochlear nuclei. Most of the axons arising in these nuclei cross to the opposite side (in the trapezoid body) and terminate in the superior olivary nucleus. (Many fibers end in the nucleus of the trapezoid body or of the lateral lemniscus). Some fibers are uncrossed.

3.   The third order neurons lie in the superior olivary nucleus present in the pons. The axons form the lateral lemniscus and reach the inferior colliculus.

4. The fourth order neurons lie in the inferior colliculus. Their axons pass through the inferior brachium to reach the medial geniculate body. (Some fibers of the lateral lemniscus reach the medial geniculate body without relay in the inferior colliculus).

5. The fifth order neurons lie in the medial geniculate body. The axons form the auditory radiation, which pass through the sublentiform part of the internal capsule to reach the auditory area of the temporal lobe.

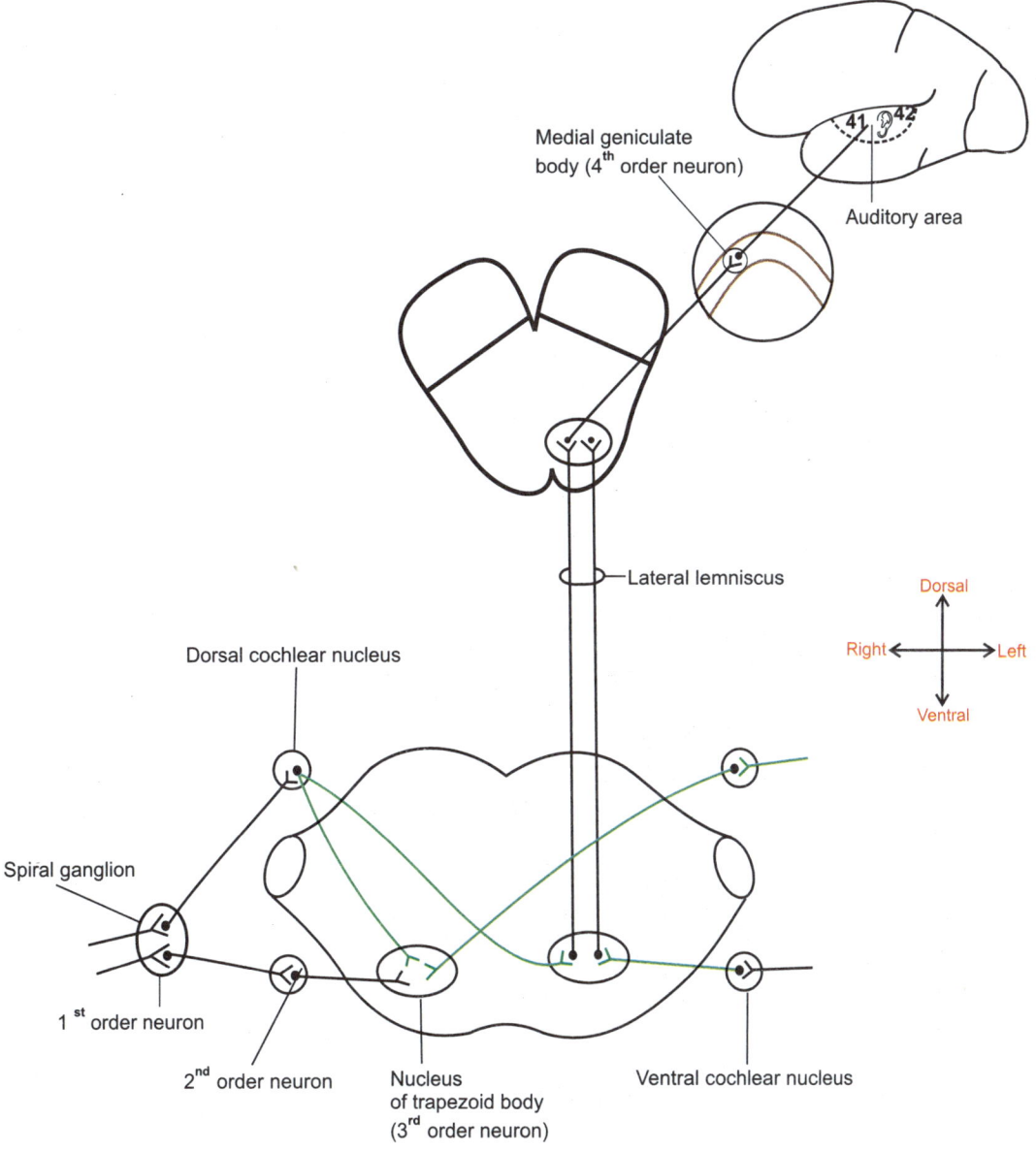

Fig. 4.81 : Auditory pathway.

SN-43   Blood supply of spinal cord

1. **The blood supply of spinal cord** is by
   A.   One anterior spinal artery.
   B.   Two posterior spinal arteries.

Table 4.25 : The table shows details about anterior and posterior arterial trunk.

	Anterior arterial trunk	**Posterior arterial trunk**
Extent	Throughout spinal cord.	
Site	Along anterior median fissure.	Posterolateral sulcus.
Number	One.	Two.
Nature	More prominent.	Less prominent.
Formation	By joining right and left anterior spinal artery branch of vertebral artery.	Posterior spinal artery branch of posterior inferior cerebellar or vertebral artery.
Joined by	Anterior radicular artery, branch of segmental artery.	
Distribution	Anterior 2/3rd of spinal cord.	Posterior 1/3rd of spinal cord.

2. **Segmental spinal branches** arise from
   A.   Vertebral artery
   B.   Ascending cervical artery   ⎫
   C.   Deep cervical artery   ⎬   Cervical segment.
                                 ⎭
   D.   Intercostal artery   Thoracic segment.
   E.   Lumbar artery   Lumbar segment.
   F.   Sacral artery.   Sacral segment.

Note : *The radicular arteries arise from vertebral, ascending cervical, intercostal, lumbar and sacral arteries. These branches anastomose with one another to form longitudinal vessels. Frequently one of the radicular arteries is larger than the remainder and is called arteria radicularis magna. It usually arises from one of the inter segmental branches of descending aorta in the lower thoracic or upper lumbar segments.*

3. **Venous drainage :**   There are about six longitudinal venous channels which drain the blood from the spinal cord. They are described as
   A.   Midline venous channel : They are two in number.
        a.   Venous channel present in the anterior median fissure.
        b.   Venous channel present in the posterior median sulcus.
   B.   Lateral venous channel : They are in two sets.
        a.   One set behind the ventral root of spinal nerve on each side.
        b.   One set in front of the dorsal root of the spinal nerve.
   All above longitudinal veins communicate with the internal vertebral plexus and drain into
        a.   Vena cava,
        b.   Azygos vein and into
        c.   Basilar venous plexus.

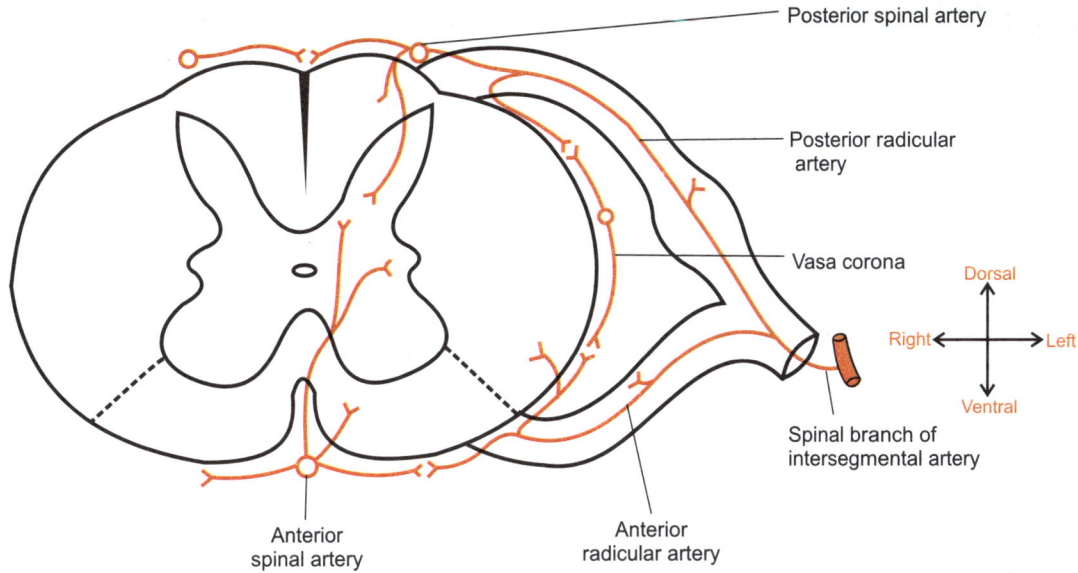

Fig. 4.82 : Arterial supply of spinal cord.

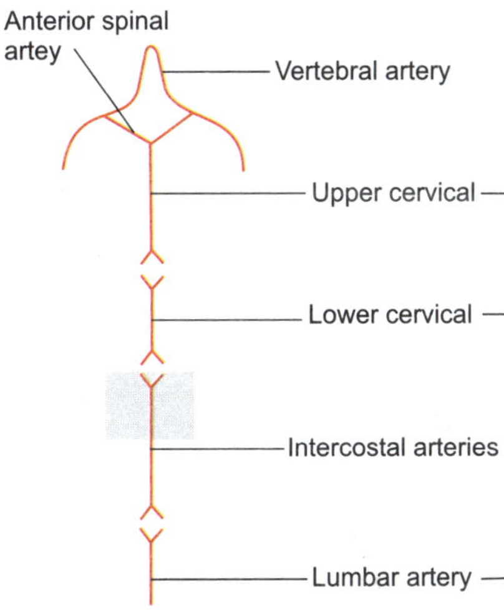

Fig. 4.83 : Formation of anterior spinal arteries in different parts of the spinal cord.

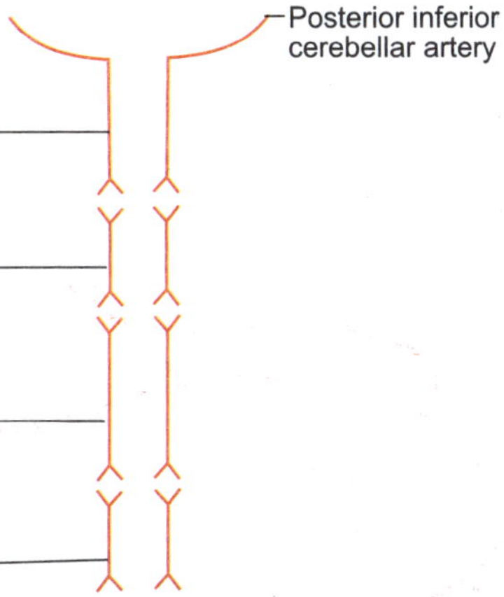

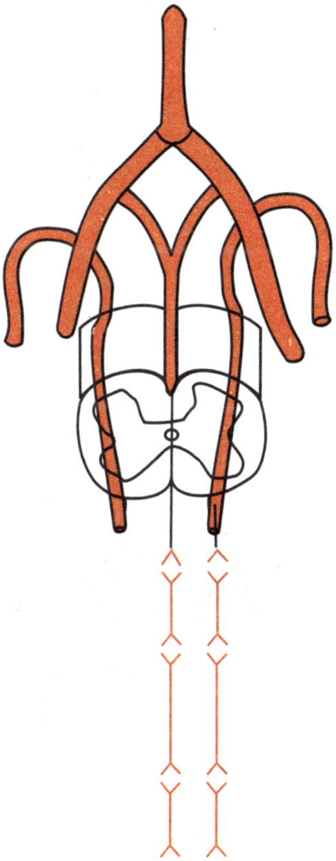

Fig. 4.84 : Formation of posterior spinal arteries in different parts of the spinal cord.

LAQ-25 Describe the blood supply of cerebral hemisphere

The blood supply of brain is divided into

1. **Arterial supply :** It is described as
    A. Cortical branches :
        a. Characters :
            I.   They supply cerebral cortex.
            II. These are not end arteries i.e. they communicate freely with the neighboring arteries.
            III. The arterial supply of the particular area is maintained in case of blockage of any one of the artery.
        b. Cortical arteries are branches of
            I.   Anterior cerebral artery, a branch of internal carotid artery. The area of distribution is
                 i. Medial surface of cerebral cortex up to the parieto-occipital sulcus.
                 ii. One inch area below the supero-medial border on supero-lateral surface.
            II. Middle cerebral artery, a branch of internal carotid artery. It supplies the area on the supero-lateral surface except :
                 .   One inch area below the supero-medial border.
                 ..   Occipital lobe.
                 ... Inferior temporal gyrus.
            III. Posterior cerebral artery, a branch of basilar artery. It supplies
                 i. Occipital lobe.
                 ii. Inferior surface of temporal lobe except temporal pole.

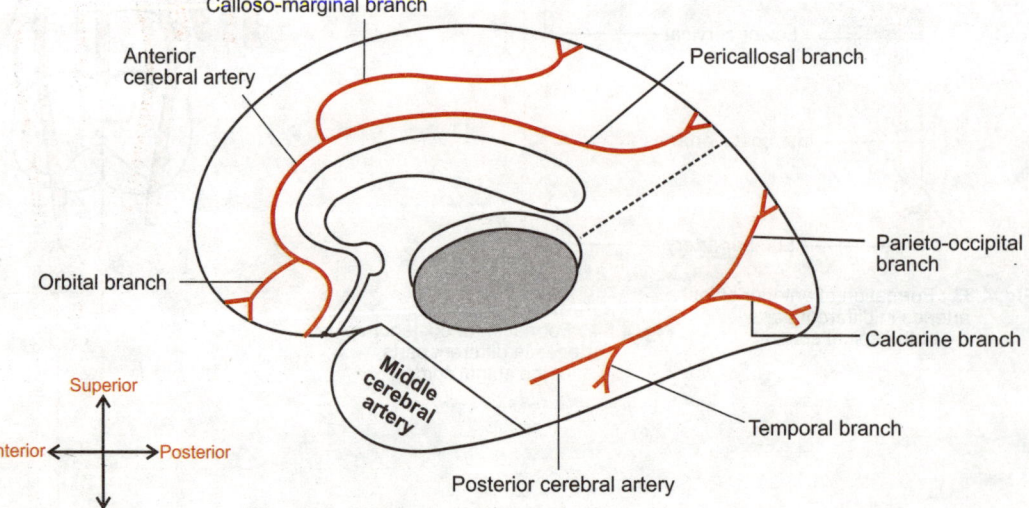

Fig. 4.85 : Blood supply of medial surface of cerebral cortex.

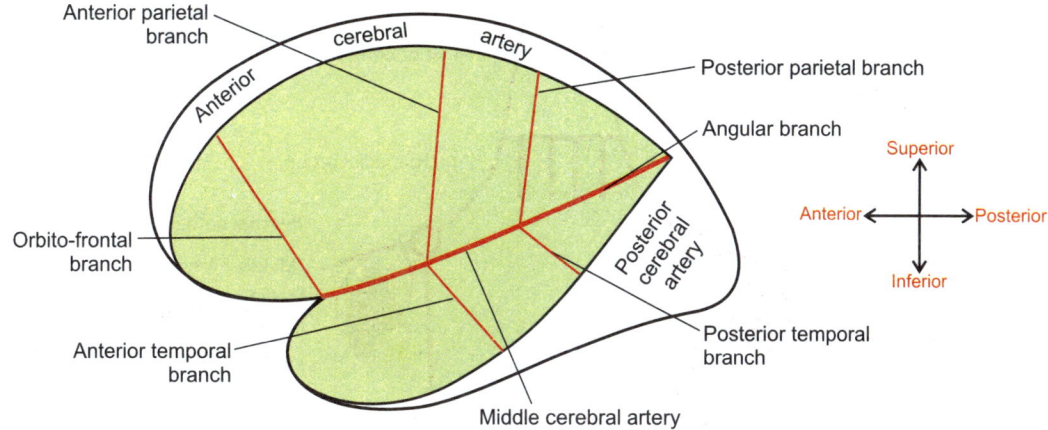

Fig. 4. 86 : Arterial supply of superolateral surface of cerebral cortex.

B. Central branches :

    a. Characters :

        I. These arteries supply central part of cerebral hemisphere.

        II. These are end arteries i.e. they do not anastomose

        III. In case of blockage of these arteries, the blood supply of the respective area is lost and the part undergoes ischemic changes.

    b. These arteries are in four groups :

Table No. 4.26 : The table shows groups of central arteries, their formation and area of distribution.

Group	Formation	Area of distribution
I. Antero-medial :	a. Anterior cerebral artery. b. Anterior communicating artery, a branch of anterior cerebral artery.	i. Anterior part of hypothalamus. ii. Preoptic and supraoptic region of hypothalamus.
II. Antero-lateral group :	a. Medial striate artery (artery of Heubner), a branch of anterior cerebral artery. b. Lateral striate artery (artery of cerebral haemorrhage), branch of middle cerebral artery.	i. Corpus striatum. ii. Internal capsule.
III. Postero-medial group :	a. Posterior communicating artery, a branch of middle cerebral artery. b. Posterior cerebral artery.	i. Medial surface of thalamus. ii. Subthalamus. iii. Hypophysis cerebri. iv. Midbrain.
IV. Postero-lateral group :	Posterior cerebral artery.	i. Caudal part of thalamus. ii Pulvinar.

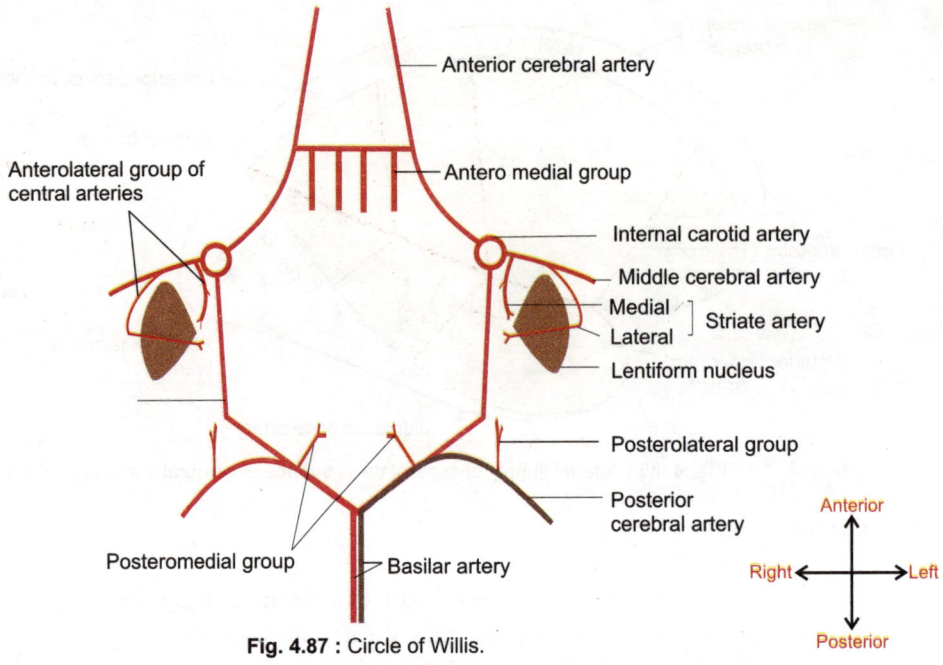

Fig. 4.87 : Circle of Willis.

2. **Venous drainage :** Veins of the cerebral cortex are grouped into
   A. Superficial veins and

Table No. 4.27 : The table shows superficial veins of cerebral cortex and the draining area.

Name	Number	Draining area	Termination
a. Superior cerebral veins.	Six to twelve.	a. Supero-lateral surface of the hemisphere. b. Medial surface of the hemisphere.	i. Superior sagittal sinus.
b. Inferior cerebral veins. i. Orbital and ii. Temporal.	Many.	a. Inferior surface of cerebral hemisphere b. Ventral part of lateral surface of hemisphere.	i. Orbital veins → superior cerebral veins. ii. Temporal veins → Cavernous sinus. iii. Occipital veins → straight sinus.
c. Superficial middle cerebral vein.	---	Around the posterior ramus of lateral surface.	i. Cavernous sinus. ii. Sphenoparietal sinus.

   B. Deep veins : They are
      a. Thalamostriate vein.
      b. Choroid vein.
         Both the veins drain into internal cerebral vein.
         Right and left internal cerebral veins drain into great cerebral vein, which drains
         into anterior part of straight sinus.

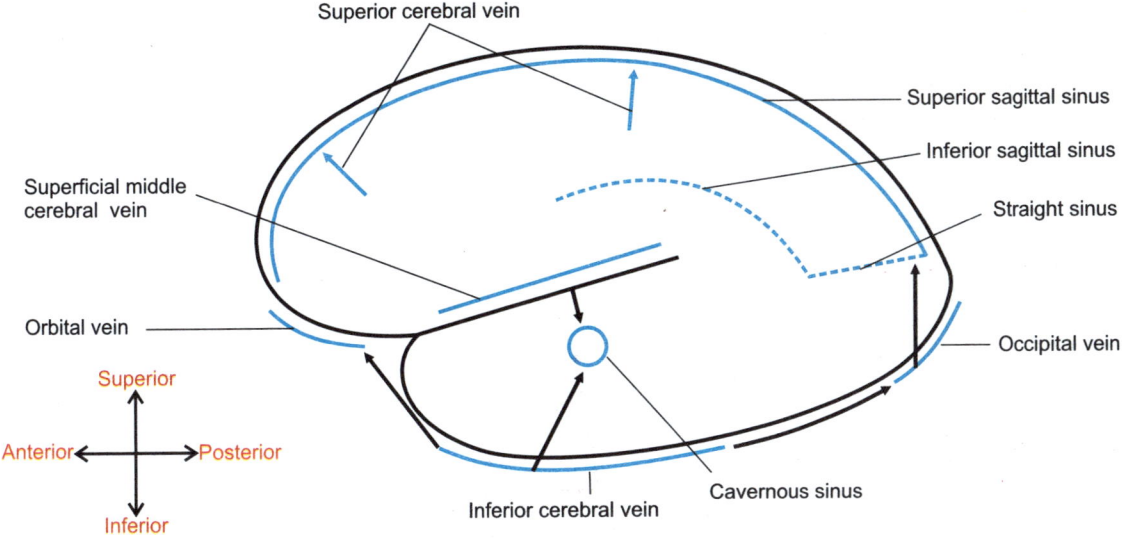

Fig. 4.88 : Venous drainage of superficial veins of cerebral cortex.

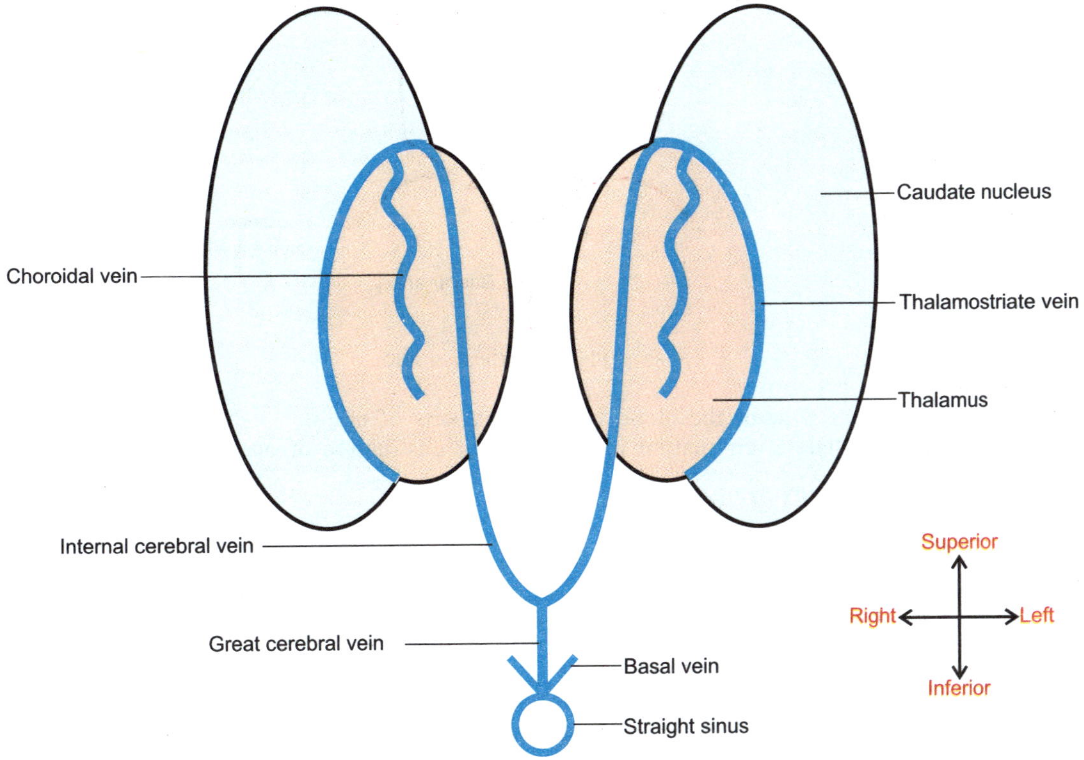

Fig. 4.88 : Venous drainage of deep cerebral vein.

SN-44 Circle of Willis

1. **Introduction :** It is a polygonal or circular anastomotic channel between two internal carotid and two vertebral arteries.

2. **Location :** At the base of brain in interpeduncular fossa. It is formed by
   A. Anterior cerebral, a branch of internal carotid artery.
   B. Posterior cerebral, a branch of basilar artery.

3. **Communicating artery :**
   A. Anterior communicating artery.
   B. Posterior communicating artery.

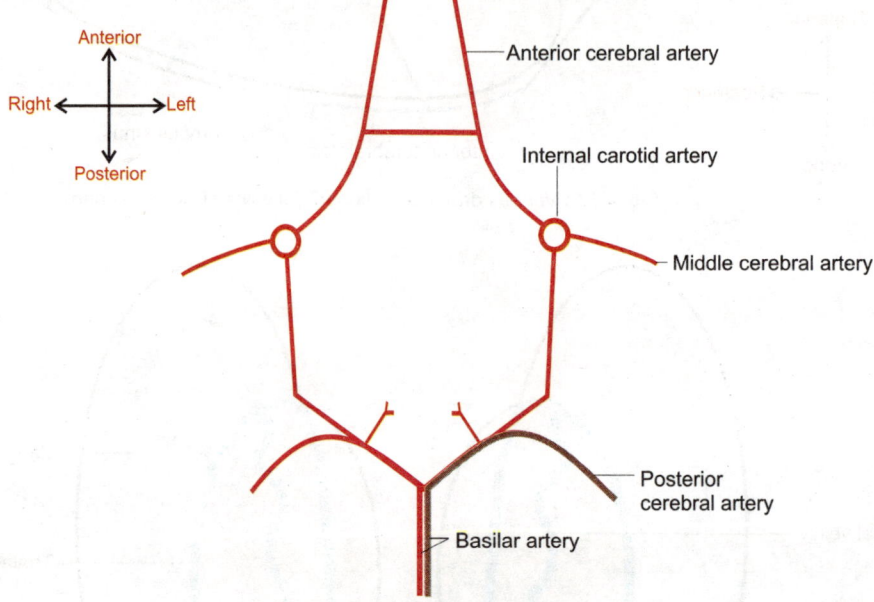

Fig. 4.90 : Circle of Willis.

4. **Importance :**
   A. It equalizes the flow of the blood to different parts of brain.
   B. It provides collateral circulation in the event of obstruction of one of its components.

5. **Nerve supply :** It is by sympathetic nerves.

6. **Branches :**
   A. The cortical branches supply cerebral cortex and they freely anastomose.
   B. The central branches penetrate the base of the brain and supply the diencephalon corpus striatum and the internal capsule. They are arranged in following groups.
      a. Anteromedial group,
      b. Paired anterolateral branches,
      c. Posteromedial branches and
      d. Paired posterolateral branches.

7. **Applied anatomy :** Circle of Willis is associated with congenital aneurysm (Berry's aneurysm, subarachnoid haemorrhage).

SN-45   **Neural crest**

1. **Introduction :** The ectoderm overlying notochordal process thickens and is called neural plate.

    Neural crest : The specialized cells situated at the junction of surface ectoderm and neural plate are called as cells of neural crest.

    Derivatives - It gives rise to following structures :   🔑   **CNS**

    <u>C</u>   Chromaffin tissue : It is similar to cells present in adrenal medulla. It is seen in relation to abdominal aorta where it forms para aortic bodies.

    <u>N</u>   Neurons of the spinal, sensory and sympathetic ganglion.

    A.   DRG (Dorsal root ganglia).

    B.   Sensory ganglion V, VII, VIII, IX & X.

    C.   Sympathetic ganglia.

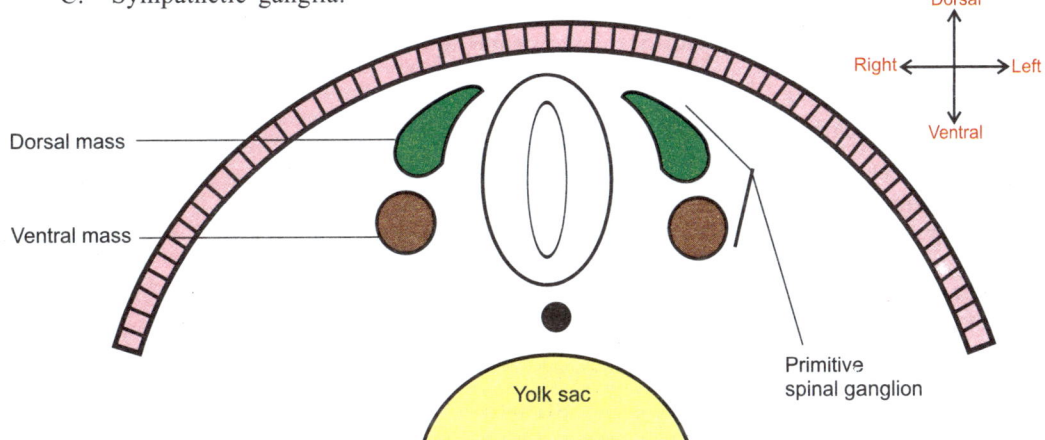

Fig. 4.91 : Formation of neural crest.

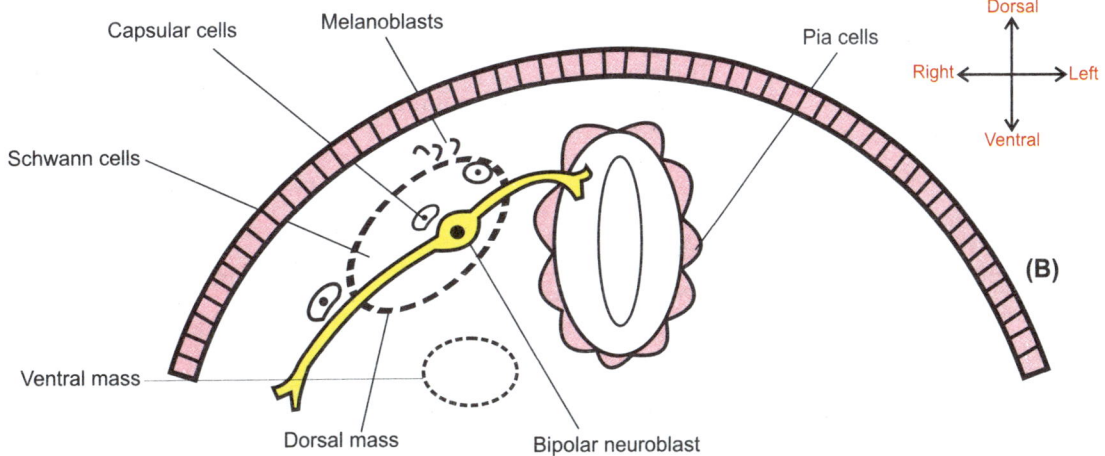

Fig. 4.92 : Structures derived from neural crest

S   A.   **S**chwann cell - forms neurolemmal sheath of peripheral nerves.
    B.   **S**pecific cells of adrenal medulla (pheochromocytes).
    C.   Pigment cells of **s**kin - (melanoblast).
    D.   Leptomeninges :
        a.   Piamater.
        b.   Arachnoid mater.
    E.   Dental papilla mesenchym.

SN-46   Neural tube

The central nervous system is developed from a hollow dorsally placed neural tube. It is derived from neuroectoderm.

The formation of neural tube is described under following heads :

1. **Chronological age :**   The closure of the neural tube starts on 21st day, in the middle part.

2. **Germ layer :** Neuroectoderm.

3. **Site :** Dorsal part of the notochord.

4. **Source :** The formation of the neural tube passes through three stages, namely neural plate, neural groove and neural tube.

   The part of the ectoderm dorsal to the notochord becomes thick and is called neural plate. It deepens along the midline and a neural groove is formed. The groove becomes further deep and the two edges of the neural plate come together and the neural groove is converted into neural tube.

Table No. 4.28 : The table shows structures developed from neural tube.

Parts	Structure	Cavity
A. Prosencephalon a. Telencephalon	I. Corpus striatum II. Cerebrum	Lateral entricle
b. Diencephalon	I. Thalamus II. Hypothalamus III. Optic stalk IV. Pars nervosa of pituitary gland	Third ventricle
B. Mesencephalon	Midbrain	Cerebral aqueduct
C. Rhombencephalon a. Metencephalon	Pons, cerebellum	IVth ventricle
b. Myelencephalon	Medulla oblongata	

5. **Anomalies :** Most defects of spinal cord result from abnormal closure of neural folds in the third and fourth weeks of development. The resulting abnormalities may involve the meninges, vertebrae, muscles and skin.
   A.   Spina bifida, a splitting of the vertebral arches.

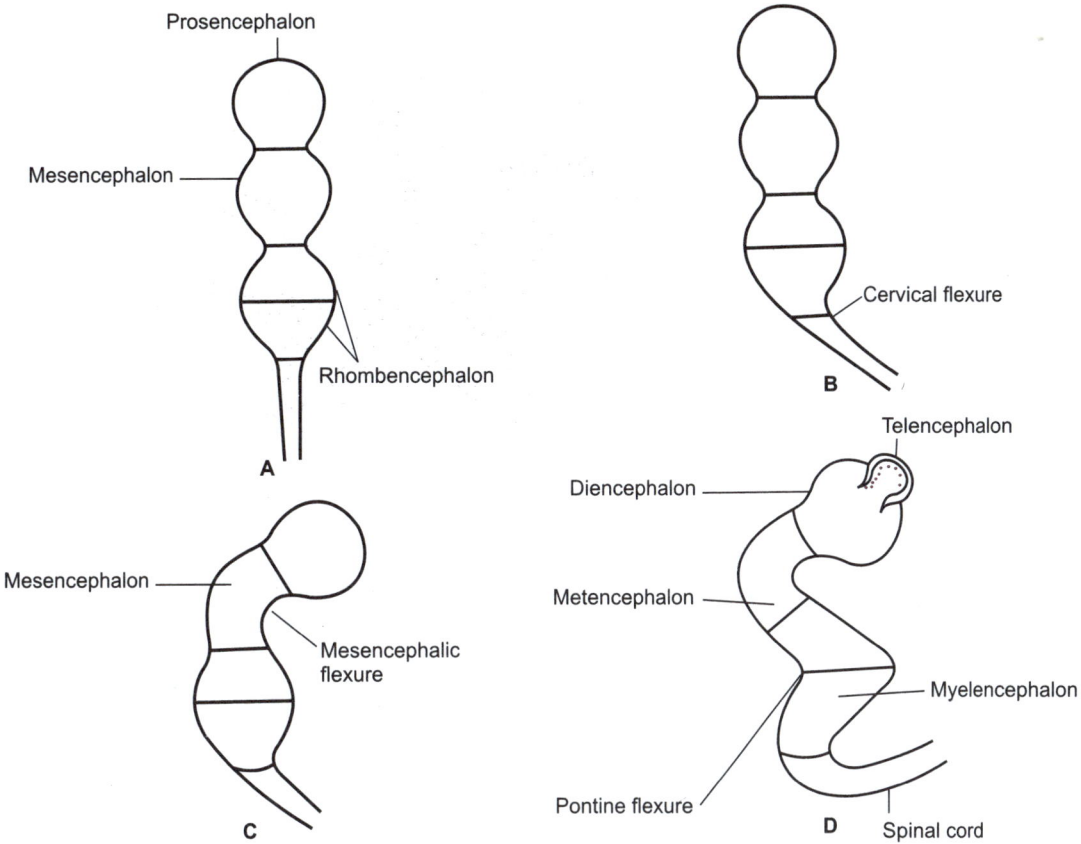

Fig. 4.93 : Structures developed from neural tube.

B.   Spina bifida occulta : It is a defect in the vertebral arches, that is covered by skin and usually does not involve underlying neural tissue.
C.   Spina bifida cystica : It is a severe neural tube defect in which neural tissue and/or meninges protrude through a defect in the vertebral arches and skin to form a cystic sac.

SN-47   Histology of cerebellum

1.   **The layers of the cerebellum :** are
   A.   The molecular layer consists of dendritic arborizations andthin axons. They run parallel to the surface. There are two types of cells, namely
     a.   Superficial stellate cells and
     b.   The deep stellate or basket cells.
   B.   A single layer of Purkinje cells.
   C.   The granular layer filled with closely packed granule cells separated by small clear zones called glomeruli.

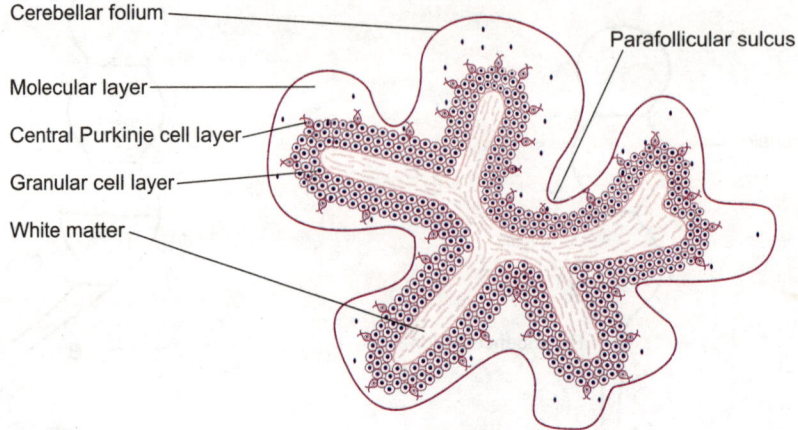

Fig. 4.94 : Histology of cerebellum.

2. **Nerve fibres in the cerebellar cortex :** Two types of afferent fibers enter the cerebellar cortex. They are
   A. The climbing fibres originating from the inferior olivary nuclear complex and ending on the dendrites of the Purkinje cells. They excite Purkinje cells.
   B. The mossy fibres are the other afferent fibres entering the cerebellar cortex. They enter the white matter where they branch repeatedly before entering the granular layer. Here they end as dilated terminals, on which the granule cell dendrites and the Golgi

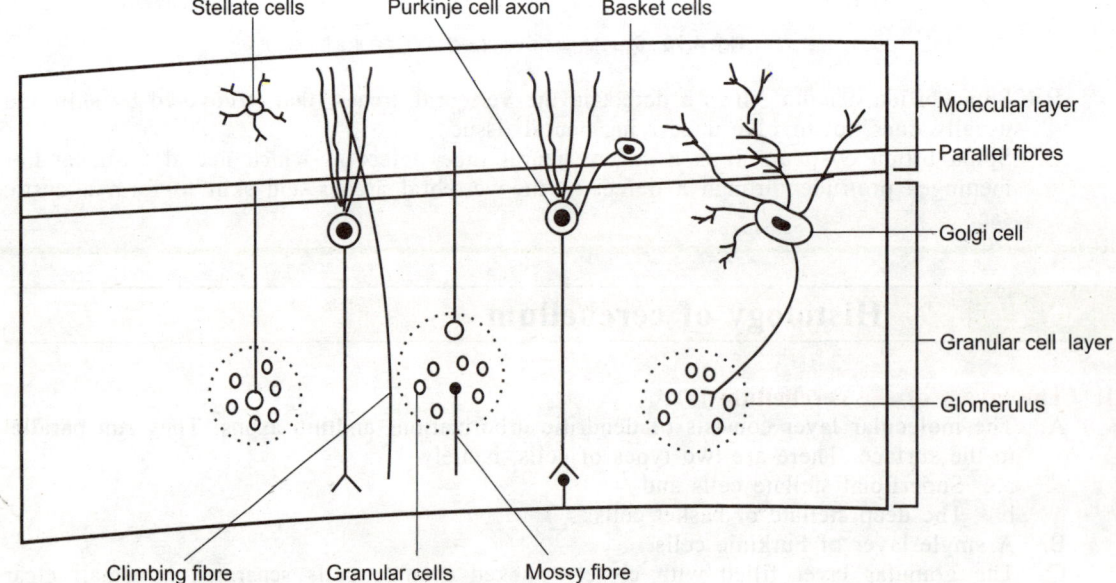

Fig. 4.95 : Structure of cerebellum.

cell axons synapse to form a rosette surrounded by glial cells. This is called a cerebellar glomerulus. The mossy fibres are excitatory to the granular cells. The Golgi cells are inhibitory to the granular cells.

The axons of the Purkinje cells are the only efferent fibres from the cerebellar cortex. They end on the cerebellar nuclei and in the lateral vestibular nuclei. All the other neurons in the cortex are inhibitory in nature.

SN-48   Cerebrum

1. **The neurons seen in the cerebral cortex can be divided into six main types:**

A. Pyramidal neurons :
    a. They are triangular cells when seen in section, the apex faces the surface of the cerebrum.
    b. The dendrites are given off from all three angles.
    c. The axon is given off from the base of the cell and goes to the deeper layers.
    d. The nucleus is large, central and vesicular with a prominent nucleolus.
    e. The Nissl substance is prominent in the cytoplasm.
    f. They are of following types
        I.   The small neurons are of 10-12 microns,
        II.   The medium sized neurons are of 40-50 microns and
        III. The large pyramidal cells are of 100 microns in diameter which are found in the motor cortex and are called the cells of Betz.

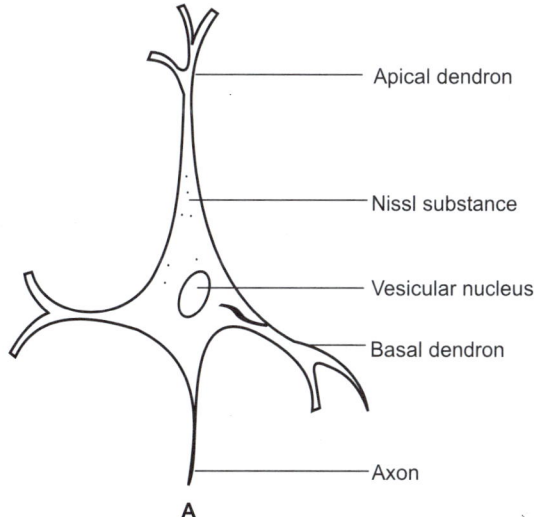

A

Fig. 4.96 : Histology of cerebellum.

B. Stellate or granular cells or small polygonal or triangular cells :
    a. They are 4-8 microns in diameter.
    b. They have a dark condensed nucleus and a very thin rim of cytoplasm.
    c. Each cell has many dendrites coming out from all over.
    d. Usually the axon is very short in Golgi type II neurons. In the larger cells the axon may be long and may enter the white matter.

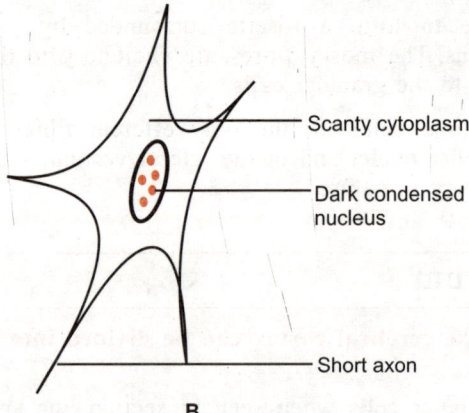

B

Fig. 4.97 : Histology of cerebellum.

C. **Fusiform cells** : Fusiform cells lie perpendicular to the surface with an axon coming out from the centre of the body. One dendron comes out from the superficial end and goes to the surface and the other goes into the deeper layers and comes out of the deep end of the cell.

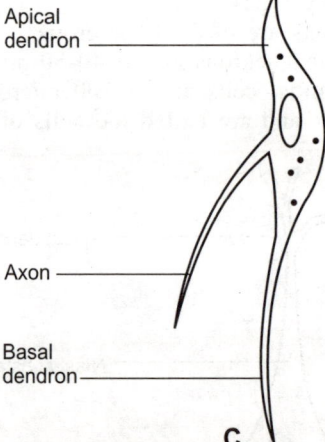

C

Fig. 4.98 : Histology of cerebellum.

D. **Horizontal cells of Cajal** : It is a spindle shaped neurons lying parallel to the surface.

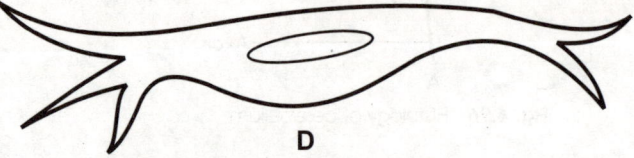

D

Fig. 4.99 : Histology of cerebellum.

E. **Cells of Martinotti or cells with ascending axons** : These are small triangular cells with axons going to the superficial layers and coming out from the apex. The dendrites are given out from the other two angles of the triangle.

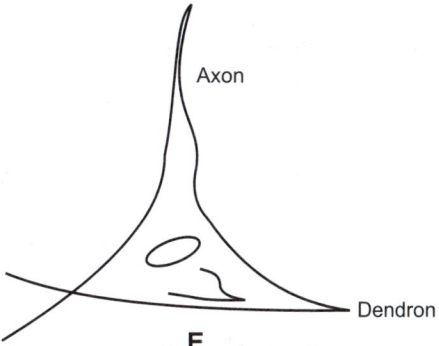

Fig. 4.100 : Histology of cerebellum.

F.   Golgi type II cells have processes ending close to the cell body.

2.   **Layers of the cerebral cortex :** From the superficial to deep

A.   Molecular or plexiform layer : Consists of few horizontal cells and Golgi type II cells. The dense tangential fibre plexus is made up of fibres from
   a.   Dendritic arborisation from deep pyramidal cells,
   b.   Fusiform cells and
   c.   Axons of Martinotti cells.

B.   External granular layer : It consists of small pyramidal cells with apical dendrites ending in the first layer. Their axons form association fibers. The fibers in this layer are called dysfibrous layer because its fibers are poorly myelinated.

C.   External pyramidal layer has two layers of pyramidal cells :
   a.   Superficial layers of medium pyramidal cells and
   b.   Deep layer of large pyramidal cells. Its axons form association and commissural fibers.
   c.   A white fibre zone called band of Kaes-Bechterew or suprastriate layer forms its superficial layer.

D.   Internal granular layer has closely packed stellate cells and white horizontal fibre layer called external band of Baillarger. These are the terminals of the thalamocortical fibers.

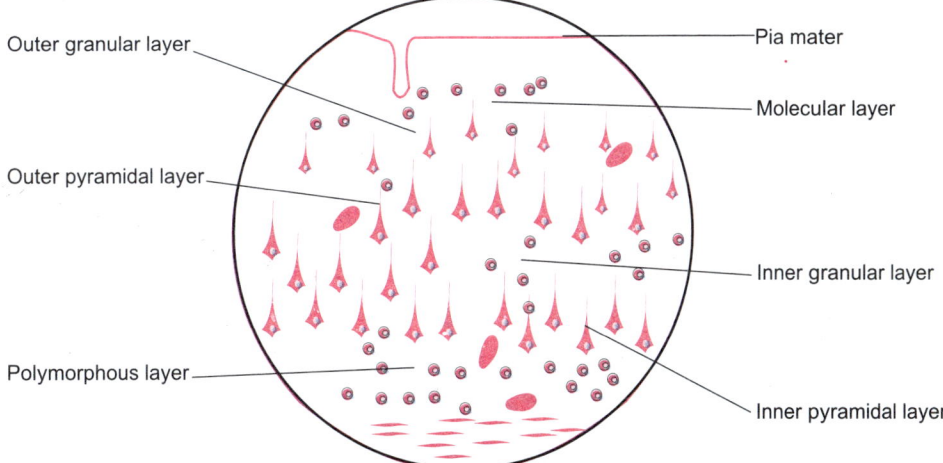

Fig. 4.101 : Histology of cerebellum.

E. Internal pyramidal or ganglionic layers : Consists of medium and large pyramidal cells intermingled with Martinotti cells. The axons form the chief projection fibers and some association fibers. Horizontal fibers in the deeper portion are called internal bland of Baillarger.

F. Multiform layer or layer of fusiform cells contains predominantly spindle shaped cells, it also contains granular, Martinotti and stellate cells.

~ ~ ~ ~ ~ ~ **Best of Luck** ~ ~ ~ ~ ~ ~

INDEX

SUPEX & THORAX

HEAD-FACE-NECK & NEURO

Feedback

The author humbly requests all the students, teachers and well wishers to point out any corrections, which will be rectified in the next edition. He is very much free for correction and welcomes all sorts of suggestions and criticism.

Name : .... Designation : ....

Name of the college : ....

Address with phone No. ....

....

....

1. About appearance of the book ....

2. Language ....

3. About text (Grammatical, typographical) ....

4. Content ....

5. Diagram ....

6. Applied anatomy ....

7. Illustration ....

8. Any other comments ....

....

....

Please mail to : --

Dr. S. N. Kazi --

60, Atlas Colony, --

Mahesh Nagar, Pimpri, --

Pune - 411 018. --

Maharashtra - INDIA. --
